D1265871

NUTRITION RESEARCH ADVANCES

NUTRITION RESEARCH ADVANCES

SARAH V. WATKINS
EDITOR

Nova Science Publishers, Inc.
New York

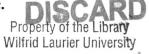
DISCARD
Property of the Library
Wilfrid Laurier University

Copyright © 2007 by Nova Science Publishers, Inc.

All rights reserved. No part of this book may be reproduced, stored in a retrieval system or transmitted in any form or by any means: electronic, electrostatic, magnetic, tape, mechanical photocopying, recording or otherwise without the written permission of the Publisher.

For permission to use material from this book please contact us:
Telephone 631-231-7269; Fax 631-231-8175
Web Site: http://www.novapublishers.com

NOTICE TO THE READER

The Publisher has taken reasonable care in the preparation of this book, but makes no expressed or implied warranty of any kind and assumes no responsibility for any errors or omissions. No liability is assumed for incidental or consequential damages in connection with or arising out of information contained in this book. The Publisher shall not be liable for any special, consequential, or exemplary damages resulting, in whole or in part, from the readers' use of, or reliance upon, this material.

Independent verification should be sought for any data, advice or recommendations contained in this book. In addition, no responsibility is assumed by the publisher for any injury and/or damage to persons or property arising from any methods, products, instructions, ideas or otherwise contained in this publication.

This publication is designed to provide accurate and authoritative information with regard to the subject matter covered herein. It is sold with the clear understanding that the Publisher is not engaged in rendering legal or any other professional services. If legal or any other expert assistance is required, the services of a competent person should be sought. FROM A DECLARATION OF PARTICIPANTS JOINTLY ADOPTED BY A COMMITTEE OF THE AMERICAN BAR ASSOCIATION AND A COMMITTEE OF PUBLISHERS.

LIBRARY OF CONGRESS CATALOGING-IN-PUBLICATION DATA

Nutrition research advances / [edited by] Sarah V. Watkins.
    p. ; cm.
  Includes bibliographical references and index.
  ISBN-13: 978-1-60021-516-2 (hardcover)
  ISBN-10: 1-60021-516-5 (hardcover)
  1. Nutrition. I. Watkins, Sarah V.
  [DNLM: 1. Nutrition. 2. Diet. QU 145 N975396 2006]
613.2—dc22
                    2006038607

Published by Nova Science Publishers, Inc. ✦ *New York*

CONTENTS

PREFACE

The taking in and use of food and other nourishing material by the body. Nutrition is a 3-part process. First, food or drink is consumed. Second, the body breaks down the food or drink into nutrients. Third, the nutrients travel through the bloodstream to different parts of the body where they are used as "fuel" and for many other purposes. To give the body proper nutrition, a person has to eat and drink enough of the foods that contain key nutrients. This new book examines new and important research in this field

Chapter I - High-fat, low-carbohydrate (ketogenic) diets (KDs) have been used clinically for the treatment of epilepsy for at least 85 years. Clinical indications for initiating such a diet, some of the side effects likely to occur during diet administration and indications for maintenance of the diet and strategies for its discontinuation are considered, largely from the perspective of treating the epileptic patient. Although the diet has most often been used for pediatric patients, recent experience has shown that it can be effective for use with adolescents and adults. The efficacy of dietary treatment of epilepsy has been extended beyond the classical 4:1 LCT (long-chain triglyceride) diet to modified Atkins and low glycemic index diets. Efficacy is most often limited by non-compliance. Among the key variables during administration of such diets are variations in the level of ketonemia, the degree of hypoglycemia and the level of hyperlipidemia. Any or all of these variables may be part of the mechanisms by which KDs reduce seizure incidence and/or severity. Several candidate mechanisms linking diet to the alteration of central nervous system excitability are identified. Lipid catabolism occurs within mitochondria and consumption of KDs leads to increased proliferation and increased size of itochondria, reflecting increased oxidative stress. Production of reactive oxygen species (ROS) under such conditions is minimized by an increased expression of uncoupling proteins (UCPs) and has consequences for calcium sequestration within the mitochondrial matrix and cytosol. All have potential for diminishing neuronal hyperexcitability. The state of oxidative phosphorylation and ATP/ADP production may affect membrane excitability by altering the activity of the Na/K ATPase or $K_{ATP/ADP}$ channels. Classical high-fat diets include elevated levels of polyunsaturated fatty acids (PUFAs), which may inhibit both Na^+ and Ca^{++} channels and activate tandem-pore potassium (K2p) channels. The net effects of any of these changes will depend upon the identity of the neuronal or glial populations most affected. For example, decreased excitation of excitatory neurons and increased excitation of inhibitory neurons would both act to reduce seizures. A working theoretical model incorporating many of the factors considered in this chapter is proposed.

Chapter II - Wernicke's encephalopathy is an acute neuropsychiatric syndrome characterized in its classical form by paralysis of eye movements, stuggering gait and mental changes, a triad not frequently encountered in clinical practice. It results from a deficiency in vitamin B1, or thiamine, an essential coenzyme in intermediate carbohydrate metabolism. Thiamine requirements are directly related to total caloric intake and to the proportion of calories provided as carbohydrates. As a consequence, high caloric and high carbohydrate oral diets increase the demand for thiamine. Moreover, genetic factors may determine the response to diet and hence influence the susceptibility to Wernicke's encephalopathy. Additional, environmental factors that may modify thiamine requirements or usefulness include prolonged cooking of foods, ethanol ingestion (which impairs thiamine transport across intestinal mucosa), post-operative intravenous hyperalimentation, the consumption of foods containing thiaminases or antithiamine compounds (e.g., the use of some raw fish and certain teas), the use of some chemotherapy agents that may impair conversion of thiamine into its active metabolite thiamine pyrophosphate, and the occurrence of magnesium depletion which may induce a refractory response to thiamine. The recommended thiamine doses for healthy adults range between 0.5 and 0.66 mg per 1000 Kcal. These doses are likely higher in children, in critically ill conditions, during pregnancy and lactation. However, the precise amount of thiamine to be given in these cases remains an important unsettled issue. Wernicke's encephalopathy may occur in chronic alcoholism, when the dietary intake of thiamine is inadequate, and may complicate any condition in which there is poor nutrition. In particular, the conditions of poor nutrition associated with Wernicke's encephalopathy include persistent vomiting, anorexia nervosa, prolonged starvation for the treatment of obesity, prolonged fasting, and the use of dietary commercial formulae, with or without thiamine, in severely ill patients. An emerging, leading potential risk factor for Wernicke's encephalopathy in susceptible individuals is the use of prolonged, apparently balanced slimming diets. Usually, these diets contain thiamine in amounts that conform to standard nutritional recommendations. Thus, the occurrence of Wernicke's encephalopathy following a slimming diet, it is not something one would predict on general principles. Common, additional supplementations to these diets include herbal preparations and certain teas. These supplements may interfere with thiamine's intestinal absorption, or act as thiamine antagonists. Moreover, another important question is "do these diets actually contain the amount of thiamine reported on the label?". These products are not well monitored by the public health authorities, and quality control can be poor as recently demonstrated by tests on other dietary formulae (e.g., a soy-based formula for infants, defective in thiamine, identified in Israel in 2003). Even when suspected, thiamine deficiency is difficult to diagnose, since the available tests for measuring thiamine activity in blood or other tissues are usually not available routinely. Wernicke's encephalopathy remains a clinical diagnosis. It is very important to make a presumptive diagnosis of this encephalopathy and treat the patient as soon as possible. Prompt vitamin B1 replenishment in suspected cases is the safest approach to prevent neurological symptoms and may be a life-saving measure.

Chapter III - For decades, research intended to reduce the incidence of criminal violence has been largely unsuccessful. Such efforts include psychoanalytic approaches, behavior modification techniques, and experimental drug therapies. One of the possible reasons for the failure is that designs do not consider biological factors such as malnutrition in the development of antisocial, violent and criminal behavior (Raine, 2002a). Although the role of malnutrition in the development of antisocial behavior has gained some attention, research has still placed little weight on this topic (Fishbein, 2001, Rutter et al, 1998). This is despite decades of the dictum "you are what you eat" which emphasized the importance of nutritional factors impacting on human being behavior. The purpose of this chapter is to provide an overview of malnutrition as a risk factor for antisocial behavior, and to identify possible brain mechanisms which may account for the malnutrition – antisocial behavior link. To better illustrate the interplay among risk factors, mechanisms and behavioral outcome, a hypothetical malnutrition–psychopathology model will be outlined to provide a conceptual framework. Using this framework, we will first review empirical research on nutrition and antisocial behavior. Three key areas of brain dysfunction due to malnutrition will then be explored. Following recent findings from Mauritius on malnutrition and externalizing behavior are briefly presented. Finally, the current limitations of nutritional research on antisocial behavior and future research direction are outlined.

Chapter IV- Research justified, that natural antioxidants and bioactive agents related to antioxidant effects could act on signal transduction pathways and/or phase II enzyme activities directly and/or indirectly. These molecules can also influence the apoptotic genes.

In the case of plant extracts, which contain several active compounds, one might consider it is impossible to discover the single mechanism of action. This problem becomes even more complicated, when we bring the obtained data of in vitro and in vivo experiments into consideration. Therefore the multifactorial actions must be analyzed in short and long term in vivo studies on redox homeostasis.

The questions are: - can the absorbed compounds of natural extracts from the gastrointestinal tract influence the changed cellular redox states in experimental bowel disease in all parts of gut, and how can these molecules act on the redox homeostasis of blood in IBD patients?

Our aim was to present the protective effect of natural polyphenols and flavonoids of the *Sempervivum tectorum* extract (2g/bwkg/day for 10 days) on alimentary induced bowel disease in rats, and the isothiocyanate-rich *Raphanus sativus* niger based granule (0.2 g/die Raphacol) in a twelvemonth clinical study in patients suffered from IBD.

The redox balance did not change significantly, when the health animals were treated with the *Sempervivum tectorum* extract. In fat rich diet induced bowel disease the treatment caused a beneficial change in reducing power of ileum and H-donating ability was significantly better in all large bowel parts. The data of scavenger capacity were better in part of short bowel and enormous changes were detected in parts of large bowel in sick animals. The *Sempervivum tectorum* treatment was beneficial. The redox concluded from these results that antioxidant compounds (after bacterial and non bacterial enzymatic transformation) take part in redox homeostasis.

Raphacol treatment did not influence the activity of IBD. Beside beneficial subjective judgement, bile acid level was elevated continuously and the values of redox parameters were decreased in the plasma during treatment. The granule diminished the erythrocyte chemiluminescence significantly and the HbA_{1c}-level moderately until the beginning of the ninth month. After this, the trend has changed until the end. Data showed, that antioxidant and isothiocyanate-rich granule could influence the redox homeostasis of IBD patients even at low dose.

Chapter V – The authors have found that the quality of nutrition during pregnancy, lactation or early ontogeny induces changes in a functioning of enzyme systems of the digestive and non-digestive organs in the adult rat posterities not only of the first generation, but also of the subsequent ones. These researches develop the ideas of academician A.M. Ugolev – a discoverer of the membrane digestion. It has been shown that protein deficiency in nutrition of pregnant or lactating rats results in significant reduction of activities of some digestive enzymes in the small intestine, and of the same enzymes in the large intestine, liver and kidney in the rat posterities of 2- and 4-months old. Activities of the enzymes in the rat posterities of 6-months old do not restore their levels in control animals, receiving a standard diet during the development. Various changes of enzymes activities in the digestive and non-digestive organs take also place in the adult posterities of the second (and the third) generations, born by rats, whose "mothers" (and "grandmothers") received a low protein diet during pregnancy or lactation. The protein excess in the diet of the lactating rats results in significant reduction of activities of the digestive enzymes in the small intestine and of the same enzymes in the large intestine, the liver and kidney in the posterities of 2- and 6-months old. On the contrary, an increase of the enzymes activities has been observed in the posterities of 4-months old. A restriction of protein in the diet of rat pups during their transition from the mixed to the definitive nutrition leads to increase of activities of some enzymes and to decrease some other ones in adult life of the rat pups and in adult life of their posterities. It has been concluded that such a stress factor, as deficiency or excess of the protein in nutrition of animals during pregnancy or lactation, and in early ontogeny as well, results in disorders of formation of enzyme systems in the digestive and non-digestive organs and in changes of their functioning in adult life of themselves and in adult life of their posterities. These processes seem to realize at genetic or epigenetic levels. The epigenetic phenomena may involve the altered packaging and activation of a variety of the genes. The unfavorable early nutrition programming of enzymatic systems of the digestive and non-digestive organs may be a key event in the disorders of various metabolic reactions, therefore promoting a development of chronic diseases.

Chapter VI - There is now some scientific evidence largely obtained from experimental animal studies that certain natural dietary and plant constituents such as Nigella sativa seed, Ginsengs, and Caffeine could have a weak therapeutic or prophylactic potential. The main advantage of these agents is their low toxicity, as they had been used as food additives for decades and centuries without the occurrence of any serious toxicity or adverse effects.

Nigella Sativa(NS) seed has been reported in researches from many countries including USA, Canada, Germany, Spain, Japan, Sweden, Eygpt,Turkey, Iran and Saudia Arabia, to have many possibly beneficial therapeutic and prophylactic effects such as anti-inflammatory effect, analgesic effect, antioxidant effect, and anti-tumor effects.NS seed has also been reported to have a protective effect against nephrotoxixity,hepatotoxicity and diabetes. In particular, there is now a rather a convincing preliminary scientific evidence that NS seed component(s) could has a beneficial adjunctive role in the management of diabetes, and also in the management of some tumors especially colonic cancer, and clinical trials are particularly recommended in these fields. The anti-leukotrienes effect can also be clinically useful as there are very few drugs have this pharmacological effect; however this effect may need more experimental studies.

The low toxicity of Nigella sativa fixed oil is evidenced by high LD50 values on experimental acute toxicity. There is no change in hepatic enzyme stability and organ integrity after 12 weeks of administration of large doses in which rats suggests a wide margin of safety for therapeutic doses of Nigella sativa fixed oil, but the changes in hemoglobin metabolism and the fall in leukocyte and platelet count must be taken into consideration when using large doses for a long time is required.

Chapter VII - Despite little literature on coffee lipids, it has been hypothesized that they lower coffee quality through hydrolysis of the triacylglycerols during storage releasing free fatty acids, which are in turn oxidized to produce compounds producing off-flavour. Coffee is stored for extended periods by small producers in Brazil to fetch better market prices. As a part of our coffee-breeding program aiming to improve the quality of Brazilian coffee, we plan to evaluate the role of lipids during storage, developing initially methods (TLC-thin layer chromatography, HLPC-LSD-high performance liquid chromatography with light sensitive detection and HPLC with refractive index detection) for their determination. In this study experiments were carried out to evaluate the variation of lipid classes (free fatty acids, fatty acids after oil hydrolysis, triacylglycerols-TAG and terpene esters-TE) during coffee storage. Three types of coffee beans (immature, random mixture and cherry) picked in Viçosa, MG, Brazil (a region traditionally considered to be a producer of low quality coffee), were dried by two widely used procedures (dryer and open air cement patio) and stored on wood shelves in a house without neither temperature nor humidity control for 19 months. We tried to reproduce storage conditions used by small farmers in Brazil. At 4, 7, 10, 13, 16 and 19 months of storage, a part of samples was withdrawn and lipid classes were analyzed using the methods developed in our laboratory. The experiment consisted of thirty-six treatments in a randomised block design with three repetitions. The following treatments (T) were used: immature coffee beans dried in a dryer (T_1) and on a patio (T_2); a random mixture of coffee beans dried in a dryer (T_3) and on a patio (T_4) and cherry coffee beans dried in a dryer (T_5) and on a patio (T_6). In these treatments, samples were stored for four months followed by analysis of lipid classes. The procedure was repeated for immature, random and cherry coffee beans after 7, 10, 13, 16 and 19 months of storage corresponding to treatments T_7-T_{12}, T_{13}-T_{18}, T_{19}-T_{24}, T_{25}-T_{30} and T_{31}-T_{36}, respectively. Lipid class data were statistically analyzed through variance and regression. The qualitative factors (type of coffee and type of drying) and the averages were compared by the Tukey test at 5% probability. The quantitative factor (months of storage) and the averages were chosen based on the significance of regression coefficients using the t test at 5% probability and determination coefficients (r^2). While apparently random variation was observed in a few cases, no effects of storage time, storage type and coffee type were found on the lipid classes. These results contradict literature studies where a small number of samples were studied utilizing short storage times.

Chaper VIII - Epidemiological studies on historical and contemporary populations indicate that the intra-uterine environment is a major factor contributing to later health and disease in the resulting offspring. These findings are supported by experimental studies which indicate that both macro and micronutrient deficiencies or excesses can have substantial long-term health implications for the offspring. In this chapter the authors will consider the extent to which changes in maternal diet, lifestyle and age can interact to substantially impact on the future health of the offspring. The impact of both increasing and decreasing maternal dietary intake, either throughout pregnancy, or at defined stages of development will be covered. Focus will be on the interaction between the maternal diet and her endocrine status with respect to placental development and later function. This will be related to key stages in development from the time of conception through to early adulthood and its impact on cardiovascular control systems, kidney development and metabolic homeostasis. Critically, they consider the extent to which a mismatch between diet in utero and that available during lactation or early childhood can mean individuals are programmed to later obesity and cardiovascular disease including diabetes.

Chapter I

DIET AND EPILEPSY

Kristopher J. Bough[1,], Douglas A. Eagles[2] and Eric H. Kossoff[3]*

[1]Food and Drug Administration, Center for Drug Evaluation and Research, Rockville, MD 20855 USA;

[2]Department of Biology, Georgetown University, Washington, DC, 20057 USA;

[3]Departments of Pediatrics and Neurology, Johns Hopkins University Hospital, Baltimore, MD USA 21287.

ABSTRACT

High-fat, low-carbohydrate (ketogenic) diets (KDs) have been used clinically for the treatment of epilepsy for at least 85 years. Clinical indications for initiating such a diet, some of the side effects likely to occur during diet administration and indications for maintenance of the diet and strategies for its discontinuation are considered, largely from the perspective of treating the epileptic patient. Although the diet has most often been used for pediatric patients, recent experience has shown that it can be effective for use with adolescents and adults. The efficacy of dietary treatment of epilepsy has been extended beyond the classical 4:1 LCT (long-chain triglyceride) diet to modified Atkins and low glycemic index diets. Efficacy is most often limited by non-compliance. Among the key variables during administration of such diets are variations in the level of ketonemia, the degree of hypoglycemia and the level of hyperlipidemia. Any or all of these variables may be part of the mechanisms by which KDs reduce seizure incidence and/or severity. Several candidate mechanisms linking diet to the alteration of central nervous system excitability are identified. Lipid catabolism occurs within mitochondria and consumption of KDs leads to increased proliferation and increased size of mitochondria, reflecting increased oxidative stress. Production of reactive oxygen species (ROS) under such conditions is minimized by an increased expression of uncoupling proteins (UCPs) and has consequences for calcium sequestration within the

---

* Correspondence concerning this article should be addressed to Kristopher J. Bough, PhD Food and Drug Administration Center for Drug Evaluation and Research, MPN1 – Room 1345, 7520 Standish Place, Rockville, MD 20855.

mitochondrial matrix and cytosol. All have potential for diminishing neuronal hyperexcitability. The state of oxidative phosphorylation and ATP/ADP production may affect membrane excitability by altering the activity of the Na/K ATPase or $K_{ATP/ADP}$ channels. Classical high-fat diets include elevated levels of polyunsaturated fatty acids (PUFAs), which may inhibit both Na^+ and Ca^{++} channels and activate tandem-pore potassium (K2p) channels. The net effects of any of these changes will depend upon the identity of the neuronal or glial populations most affected. For example, decreased excitation of excitatory neurons and increased excitation of inhibitory neurons would both act to reduce seizures. A working theoretical model incorporating many of the factors considered in this chapter is proposed.

Keywords: ketogenic diet, epilepsy, seizure, fat, energy, metabolism, hippocampus

INTRODUCTION

History of a Dietary Treatment for Epilepsy

"When one wanted to turn a clouded mentality to a clear one, it could almost always be done with fasting" (Geyelin, 1921). This remains true to date 85 years after Dr. H. Rawle Geyelin, an endocrinologist at the New York Presbyterian Hospital, reported his results with fasting to treat epilepsy at the annual meeting of the American Medical Association in 1921. Fasting was the initial basis for the eventual ketogenic diet (KD), and children were often fasted for up to three weeks with good results; however, seizures then would often return (Geyelin, 1921; Lennox and Cobb, 1928; Talbot et al., 1927; Weeks et al., 1923). The reason why fasting worked was unclear, and Dr. Hugh Conklin, an osteopathic physician and one of the first to publish on this therapy, believed fasting purged the body of toxins secreted from the Peyer's glands into the lymphatic system (Conklin, 1922).

Fasting could not be maintained for long periods of time, and seizures would often return after food was reintroduced. To solve this dilemma, Wilder (Wilder, 1921), at the Mayo Clinic, created a high fat, low carbohydrate diet to induce ketosis and treat epilepsy long-term. The KD in use today is nearly identical to that used by Dr. Wilder. The diet became widely used for both children and adults in the 1920s and 1930s until phenytoin was discovered in 1938 (Merritt and Putnam, 1938a; Merritt and Putnam, 1938b) and anticonvulsant medications became the treatments of choice for epilepsy. In comparison, the KD was perceived as restrictive, unpalatable, and expensive. As research increased dramatically for anticonvulsants over the next several decades, most neurologists also perceived the KD as unproven and ineffective.

In 1994, a 2-year-old boy named Charlie Abrahams was treated at the Johns Hopkins Hospital for intractable epilepsy that had not responded to either medications or surgery. After Charlie became both seizure-free and developmentally improved after treatment with the KD, his father created the Charlie Foundation to inform both parents and physicians about the important role that could be served by the KD. Since that time, clinical interest in the diet has skyrocketed and books have been written on the subject (Freeman et al., 2000). Today, nearly all major cities and epilepsy centers in the United States offer the KD. In an email survey, clinics in 41 countries reported using the diet, and that number is increasing annually (Kossoff and McGrogan, 2005). From nearly 100 years of clinical use, it is clear that a KD can have dramatic effects on cognitive health. The goal of this chapter is to examine how diet influences cognitive function and possible mechanisms responsible for seizure resistance. It is divided into two primary sections. The first section is geared toward understanding clinical use of a KD and key variables related to its implementation and effectiveness. In the second section, we review experimental studies focused on understanding *how* diet affects neuronal (dys)function.

CLINICAL USE OF A KETOGENIC DIET

The KD is a high fat, moderate to low protein, and very low carbohydrate diet. The diet is calculated to provide either a 3:1 or 4:1 ratio of fat to combined carbohydrate and protein (by weight). Higher ratios are typically associated with higher levels of ketosis, and therefore theoretically greater efficacy. Commonly, infants and adolescents are started on a 3:1 KD ratio, in order to be able to provide extra protein and to allow adolescents increased choices of foods (Freeman et al., 2000). Most other children are started on a 4:1 ratio. However, lower ratios, even 2:1 or lower, have been successfully used in India, China, and other nations in which rice is difficult to restrict in diets (Kossoff and McGrogan, 2005). A modified version of the Atkins diet, under current investigation, is likely a 1.5-2:1 ratio KD (Kossoff et al., 2003).

Fats are provided in both saturated and polyunsaturated forms, and traditionally as large-chain triglycerides (LCT), comprising 85-90% of calories. High fat foods used with the diet include 36% heavy whipping cream, butter, oils (canola, olive), and mayonnaise. A version of the KD using medium chain triglyceride (MCT) oil has been used in some centers since the 1960s to allow more carbohydrates, but can be associated with abdominal distention, cramps, and diarrhea (Huttenlocher, 1976; Schwartz et al., 1989b). There is no evidence of superiority of this diet over the traditional LCT diet, and a current randomized trial of 120 patients comparing the two diets again is nearing completion in London (personal communication, Helen Cross). The daily protein amount is based on requirements for age and size (typically 1 gram/kg/day); carbohydrates are typically fewer than 10 grams per day, with the remainder of calories then calculated as fat.

Calories are restricted to 75% of the estimated daily requirement; however, children with unusually high or low metabolic needs may receive an adjusted percentage. In general, most dietitians target a body mass index (BMI) for age of 50%. Fluids are traditionally also restricted to 80% of the recommended daily intake, although there is no evidence to support this restriction. In our experience, children may actually be receiving fewer fluids prior to the diet normally, and the fluid "restriction" is actually an increase. In children with risk factors for kidney stones (carbonic anhydrase inhibitor anticonvulsant medications, prior history of renal stones or disease, strong family history of kidney stones), fluids are often not restricted (Kossoff et al., 2002a). Meals are computer-calculated and foods are carefully weighed using a gram scale by parents at home. Snacks are often provided as well in order to satisfy hunger and spread fat calories (and therefore maintain constant ketone levels) throughout the day and evening.

Administration of a Ketogenic Diet

Beginning the Diet

The decision by a family to begin the KD for their child is a complicated one. Unless families must travel a great distance to our center, we universally will discuss the advantages and disadvantages of the diet in person before any admission is scheduled. Our center routinely asks both parents to handwrite their goals and expectations for the diet beforehand in order to facilitate communication between the KD team and families. When these letters were evaluated, although seizure and anticonvulsant reduction were the two highest expectations, cognition and alertness improvement were also very important to 90% of families (Farasat et al., 2006). Achieving the pre-diet parental goals for cognition correlated with eventual diet duration, unlike goals for seizure and anticonvulsant reduction. Most families were very realistic about the likelihood of freedom from seizures or medications.

Children are often admitted in groups of 3-4 in order to facilitate nursing management and education. All children have baseline metabolic testing done to ensure no contraindications exist to the use of the diet. These would include pyruvate carboxylase deficiency, fatty acid oxidation defects, carnitine deficiency, and some mitochondrial disorders.

Most KD centers admit children to the hospital for a 3 to 5-day period, during which the KD is gradually advanced after a 24-48 hour fast. The specific protocol used at the Johns Hopkins Hospital during the admission period is described in Table 1. Although there is good evidence to suggest that long-term outcomes may be similar for children started gradually on the diet without a fast, we have found the short-term benefits of the fast can be very reassuring to families (Bergqvist et al., 2005; Freeman and Vining, 1999; Kim et al., 2004; Wirrell et al., 2002). For some children, the initial fast can provide an immediate improvement in seizure control that can be motivating to the patient and family. In addition, a repeated, brief outpatient fast is a useful therapy physicians can recommend if a child is ill and has lower ketosis. In our experience, the side effects of fasting are minimal, transient, and easily treatable (hypoglycemia, vomiting, and occasional acidosis). Even centers that do not fast children typically will admit them for several days, as the hospitalization is a valuable opportunity to watch for any acute worsening on the diet (as might be seen in an unrecognized metabolic disorder) and to provide adequate education for the families. The admission period also allows for the child's medications to be reviewed, ensuring that they are as free of carbohydrates as possible (Lebel et al., 2001). Many suspension forms of anticonvulsants contain carbohydrates or sugar alcohols that can disrupt ketosis. The use of tablets, sprinkles, or orally ingested intravenous preparations (e.g. phenytoin and phenobarbital) is usually recommended.

Diet Maintenance and Discontinuation

The management of children on the diet is unique to each individual center and non-standardized. Several common practices do exist, however. All children should be discharged home with prescriptions for daily multivitamin and calcium supplements, either Unicap M™ and Calcimix™ or other products lacking carbohydrates. Urine ketones are checked several times per week by parents, often at the same time each day. It is important to remember than urinary ketosis may reflect dietary intake over 1-2 days, and sudden dietary changes should not be based on these results. Some centers have found serum BHB levels checked with a hand-held ketone meter to be helpful in some situations as well (Gilbert et al., 2000). Weight, height, laboratory values (urine calcium and creatinine, urinalysis, fasting complete lipid profile, electrolytes, liver function tests, and a complete blood count) are often checked every 3-6 months along with outpatient KD clinic visits. Infants are often seen more frequently, occasionally monthly. Some centers either start carnitine initially or monitor acyl-carnitine levels while the child is on the diet. Evidence for the clinical benefit of carnitine is lacking, however, and the addition of this supplement to the diet can be costly (Berry-Kravis et al., 2001a).

Table 1. Ketogenic diet protocol at Johns Hopkins Hospital

Day prior to admission (Sunday)
- Reduced carbohydrates for 24 hours
- Fasting starts the evening before admission

Day 1 (Monday)
- Admitted to the hospital
- Fasting continues
- Fluids restricted to 60-75 cc/kg
- Blood glucose monitored every 6 hours
- Use carbohydrate-free medications
- Parents begin educational program (diet overview)

Day 2 (Tuesday)
- Dinner given as 1/3 of calculated diet meal as "eggnog"
- Blood glucose checks discontinued after dinner
- Parents begin to check urine ketones periodically
- Education continues (calculating and weighing foods)

Day 3 (Wednesday)
- Breakfast and lunch given as 1/3 of diet
- Dinner increased to 2/3 (still eggnog)
- Education continues (maintenance, checking ketosis)

Day 4 (Thursday)
- Breakfast and lunch given as 2/3 of diet allowance
- Dinner is first full ketogenic meal (not eggnog)
- Education completed (handling illnesses)

Day 5 (Friday)
- Full ketogenic diet breakfast given
- Prescriptions reviewed and follow-up arranged
- Child discharged to home

Many families request a tapering or discontinuation of anticonvulsant medications almost immediately after beginning the diet (Kossoff et al., 2004b). Typically, anticonvulsant medications are not changed immediately after starting the diet; however, they can be tapered and discontinued rapidly if side effects are significant and drug efficacy is questionable. Recent evidence suggests that although this is generally safe and seizures do not become more prevalent, the families' long-term compliance with the diet is not improved by an immediate medication taper. Patience is advised.

Most children on the diet remain on at least one anticonvulsant medication. To date, there is no clear evidence that any single anticonvulsant medication is more efficacious when used in combination with the diet. There is also no evidence that any medication is unsafe. Topiramate and zonisamide, medications that can also lead to acidosis and kidney stones, do not increase the risk above that of the diet alone (Kossoff et al., 2002a; Takeoka et al., 2002). Valproate also appears to be unlikely to cause adverse effects when used with the diet (Lyczkowski et al., 2005). Interestingly, another non-pharmacologic therapy, vagus nerve stimulation (VNS), in anecdotal experience appears to work well in combination with the diet and is under investigation.

The decision to discontinue the diet is individualized and based on physicians' and parents' combined experiences for the child. If the diet is unsuccessful in seizure or medication reduction, despite elevated ketosis and absence of other confounding factors (e.g. illness, surgery, cheating), most families discontinue the diet by 6 months (Freeman et al., 1998). Approximately 50% of the children started on the diet remain on it for one year. Children are maintained on the KD for as long as it is beneficial, but typically 1-2 years if it is successful, in a manner similar to anticonvulsants. A significantly higher number of children that failed to respond to the diet will have seizure improvement 3-6 years later if surgery or VNS has been tried (as opposed to more anticonvulsants). Even for children who do not become completely seizure-free, the diet has often been more successful than were any medications. In this situation, children may be maintained on the diet indefinitely. There is no mandatory recommendation to discontinue the diet; however, if side effects become problematic then the utility of the diet needs to be carefully assessed.

At the Johns Hopkins Hospital, 28 children, approximately 5% of those started on the diet at our institution since 1993, have been in ketosis for 6-12 years (Groesbeck, et. al., unpublished data). For these families, 24 (86%) children experienced >90% reduction in seizures and, of these, 22 (96%) parents reported satisfaction with the diet's efficacy. The diet was perceived as "easy" for 91% of parents responding to a phone questionnaire. As a result, only about half the patients on the diet felt the need to monitor urinary ketosis more often than once per month.

When the decision is made to discontinue the diet, in a manner similar to that practiced with anticonvulsant drugs, the diet is not stopped abruptly. The diet is traditionally tapered over 1-2 months by lowering the fat to protein and carbohydrate ratio (e.g., from 4:1 to 3:1 then 2:1), then relaxing restrictions on weighing foods and measuring carbohydrate intake. During this process, ketones can be checked and if seizures worsen, the diet ratio increased. When the diet is perceived to be harmful or families request the diet to be discontinued more rapidly, 36% heavy cream can be changed immediately to whole-milk, then 2% milk, and, eventually, skim milk over a period of several days. In some situations, such as during inpatient hospitalizations following seizures, the diet can be discontinued immediately while intravenous anticonvulsants are administered.

Side Effects

The KD is a serious medical therapy with potential side effects and complications (Wheless, 2001). References to the diet as "alternative" or "all-natural" are erroneous. However, the side effects of the diet are very predictable and rarely lead to diet discontinuation.

Complications of the diet are best divided into common and expected, occasional, and rare (case reports). The common side effects include a lack of weight gain or a weight loss (sometimes this is planned), constipation, low-grade acidosis (which can worsen with concurrent illnesses), and transient hypoglycemia during the fasting period (Ballaban-Gil et al., 1998; Kang et al., 2004; Kim et al., 2004). All of these side effects are manageable, and small changes in caloric restriction or fluid allotment can lead to improvement.

Occasional complications include kidney stones (6%), dyslipidemia (changes in cholesterol, triglycerides, HDL and LDL), and diminished growth (Furth et al., 2000; Kwiterovich et al., 2003; Liu et al., 2003; Peterson et al., 2005; Vining et al., 2002; Williams et al., 2002). Kidney stones are clinically obvious and can be associated with hematuria and pain. We routinely screen the urine calcium to creatinine ratio every 3-6 months and begin oral alkalinization (Polycitra K™, 2 Meq/kg/day divided twice daily) if the ratio is higher than 0.2. Unless there is a personal or family history of renal stones, there is no evidence that anticonvulsants with carbonic anhydrase inhibition properties (topiramate, zonisamide, and acetazolamide) increase the risk of stones and should be avoided (Kossoff et al., 2002a). Growth tends to be most affected in children under age 2 and, possibly, in those on the KD for prolonged periods or with higher levels of ketosis (Peterson et al., 2005; Vining et al., 2002). Blood lipids are typically increased 130% after 6 months on the diet, but do not continue to increase in the majority of the patients after that point (Kwiterovich et al., 2003). Significant dyslipidemia can be treated by lowering the diet ratio or by substituting polyunsaturated fats or MCT oil. None of the above mentioned side effects should necessitate diet discontinuation and can be treated with diet modifications or supplemental medications. Rare, typically single case-report only, side effects include vitamin and mineral deficiencies (prevented with typical supplementation), selenium deficiency, pancreatitis, cardiomyopathy, bruising, basal ganglia change, and prolonged QT intervals (Ballaban-Gil et al., 1998; Bergqvist et al., 2003; Berry-Kravis et al., 2001b; Best et al., 2000; Erickson et al., 2003; Hahn et al., 1979; Stewart et al., 2001).

Long-term side effects of the diet (e.g., fractures, atherosclerosis, and growth deficiencies) remain to be formally identified. In a recent study by our center of 28 children on the diet for 6-12 years duration, 25% had fractures, and 21% had kidney stones (Groesbeck et. al., unpublished data). Nearly 80% were <10% for age in their heights and weights, although 36-50% were <10% in these growth parameters, respectively, at the time the diet was started. On the other hand, no family discontinued the diet for these reasons and nearly all had a >90% improvement at the most recent follow-up. In addition, cholesterol and other lipids were not abnormally elevated. After 6 years, mean cholesterol was 201 mg/dl, HDL 54 mg/dl, LDL 129 mg/dl, and triglycerides 97 mg/dl.

Use of a Ketogenic Diet for Epilepsy

For the majority of the clinical use of the KD in history, it has been used to treat intractable childhood epilepsy. However, both recent as well as older studies have questioned this traditional indication for all three components: "intractable", "childhood", and "epilepsy." Research exists to support the clinical use of the diet for the care of both relatively new onset childhood seizures, difficult-to-control epilepsy in infants, adolescents, and adults, and medical conditions other than epilepsy. These will be all discussed in detail later in this review.

The most common usage of the diet in regards to seizure types is for children with symptomatic generalized epilepsies such as Lennox-Gastaut syndrome. This syndrome is one of the more common conditions to be investigated in both retrospective and prospective studies of the diet (Freeman et al., 1998; Kinsman et al., 1992; Vining et al., 1998). In this condition, children will often have multiple seizure types including atonic, tonic, myoclonic, and atypical absence seizures. The EEG will commonly reveal slow (2-2.5 hertz) spike-wave discharges with an abnormal background.

One other epilepsy syndrome that has been effectively treated by the KD includes infantile spasms. In this condition affecting infants ages 3-6 months at onset, a high voltage, chaotic multifocal spike and slow wave pattern is recognized on the EEG in association with clusters of head drops and arm extensions. Infants often have developmental delay in association with this condition. Effective therapies include ACTH (adrenocorticotropin hormone) and vigabatrin, but both have significant side effects and vigabatrin is no longer available in the United States (Appleton et al., 1999; Vigevano and Cilio, 1997). Two publications have described the benefits of using the KD for intractable infantile spasms, one for this disorder specifically (Kossoff et al., 2002b; Nordli et al., 2001). In one study, approximately half of 23 infants had a 90% improvement in spasms, development, and EEG after 12 months. A recent abstract presentation at the American Epilepsy Society in 2004 reported similar results from South Korea (Eun et al., 2004). Interestingly, the diet appears to be most effective in infants treated before the age of 1 year and prior to attempting three anticonvulsants, raising the theoretical possible benefit of using the KD as first-line therapy (Nordli et al., 2001).

Other generalized seizure types such as myoclonic, atonic, and tonic seizures have been treated effectively with the diet, especially those affecting infants or very young children (Caraballo et al., 2005). Myoclonic-astatic epilepsy (Doose) has been reported to be amenable to the KD as well (Laux et al., 2004). Most epileptologists do not believe the diet is as effective for partial-onset epilepsy. In a study of 150 children placed on the diet by Johns Hopkins Hospital, the diet was equally effective for all seizure types, including partial epilepsy (Freeman et al., 1998); however, others have found it less effective in this situation (Maydell et al., 2001). When 18 children that had an early, dramatic response (seizure-free within 2 weeks) to the KD were compared to the overall population, none had partial epilepsy (Than et al., 2005). Our experience suggests that the KD is very helpful in managing partial onset epilepsy, and occasionally delays the time until resective surgery is performed, but rarely represents a cure.

Other conditions for which the KD has been beneficial include tuberous sclerosis complex (TSC) and Rett syndrome (Kossoff et al., 2005); ((Liebhaber et al., 2003). After 6 months, 11 (92%) of the combined 12 children treated with the diet for intractable seizures associated with TSC at Johns Hopkins Hospital and Massachusetts General Hospital were over 50% improved, and 8 (67%) were >90% improved (Kossoff et al., 2005). Five children had seizure-free periods of at least 5 months duration. For this syndrome, typically associated with focal epilepsy (due to cortical tubers), the efficacy was surprisingly high.

Another population worth discussion is children with epilepsy that have gastrostomy tubes in place for nutrition. Two recent publications demonstrated impressive results when children are provided the diet solely as a formula (Hosain et al., 2005; Kossoff et al., 2004a). This can be provided using either modular components such as Microlipid™, Ross Carbohydrate-Free™, and Polycose™, or as a pre-packaged 4:1 powdered form (SHS KetoCal™). Patients on formula-only diets have guaranteed compliance along with excellent tolerability. In a study from Johns Hopkins of 61 children formula-fed (30 had gastrostomy tubes), 59% had a >90% seizure reduction at 12 months, which is nearly double that of the overall population treated with the diet (Kossoff et al., 2004a).

Newer Onset Epilepsy

Is there a role for the diet prior to treatment (and failure) with several anticonvulsant drugs? As with most medications, the diet is more effective when used early in the course of epilepsy treatment (Freeman and Vining, 1998; Kossoff, 2004). However, most neurologists still use the diet only after typically 4-5 anticonvulsants have been tried and have failed (Hemingway et al., 2001). In 2001, *Epilepsy and Behavior* published "The Expert Consensus Guidelines," in which 100 epileptologists reviewed clinical case scenarios and provided their treatment options in order of preference (Karceski, 2001). For idiopathic generalized epilepsy, the diet ranked 15th in a list of possible therapies; seventy-four percent of the physicians considered it an appropriate choice, but only as a third-line therapy. Even in symptomatic generalized epilepsies (e.g., Lennox Gastaut syndrome), the diet ranked no higher than 9th place. For partial epilepsy, it barely made the list.

The KD was one of the only therapies for epilepsy in the early part of the 20th century, before anticonvulsants such as phenytoin and carbamazepine were developed. In one of the earliest reports of the diet, the Mayo Clinic reported 17 children in which 10 (60%) were seizure-free, and four (23%) were >90% improved (Peterman, 1924). These children were likely less intractable. Since 1994 at Johns Hopkins Hospital, the KD has been used either as the first or second therapy for epilepsy in approximately 3% (13 of 460) of patients (Rubenstein et al., 2005). In these 13 children, 60% had a >90% seizure reduction at 6 months and 100% had a >90% reduction at 12 months. Many had infantile spasms and several had family members who had epilepsy and a beneficial response to the diet previously.

No neurologist or parent would deny that it is easier to swallow a pill or drink a suspension than completely alter a child's eating habits and lifestyle. However, many families, if given the choice, would prefer to try. The increasing research into less restrictive and more tolerable diets such as a modified Atkins and low-glycemic index may result in dietary therapies for epilepsy being used earlier (Kossoff et al., 2003; Pfeifer and Thiele, 2005).

Ages outside Childhood

Use of the KD is perhaps increasing most rapidly for infants. Earlier recognition of the severe infantile epilepsies by both advanced EEG monitoring and genetic testing has led to neurologists using non-pharmacologic approaches sooner for affected infants. The diet has been reported as beneficial to those as young as 2 months, including those affected by the specific seizure syndromes of West and Dravet syndrome (Caraballo et al., 2005; Klepper et al., 2002; Kossoff et al., 2002b; Nordli et al., 2001). Providing the diet is relatively easy; substitution of formula or breast milk for either SHS KetoCal™ or modular formulas can be done immediately or after a brief fasting period. As discussed earlier in this review, there is evidence for its value for infantile spasms, and using a formula-only KD assures compliance as well (Hosain et al., 2005; Kossoff et al., 2004a; Kossoff et al., 2002b; Nordli et al., 2001). However, although the diet can be easily provided to this population, impaired growth appears to be more prevalent in children under age 2, so it must be carefully monitored (Vining et al., 2002).

Adolescents have also been successfully managed with the KD, despite a common misperception that the diet is intolerable for children in high school due to social factors and restrictiveness. A retrospective study from Johns Hopkins Hospital and the University of Texas at Houston reported on 45 patients aged 12-19 years (Mady et al., 2003). Despite the concerns of possible restrictiveness, seizure improvement and tolerability were remarkably similar to those in more typical school-age children. At 12 months, 20 (44%) of 45 remained on the diet, with 13 (65%) achieving >50% seizure reduction.

The use of the diet for adults has been described in the literature as early as 1930, in which 100 adults were treated (Barborka, 1930). In this study from the Mayo Clinic, 56% had a >50% response and 12% were seizure-free, an outcome remarkably similar to those reported for children. Interestingly, the authors commented that "there seems to be no question but that the patient who can be afforded the best opportunity for treatment is the child or young adult whereas older patients are the least likely to be benefited" (Barborka, 1930). One suspects they were comparing their results to the very high efficacy reported by Peterman five years earlier (Peterman, 1924). Although not systematically monitored, cholesterol increased in several patients; amenorrhea occurred in 12 (21%) of the 56 women treated, an occurrence also seen in a recent study of adolescents (Mady et al., 2003).

With the advent of new anticonvulsants, other than reports from a single center (Jefferson Comprehensive Epilepsy Center, Philadelphia, PA), the KD for adults has not been studied (Sirven et al., 1999). Fifty-four percent had a >50% response, and the 12 patients with symptomatic generalized epilepsy had the best outcome, with 73% having a >50% response, compared with only 27% of the 11 adults with partial epilepsy. Diet duration was relatively short for these adults (seven months average). Weight loss was notable, with a mean decrease of 6.7 kg. Several patients were placed on a modified Atkins diet, with efficacy correlating with level of ketosis (Kossoff et al., 2003). A prospective trial of a modified Atkins diet (15 grams of carbohydrates per day, with encouragement of fat intake) for adults is underway at the Johns Hopkins Hospital.

What is the Evidence for Efficacy?

Since the diet has been available, many large studies have been published regarding its benefits (Table 2) (Coppola et al., 2002; Francois et al., 2003; Freeman et al., 1998; Hopkins and Lynch, 1970; Kim et al., 2004; Kinsman et al., 1992; Klepper et al., 2003; Kossoff et al., 2002b; Mady et al., 2003; Nordli et al., 2001; Schwartz et al., 1989a; Vaisleib et al., 2004; Vining et al., 1998). One of the earliest retrospective studies was by Peterman (Peterman, 1924) from the Mayo Clinic in Rochester, Minnesota in 1924. In this study including 17 children, 10 (60%) were seizure-free and four (23%) were significantly (>90%) improved. Few prospective or large studies followed over the next 70 years until 1998, when the largest prospective study up to that time was published (Freeman et al., 1998). In this study, 150 children aged 1-16 years with more than two seizures per week that had failed at least two anticonvulsants were followed for 1 year. At six months, 71% remained on the diet. Fifty-one percent had a >50% improvement and 32% had a >90% reduction. No specific seizure type preferentially improved, but the diet was less effective in children older than eight years. These children were then followed for an additional 3-6 years, and 44% had >50% improvement (Hemingway et al., 2001).

Table 2. A summary of published retrospective and prospective* efficacy studies of the ketogenic diet including over 20 patients, 1970-present

Reference	Year	No. of patients	Age Range (yrs)	>90% improvement rate at 6 months	>50% improvement rate at 6 months
Hopkins and Lynch	1970	34	1-13		71%
Sills et al.	1986	50	2-15	24%	44%
Schwartz et al. *	1989	59	<54	41%	81%
Kinsman et al.	1992	58	0.2-7	29%	67%
Vining et al. *	1998	51	1-9	29%	53%
Freeman et al. *	1998	150	1-16	32%	51%
Hassan et al.	1999	52	2-9		67%
Kankirawatana et al.*	2001	35	0.2-13	75%	
Nordli et al.	2001	32	0.5-1.5		55%
Kossoff et al.	2002	23	0.5-2	39%	72%
Coppola et al. *	2002	56	1-23		27%
Francois et al.	2003	29	0.3-12.5		41%
Mady et al.	2004	45	12-19	29%	50%
Kim et al.	2004	124	2-7	53% (3 mos)	76% (3 mos)
Klepper et al.	2004	111	0.1-18	17%	31%
Vaisleib et al.	2004	54	2-14		65%

In 2000, an article written for the Blue Cross Blue Shield insurance company reviewed all studies to date and concluded the diet led to a "significant reduction in seizure frequency" and that "it is unlikely that this degree of benefit can result from a placebo response and/or spontaneous remission" (Lefevre and Aronson, 2000). In all studies combined, 16% were seizure-free, 32% improved by more than 90%, and 56% improved by more than 50%. In another recent review, similar improvements were found (**Figure 1**).

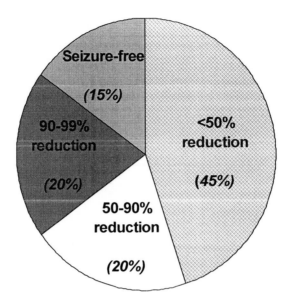

Figure 1. Percentage improvement in seizure control after six months of treatment with ketogenic diet in combined studies to date.

Despite more than 85 years of clinical experience, however, the diet has not yet been proven to be effective in a randomized, blinded, placebo-controlled study. A Cochrane Library meta-analysis in 2003 concluded "there is no reliable evidence from randomized controlled trials to support the use of KDs for people with epilepsy" (Levy and Cooper, 2003). However, the reviewers judged the diet as a "possible option" due to the observation that "a small number of observational studies lend some support for a beneficial effect."

The lack of randomized studies noted in 2003 is no longer accurate. A study randomizing patients to either a fasting period or gradual introduction of the diet by the Children's Hospital of Philadelphia revealed no long-term differences in efficacy but fewer side effects (Bergqvist et al., 2005). A randomized, double blind, placebo-controlled trial of 20 patients (glucose versus saccharin solution given sequentially during an initial fasting period) has been completed at the Johns Hopkins Hospital and is being analyzed. In addition, a study examining the MCT and LCT diets, with a 4-week waiting period for each arm serving as a control, is being completed at Great Ormond Street Hospital in London (Helen Cross, personal communication). Each arm is also then randomized with an additional 12-week control period.

Other than seizure reduction, there are financial benefits to the diet. Medications can be very costly, and the diet may be far less expensive than newer medications (Gilbert et al., 1999). In one study of children who remained on the diet for 12 months, medication costs were reduced by 70%.

Other Types of Diets Control Seizures Too

The KD in use today is remarkably similar to that created 85 years ago. Do we need to change it? There are clearly drawbacks to the KD other than the side effects previously discussed. Meals must be carefully computer-created, with grams of foods measured carefully by the parents in advance and prepared. The ability to eat outside the home can be very difficult. Due to these factors, cheating can be an obstacle, especially for adolescents. In addition, the time and resources required to manage a KD center can be considerable, and financial reimbursement by insurance companies for the time spent is often poor. The majority of centers start the diet during a one-week admission period; this can be disruptive and costly for working parents as well as children in school. The advantages of diets that could be started as an outpatient, with fewer restrictions on food choices, have led to the creation of two current alternative dietary therapies for epilepsy.

Modified Atkins Diet

Created for weight loss in the 1970s by the late Dr. Robert C. Atkins, the Atkins Diet was often mistaken for the KD by our patients during the recent low-carbohydrate trend of the past decade (Atkins, 2002). There are many reasons for this common misconception. Both diets encourage significant fat intake, restrict carbohydrates, and can induce weight loss. Foods eaten tend to be very similar. There are significant differences however (**Table 3**).

Table 3. Differences between the ketogenic and a modified Atkins diet

	Ketogenic Diet	*Modified Atkins Diet*
Fat	80%	60%
Protein	15%	30%
Carbohydrates	5%	10%
Calories (%RDA)	Restricted (75%)	Unrestricted
Fluids	Restricted (80%)	Unrestricted
Diet Initiation	Inpatient (3-5 days)	Outpatient
Fasting Period	Typically (~36 hours)	None
Meal Plan Computer-created	Yes	No
Foods Weighed and Measured	Yes	No
Ability to eat outside the home	Limited (if pre-made)	Yes
"Low carbohydrate" Store-bought Products (e.g., shakes, chocolates)	Not used	Allowed-sparingly
Published Evidence for Efficacy	Yes	Very Limited

Perhaps the most important similarity is the ability of a modified Atkins diet to create and maintain long-term ketosis. This has been described in Atkins paperbacks as an additional method to monitor weight loss (Atkins, 2002). However, diet-induced ketosis appears to be effective for weight loss, and when a modified Atkins diet (10 grams of carbohydrates per day) was used in 6 patients (aged 7-52), half became seizure-free or had only brief auras (Kossoff et al., 2003). Success tended to correlate with the level of urinary ketosis. Following this preliminary study, a prospective trial of the Atkins Diet was recently completed. Twenty children (aged 3-18 years) who had: (1) more than 3 seizures per week, and (2) failed two or more anticonvulsants, were enrolled. Carbohydrates were limited to 10 grams per day and anticonvulsants were not changed for the first month. Thirteen of the 20 children (65%) had a >50% seizure reduction, seven of which (35%) exhibited a >90% improvement, and four (20%) became seizure-free; nine children were successfully able to reduce anticonvulsant medications (Kossoff et al., 2006). Side-effects were minimal and the majority of patients gained weight over the six-month period.

Low-glycemic Index Diet

Another dietary therapy for epilepsy is perhaps even less restrictive than a modified Atkins diet. The center at Massachusetts General Hospital has been investigating a "low glycemic index" diet in which carbohydrates are restricted to 40-60 grams per day, and high glycemic index carbohydrates are avoided. In this diet, ketones are not routinely measured. In addition, a high fat intake is not recommended. In a recent abstract presentation at the 2005 American Epilepsy Society annual meeting, 50 children and adults over a 2-year period were presented. Fifteen (30%) had a >90% seizure reduction; and several were able to increase carbohydrates to as high as 100 grams per day (Pfeifer and Thiele, 2005).

KEY VARIABLES OF KETOGENIC DIET TREATMENT

Because different diets similarly improved seizure control, one asks: what key features do these diets have in common? Which aspects of diet treatment are most important to seizure protection? Given the long-standing history of efficacy of the diet, surprisingly few experimental studies have carefully identified critical variables of KD related to efficacy. Within the past decade, however, this has begun to change; both clinical and basic research into the diet has increased substantially. A PubMed search from 1965-1995 reveals 45 publications with "ketogenic diet" in the title. When a similar search is done from 1995-to-present, 208 articles have been published. In the past 12 months alone, 40 articles have been written. The first textbook devoted entirely to the KD and written by both basic scientists and clinical pediatric epileptologists, entitled *"Epilepsy and the Ketogenic Diet"*, was published in 2004 (Stafstrom and Rho, 2004).

Early studies employed a wide array of methodologies; generalizations proved difficult. Diverse variables such as ketonemia (Huttenlocher, 1976), hyperlipidemia (Dekaban, 1966), hypoglycemia (Greene et al., 2001), have been correlated to seizure protection. Over the last few years, however, studies have more clearly defined the role of several key variables related to KD. In this second section of this book chapter, we review information gleaned from studying different dietary regimens and propose a novel hypothesis based on emerging evidence from others and us on how these pieces fit together.

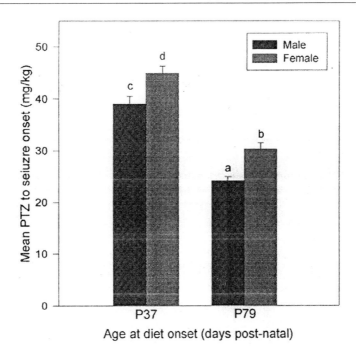

Figure 2. Female rats (light grey bars) exhibited an increased resistance to pentylenetetrazole (PTZ)-induced seizures compared to male rats (black bars) when evoked at age 37- (P37) or 79-post-natal days (P79; p<0.05, ANOVA).

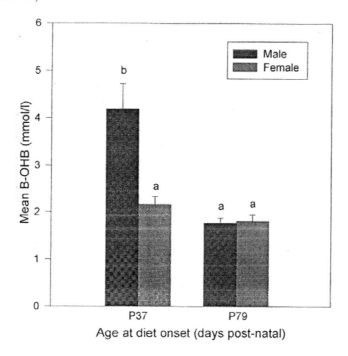

Figure 3. Blood levels of beta-hydroxybutyrate (B-OHB) are reduced (age 37 days post-natal, P37) or similar (P79) in female compared to male rats, despite an increased resistance to pentylenetetrazole (PTZ)-induced seizures in female rats Error bars are + SEM. (please see also Figure 2 above).

Ketonemia

Ketosis is the foremost, measurable result of the KD regimen. Perhaps because of this and the previous clinical observation that rapid loss of ketosis (in one child) led to rapid loss of seizure control (Huttenlocher, 1976), the most common and widely considered mechanism of action is related to ketosis. But it is still not clear whether ketosis is solely responsible for the anticonvulsant actions of the diet. Some clinical studies describe patients with higher levels of ketosis as having better seizure control, and note that a loss of ketosis rapidly results in loss of seizure control (Gilbert et al., 2000; Kossoff et al., 2003). However, many patients appear to do just as well with lower levels of ketosis over time; the modified Atkins and low-glycemic index diets both exhibit improved seizure protection with low levels of ketosis.

Recent experiments using rodents (Eagles et al., unpublished) have shown a similar disparity between ketonemia (as BHB) and seizure threshold. Normal male and female rats, for example, show different susceptibility to seizures induced by tail vein infusion of pentylenetetrazole (PTZ), with females having the higher thresholds (Figure 2). If BHB levels were the key to seizure resistance, it would be expected that the females would have the greater blood concentrations of this ketone body but, as shown in Figure 3, they have much lower levels of BHB than do the males. Another disparity is also shown in Figure 4. This figure represents the BHB levels observed in male rats fed different diets. The first bar in each set of three represents the BHB levels seen in animals fed, ad libitum, a normal (chow) diet, a high-fat (ketogenic) diet and a high carbohydrate diet. The second and third bars in each set of three show the BHB levels in animals fed the respective diets, but on an intermittent schedule: fed ad libitum one day and fed nothing at all the next. BHB levels were low in rats fed the normal and high carbohydrate diets, compared to those fed the KD, and did not rise with intermittent feeding of either diet. Rats fed the KD, by contrast, showed marked elevation of BHB level with intermittent feeding. Seizure thresholds, however, were elevated by intermittent feeding of the normal diet (at least on one of the measures) and of the high carbohydrate diet relative to the thresholds seen with ad libitum feeding of each diet and equaled the threshold seen in animals fed the KD. Curiously, intermittent feeding did not elevate seizure threshold in rats fed the ketogenic diet. Clearly, there is a disparity between the levels of ketonemia (as BHB) and the seizure threshold for animals fed these several diets and regimens. Rats fed a KD show wide disparity in the level of ketonemia attained and in the seizure threshold produced. As shown in Figure 5 [modified from (Bough et al., 2000b)], only approximately 4% of the level of BHB in blood correlated with the elevation of seizure threshold.

Dietary fatty acids are metabolized via beta-oxidation into two-carbon acetyl CoA molecules. During KD treatment (or fasting), when glucose concentrations are limited, acetyl CoA molecules cannot enter the TCA cycle because of low availability of oxaloacetate (which is formed primarily from glucose) (Nordli and De Vivo, 1997). As a result, two-carbon acetyl CoA molecules are condensed into four-carbon ketone bodies, BHB and acetoacetate (McGarry and Foster, 1980). Because the liver lacks the enzymes necessary to metabolize ketones, BHB and acetoacetate are released into the blood where the brain can use them as a supplemental energy source.

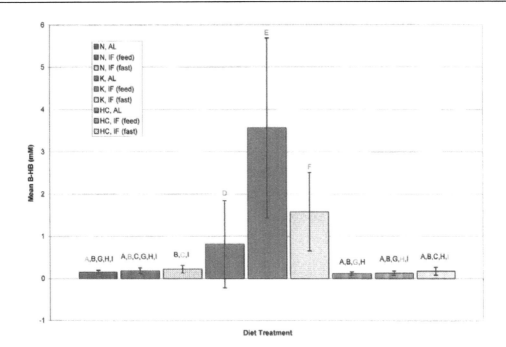

Figure 4. Plasma levels of beta-hydroxybutyrate (BHB) measured in male rats maintained on various feeding schedules and administered different diet treatments. N, AL=normal chow, ad libitium; N, IF=normal chow, intermittent feeding; K, AL=ketogenic diet, ad libitum; K, IF= ketogenic diet, intermittent feeding; HC, AL =high-carbohydrate chow, ad libitum; HC, IF=high carbohydrate chow, intermittent feeding; see text for additional details. Error bars represent + SEM.

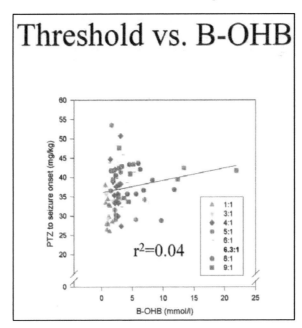

Figure 5. Plasma levels of beta-hydroxybutyrate (B-OHB) are not positively correlated with seizure protection when age at diet onset as a variable is held constant. Rats were fed increasing ketogenic diets of greater fat:(protein+carbohydrate) content (e.g., 4:1 = 4 parts fat to 1 part protein + carbohydrate). Each point represents the result from a different animal.

Three different ketone bodies are generated during KD treatment, adding to the complexity of studying KD-ketonemia relationships. In addition to BHB, both acetoacetate and acetone are produced, both of which have some anticonvulsant actions. Most studies of KD measure only BHB. Whereas a correlation between BHB and seizure protection is lacking (Bough et al., 1999; Bough et al., 2000b; Likhodii et al., 2000), acetoacetate has been shown to protect rabbits from chemically-induced seizures (Keith, 1933). This finding was extended to an 'epileptic' mouse model (i.e., the Frings mouse model), when Rho and colleagues (Rho et al., 2002) reported that acetoacetate and acetone – but not BHB – protected audiogenically-susceptible mice from seizures. Like acetoacetate, the anticonvulsant properties of acetone were initially described in the 1930's (Helmholz and Keith, 1930). Acetone was shown to induce seizure protection across a variety of different evoked seizure types (Likhodii et al., 2003), perhaps owing to its actions as a general anesthetic. A more recent report in humans, however, found neither intra- nor inter-subject associations between breath acetone and seizure frequency (Musa-Veloso et al., 2006).

Whereas acetone may contribute to seizure resistance, BHB and acetoacetate do not act to directly confer seizure control. Evidence indicates that neither BHB nor acetoacetate acts directly to limit excitability in vitro. Acute application of ketones did not alter whole-cell currents induced by application of kainate, GABA, or glutamate in cultured hippocampal neurons; fast excitatory (AMPA), slow excitatory (NMDA), and fast inhibitory (GABA) autaptic currents (i.e., synapses formed by an axon onto its own somatodendritic domain) were unaffected by ketones (Thio et al., 2000) and neither ketone affected hippocampal field potential excitability nor inhibited 4-aminopyradine-induced epileptiform bursting (Thio et al., 2000). Although these experiments were performed in vitro and in "non-epileptic" tissue, these data indicate that neither BHB nor acetoacetate directly affect neuronal excitability via direct modulation of ionotropic receptors.

Ketonemia appears within a few hours after KD implementation (Bough et al., 2006). Maximal seizure protection, however, is not observed for 10-14 days in rodents (Appleton and DeVivo, 1974) (Bough et al., 2006) or at least 2-3 days post-ketosis in humans (Freeman and Vining, 1999). The MCT diet induces higher levels of ketonemia than the "conventional" LCT diet, but does not confer as robust seizure protection either in humans (Huttenlocher, 1976) or in rodent models (Thavendiranathan et al., 2000).

These data collectively suggest that ketones are "necessary but not sufficient" for seizure protection. Rather, slowly developing changes – perhaps because of chronic ketosis – seem more likely to underlie the anticonvulsant effects of the KD.

Hypoglycemia

It is well known that the brain is dependent upon glucose almost exclusively for its energy supply. When consumption of carbohydrates is low and protein and/or fat consumption is high, or when animals are fasting, ketone bodies are elevated and contribute significantly to the brain's energy supply. The brain, however, is *never* independent of glucose. It continues to use glucose even when levels are depressed to a "low-normal" range during consumption of high-fat diets. Sokoloff (unpublished) reported that cultures incubated with no glucose die rapidly, even if supplemented with ketone bodies. This observation has led Greene et al. (Greene et al., 2001; Greene et al., 2003) to argue that low glucose levels, not elevated ketones, are essential to seizure protection. They hypothesized that a simultaneous reduction in brain glucose metabolism and increase in brain ketone metabolism is essential to the process by which the KD, calorie restriction, and fasting act in common to inhibit seizures. Their findings, based upon calorie restriction of a normal rodent chow diet in the EL mouse (an epileptic strain), show that seizure protection is inversely correlated with blood glucose (Greene et al., 2001). Indeed, as with ketosis, there is a temporal disconnection between a drop in blood glucose (<6 hours) and elevation in seizure threshold (>7 days) (Bough et al., 2006).

Calorie restriction by itself can result in seizure protection (Bough et al., 2000b). If hypoglycemia were mechanistically related to seizure control after KD, one would expect that calorie-restricted diets – of any type – would be equally seizure protective. At equal degrees of calorie restriction, however, a KD provides approximately 50% greater seizure protection over the same degree of calorie restriction alone (Bough et al., 2000a). This suggests that the anticonvulsant effects of calorie restriction and the consumption of fatty acids are additive or synergistic. In view of data showing that brain glucose levels remain constant after KD (Al-Mudallal et al., 1996), these data support the view that KDs that elevate ketone/glucose ratios should be calorie-restricted to enhance efficacy (Freeman et al., 2000).

Hyperlipidemia

Because the KD is largely fat, another common mechanistic theory relates to the role of fatty acids within the diet. It has been hypothesized that fatty acid incorporation into neuronal cell membranes may stabilize neuronal function and limit hyperexcitability (Yehuda et al., 1994). The KD currently provides mixed quantities of various fats, and changes in their components are only made for tolerability purposes. Although chain lengths (i.e., MCT vs. LCT) or types of fatty acids do not appear to affect diet outcome (Dell et al., 2001; Thavendiranathan et al., 2000), it is still possible that fatty acids with differing degrees of saturation could be more critically involved in the anticonvulsant actions of the diet. Thus, although there is no apparent relationship between chain length and efficacy of the diet, there maybe an important role for PUFAs in the anticonvulsant nature of the KD.

A dietary deficiency of n-3 PUFAs has been suggested as a basis for the refractoriness of some seizures (Yuen and Sander, 2004). In two rat models, diets enriched with PUFAs were protective against several different types of evoked seizures (Voskuyl et al., 1998; Yehuda et al., 1994). After KD consumption, changes in fatty acid metabolism resulting in an increase in brain polyunsaturates, particularly docosahexanoic (DHA), eicosapentanoic (EPA), or arachidonic acid (AA), may help limit seizures. Clinical studies have shown that dietary supplementation with sources of PUFA (e.g., margarine) results in increased blood levels of DHA and AA (Uauy et al., 2003). Circulating levels of AA and DHA were elevated after KD in children and seizure control paralleled serum levels of AA (Fraser et al., 2003), possibly reflecting the inhibitory effect of AA upon sodium currents seen in vitro (Fraser et al., 1993).

The time course for the development of hyperlipidemia (Dekaban, 1966) is similar to the development of the anticonvulsant actions of the KD (Appleton and DeVivo, 1974) (Bough et al., 2006); both peak at approximately two weeks. Dell et al. (Dell et al., 2001) found that linoleic acid and α-linolenic acid were both elevated in depot fat relative to diet when a MCT diet was fed to rats and speculated that depot reservoirs of these two PUFAs were spared during beta-oxidation of the shorter-chain fatty acids found in the MCT diet. Dietary treatment with a 4:1 fatty acid mixture of linoleic: alpha-linolenic acid increased the resistance to a variety of evoked seizures in rats (Yehuda et al., 1994). Intravenous administration of PUFAs to rodents also increased seizure resistance. DHA, EPA, linoleic, and oleic acid were shown to increase the resistance to cortically-evoked seizures, although linoleic acid was less effective than either DHA or EPA (Voskuyl et al., 1998). A recent study in 57 patients showed that dietary supplementation with EPA and DHA transiently reduced seizure frequency over the first six weeks of treatment, but the anticonvulsant effect was not sustained (Yuen et al., 2005). Whereas EPA and DHA concentrations were significantly elevated after supplementation, AA and linoleic acid levels were decreased (Yuen et al., 2005).

Interestingly, however, it has been demonstrated that low micromolar concentrations of DHA suppress inhibition mediated by GABA (Hamano et al., 1996) and, at higher concentrations, enhance NMDA responses (Nishikawa et al., 1994); both actions would be likely to *increase* neuronal excitability. However, because of the anticonvulsant effects of PUFAs in vivo and earlier studies that showed DHA and EPA were especially effective at reducing voltage-gated Na^+ and Ca^{++} currents in hippocampal neurons (Vreugdenhil et al., 1996), Voskuyl hypothesized that the anticonvulsant effects of PUFAs were mediated by their ability to stabilize Na^+ and Ca^{++} channels in the inactivated state. The effect of PUFAs on Na^+ and Ca^{++} channels was linked to the degree of saturation (Kang et al., 1995; Vreugdenhil et al., 1996), in accordance with their findings in vivo (Vreugdenhil et al., 1996).

Not surprisingly, a diet enriched in PUFAs has been proposed. In human patients, a recent report of five patients from Israel reported success in treating epilepsy by providing five grams of a special spread containing 65% n-3 PUFAs (Schlanger et al., 2002). All five patients, aged 12-26 years, had severe mental retardation and were on other anticonvulsants at the time. At least a 75% reduction in seizures was noted over 6 months in this small case series. Although taste was not discussed, 16 patients refused to eat the spread and were disqualified. A double-blind, randomized, placebo-controlled trial providing DHA and EPA supplements to patients with epilepsy over a week period showed that seizure frequency was reduced over the first six weeks of treatment in the supplement group, but, somewhat surprisingly, this effect was not sustained.

Summary – Key Variables

An increase in the ketone/glucose ratio seems "necessary but not sufficient" for seizure protection. Ketonemia must be chronically maintained for at least 10-14 days before seizure resistance becomes maximally effective experimentally. Seizure protection is independent of diet type, as different types of ketogenic fats or proteins are equally effective. Calorie restriction enhances outcome, as does dietary supplementation with PUFAs. In particular, fatty acids with greater degrees of unsaturation (e.g., DHA and EPA) may enhance the anticonvulsant nature of the diet. Collectively, these studies identify means of optimizing the administration of a KD for the treatment of epilepsy and offer potential insights into the underlying actions of the KD.

DIETARY MECHANISMS OF SEIZURE PROTECTION

Diverse genetic and/or biochemical abnormalities produce various types of seizure disorders, which vary from individual to individual and, likely, episode to episode. The KD, by comparison, can be used effectively across dissimilar, medically-intractable epilepsies. We argue here, at the core, all epilepsies can be linked to metabolism. Available evidence paints an interesting picture of how diet can modify gene expression and cellular metabolism. We conclude that the KD activates endogenous genetic programs related to adaptive thermogenesis to limit neuronal hyperexcitability. Below, we highlight several disparate theories of mechanism of how the KD may control the epilepsies. This hypothesis is summarized in Figure 6.

Chronic Oxidative Stress is the Key First Step in the Anticonvulsant Action of the KD

The brain has a high metabolic rate. Although it comprises only 2% of body weight, the brain accounts for approximately 20% of basal oxygen consumption in adults and up to 50% in children (Shulman et al., 2004). Not surprisingly, metabolic dysfunction has been associated with epilepsy and the regions of hyperexcitability within the brain. Impairment of mitochondrial function has been observed in the seizure focus of both human and experimental epilepsy (Kudin et al., 2002) and severe metabolic dysfunction is noted in both human and rat hippocampal tissue during periods of sustained neuronal activity (Kann et al., 2005). Kudin et al. (Kudin et al., 2002) demonstrated that seizure activity downregulates mitochondrial enzymes involved in oxidative phosphorylation. In an earlier study, the same group demonstrated a specific deficiency in complex I activity and mitochondrial ultrastructural abnormalities within the hippocampal CA3 region of epileptic tissue resected from 57 human patients (Kunz et al., 2000). These findings led the authors to conclude that reduced hippocampal levels of phosphorylation in both rat and human were not attributed to alterations in oxidative enzymes, but rather reflected a decrease in mitochondrial DNA copy number in epileptic tissue (Kunz et al., 2000). In sum, metabolic hypofunction has been frequently observed in epileptic tissue. Whether or not this deficiency contributes to the epileptic phenotype or is a result of it (or both?) is still unclear.

Surprisingly, however, chronic oxidative *stress* produces seizure protection. Through homeostatic biochemical and genetic programs, a 'priming-like' reaction to chronic oxidative stress increases resistance to seizures. Oxidative stress via diet and concomitant seizure control can be achieved in a variety of ways. Fasting reduced seizures in rodents (DeVivo et al., 1975) and humans (Peterman, 1924). Calorie restriction (CR), in reductions of as little as 15% from recommended daily allowances, produced seizure protection in both epileptic EL mice (Greene et al., 2001) and in rats (Eagles et al., 2003). Alternate-day feeding, which is thought to approximate ~40% CR (Anson et al., 2003), also increased the resistance to seizures (Eagles et al., 2003). Most notably, seizure protection was *irrespective* of diet type. Calorie restriction of normal rodent chow, a high-fat KD, or even CR of an *anti-ketogenic,* high-carbohydrate diet elevated PTZ seizure threshold (Eagles et al., 2003).

Chronic oxidative stress via food restriction activates the sympathetic nervous system and promotes NE release in the brain. The KD might act similarly. NE levels are elevated in brain after food restriction (Paez et al., 1993) and CR is known to potentiate carbohydrate consumption (Tempel and Leibowitz, 1993). After CR, mice maintained on a reduced calorie diet (~40%) exhibited significantly greater concentrations of the neurotransmitters 5-HT and NE after 7-11 months (Kim and Choi, 2000). Further, exercise significantly increases NE release in the brain (Dalsgaard et al., 2004).

NE is anticonvulsant in a variety of experimental models of epilepsy (Giorgi et al., 2004). Whereas diet and NE may act to promote the release of anticonvulsant orexogenic peptides such as neuropeptide-Y (NPY) or galanin, there was no evidence for enhanced transcription of either of these peptides in the brain, suggesting that neither NPY nor galanin contribute significantly to the anticonvulsant actions of KD (Tabb et al., 2004). Of significant interest, however, is the observation that mice lacking the ability to produce NE (DBH2-knockout mice) do not exhibit an increased resistance to seizures when fed a KD (Szot et al., 2001). Further, mice lacking the NE transporter gene (*Slc6a2*) responsible for NE re-uptake and termination of NE activity exhibited similar protection from seizures compared to KD-fed controls and the protection was additive in KD fed knockouts (Martillotti et al., 2005). These data suggest that the KD, via an alteration in diet and caloric intake, acts to increase the release of NE in the brain, changes that are required for the anticonvulsant action.

The findings of Szot et al. (Szot et al., 2001) showing the failure of DBH-2 knockout mice to gain seizure protection from the KD may relate to the absence of NE in these animals. In mammals, NE (and epinephrine) act upon adipocytes by binding to α-2 and β-1,2,3 receptors. In rodents, there are very few α-2 receptors. Thus, the action of NE/epinephrine is mediated by β-receptors. Beta receptors are coupled to Gs (stimulatory G proteins) which activate adenylyl cyclase, producing cAMP, which, in turn, activates protein kinase A (Figure 6). Protein kinase A activates hormone-sensitive lipase, the enzyme responsible for releasing the two terminal fatty acids from triglyceride. The fatty acids leave the adipocyte, bind to circulating albumin, and are transported to the liver, where β-oxidation takes place and, ultimately, ketone bodies are produced. Elsewhere in this chapter we have argued that ketonemia is not correlated with seizure protection (threshold elevation), however, that does not preclude a role for ketone bodies or fat catabolism in elevation of seizure threshold. It may be that stresses due to starvation, calorie restriction and carbohydrate restriction, coupled with resultant elevation of NE levels and their role triglyceride catabolism, are required for the KD to be effective, as previously suggested (Szot et al., 2001).

Larger mammals, including humans, employ the same pathway for the action of NE, with one major modification. The α-2 receptor is expressed and has an important role, though it is less abundant than the β-receptors. The α-2 receptor is coupled to Gi (inhibitory G protein) and suppresses adenylyl cyclase activation. This consequently inhibits triglyceride catabolism. The binding affinity of the α-2 receptor is greater than that of any of the β-receptors so, when NE levels are low, fat catabolism is suppressed. As NE levels rise, the α-2 become saturated and the β-receptors bind appreciable amounts of NE and their greater number drives a net stimulatory effect on the lipid catabolic pathway.

Fat catabolism is also regulated by a mechanism independent of NE/epinephrine, the malonyl-CoA pathway first described by McGarry and Foster (McGarry and Foster, 1980). β-oxidation of fatty acids occurs in the mitochondrial matrix. A key control point is carnitine acyl transferase I, an enzyme mediating the transport of fatty acids (as fatty acyl carnitine) across the outer mitochondrial membrane. Malonyl-CoA inhibits carnitine acyl transferase I, preventing uptake of fatty acids by mitochondria. In a well-fed animal malonyl-CoA is constitutively produced from acetyl-CoA by the action of acetyl-CoA carboxylase. When calories, especially as carbohydrates, are low, insulin levels fall and glucagon levels rise. Glucagon activates protein kinase A, leading to the phosphorylation of acetyl-CoA carboxylase, inactivating it, stopping production of malonyl-CoA and relieving its inhibition of carnitine acyl transferase I, permitting fatty acid transfer into the mitochondrial matrix for β-oxidation.

By these mechanisms, adrenergic activation and release of NE potentiates the release of fatty acids and enhances ketogenesis (Bahnsen et al., 1984). This would be in addition to the noted increase in serum free fatty acids (Dekaban, 1966; Dell et al., 2001; Theda et al., 1993) and PUFAs (Fraser et al., 2003) after KD. Whereas some neuroactive PUFAs such as AA and DHA can be reduced in plasma, they are increased in brain by 15% after consumption of a KD (Taha et al., 2005). Polyunsaturated fatty acids in particular can regulate transcription of genes linked to energy metabolism, whereas saturated and monounsaturated fatty acids do not (Sampath and Ntambi, 2005). This is accomplished in large part through activation of peroxisome proliferator activated receptor alpha (PPARα), where KD is thought to reprogram cellular metabolism (Cullingford, 2004).

PPARα plays a vital role in metabolic adaptation (Nakamura et al., 2004). Genes related to carbohydrate metabolism are repressed, while genes related to oxidative phosphorylation and ketogenesis are induced (Nakamura et al., 2004). Whereas there is no direct evidence for an induction of PPARα in the brain after KD, at least two reports have theorized that KD may act via this pathway to produce seizure protection (Cunnane, 2004; Veech, 2004).

PUFAs Act both Directly and Indirectly to Reduce Seizures

PUFAs such as DHA, AA, and EPA have been implicated in the prevention of various human diseases, including obesity, diabetes, coronary heart disease and stroke, and neurologic diseases such as epilepsy. As noted above, hyperlipidemia develops after KD. According to one report, hyperlipidemia develops gradually over the course of approximately 2-3 weeks (Dekaban, 1966), temporally correlating with the anticonvulsant effects of the KD in rats (Appleton and DeVivo, 1974). Poly-unsaturated fatty acids (PUFAs), in particular, are elevated after the KD (Fraser et al., 2003) and can easily cross the blood-brain barrier and increase in concentration in neuronal membranes (Cunnane, 2005; Rapoport, 2001; Rapoport, 2003). Mechanistically, dietary PUFAs may act directly and/or indirectly to help stabilize neuronal activity and reduce seizures.

Direct Actions

First, one direct action PUFAs may have is by direct inhibition of voltage-gated Na^+ channels. Omega-3 PUFAs, specifically EPA (C20:5ω3) and DHA (C22:6ω3), have been shown to reduce neuronal membrane excitability in animals, whereas saturated and monounsaturated fatty acids do not (Xiao and Li, 1999). PUFAs inhibited both Na^+ and Ca^{2+} currents in a concentration-dependent manner in CA1 hippocampal cells (Xiao and Li, 1999) and significantly reduced hippocampal CA3 bursting induced by either glutamate or PTZ (Xiao and Li, 1999). From analogous studies in the heart, both EPA and DHA PUFAs acted directly on Na^+ and Ca^{2+} channels (Kang and Leaf, 1996) to increase the recovery time from inactivation in neurons (Vreugdenhil et al., 1996). Further, in recordings from CA1 pyramidal cells in vitro, DHA inhibited bursting induced by either bicuculline or 0 mM Mg^{2+} (Young et al., 2000) and caused a slight hyperpolarization of the resting membrane potential (Leaf et al., 1999; Xiao and Li, 1999). Importantly, because of the activity dependent nature of these PUFA-induced effects, "non-hyperexcitable" neurons would not be appreciably affected and would continue to function normally.

Second, PUFAs may act directly to limit hyperexcitability and seizure activity by activating the K2p potassium channel. Recently described K2p channels appear to be the persistent "leak" currents recognized long ago by Hodgkin and Huxley (Hodgkin and Huxley, 1952). Variants within this family are prominent in excitable cells and tissues. For example, K2p channels are found in myocardial tissue (Tan et al., 2004), cells within the adrenal cortex (Enyeart et al., 2004), and TREK (Miller et al., 2004) and TRAAK (Kim et al., 2001) are types of K2p channels found in brain. Members of this family of channels found in spinal cord and brain have attracted attention because they are also activated by anesthetics such as halothane and isoflurane (Heurteaux et al., 2004; Liu et al., 2004). It would be of interest to know whether there are interactions between K2p channels and acetone given previous findings that acetone (Bough et al., 2003; Likhodii et al., 2003) may be anti-ictal. K2p channels are strongly activated by PUFAs (Fink et al., 1998). Because the KD elevates PUFAs, these findings suggest that KD may act to stabilize or even hyperpolarize the neuronal membrane nearer to the potassium equilibrium potential. Indeed, one study has reported that DHA and EPA both hyperpolarize CA3 pyramidal cells (Xiao and Li, 1999).

Third, PUFAs have the potential to activate (open) K_{ATP} channels, hyperpolarize neurons (and/or glia), limit neuronal excitability (and/or improve K^+ buffering) and dampen seizure activity (Vamecq et al., 2005). Part of this reasoning stems from the observation that glibenclamide, which specifically blocks K_{ATP} channels, inhibits the neuroprotection afforded by the PUFA linolenic acid (Blondeau et al., 2002).

Finally, there is a "membrane pacemaker theory of metabolism" that relates membrane lipid composition to activity of the Na/K ATPase (Wu et al., 2004). Interestingly, high levels of ω-3 PUFAs in cell membranes increase the activity of the Na/K ATPase (Wu et al., 2004).

This indicates that the KD-induced elevation in PUFAs in the brain (Cunnane, 2005) may lead to neuronal and/or glial membrane hyperpolarization, even if energy is increased on such diets. If PUFAs were more prevalent in the neuronal and/or glial cell membranes after KD treatment, enhanced metabolic rate may lead to greater PUFA liberation from cell membranes and may account for differences in the activity of Na/K ATPase, even when the density of the pumps is similar (Wu et al., 2004).

Indirect Actions

Whereas direct modulation of synaptic transmission may play an important part of the anticonvulsant nature of the KD acutely, PUFAs may also act indirectly to induce longer-lasting changes in membrane lipid composition (cellular and mitochondrial?), cellular metabolism, signal transduction, and gene expression that result in seizure protection. Because the anticonvulsant efficacy develops over the course of ~2 weeks, potential anticonvulsant actions of PUFAs are likely to occur, in large part, through inducing a 'switch' in gene expression. PUFAs regulate the expression of genes in various tissues, including the liver, heart, adipose tissue, and brain. The role of transcription factors such as SREBP1c and nuclear receptors such as PPARα (along with its co-activator, PGC-1), HNF-4α, and LXRα are important in mediating the nuclear effects of PUFAs (Sampath and Ntambi, 2004).

UCPs, Mitochondrial Biogenesis, and Enhanced Oxidative Phosphorylation

One way in which PUFAs may induce a long-term metabolic switch is through transcriptional and biochemical activation of uncoupling proteins (UCPs). Uncoupling proteins are homodimers within the inner mitochondrial membrane. As reducing equivalents from glycolysis and the TCA cycle are passed down the electron transport chain and "handed off" to oxygen, protons are pumped out of the mitochondrial matrix. This proton motive force established across the inner mitochondrial membrane is subsequently harvested by mitochondria to produce ATP. Uncoupling proteins allow for proton escape back into the mitochondrial matrix. This reduces the proton motive force, and 'uncouples' electron transport from ATP production, which, in turn, reduces reactive oxygen species (ROS) generation and increases local heat production (thermogenesis).

Uncoupling proteins are activated by both free fatty acids and (in a feedback manner) ROS (Jaburek et al., 1999). PUFAs, through induction of the PPAR and its co-activator PGC-1, induce the expression of mitochondrial UCPs and activate these proteins directly (Diano et al., 2003). Indeed, recent evidence suggests that fatty acids, PUFAs in particular, are required for the UCP-mediated uncoupling mechanism of shunting protons across the inner mitochondrial membrane (Garlid et al., 2001). One might think that a chronic increase in expression of UCPs would result in diminished long-term energy production and reduced energy reserves. However, a chronic induction of UCPs in the inner mitochondrial membrane triggers mitochondrial proliferation and enhanced ATP production within the cell (Diano et al., 2003).

Uncoupling proteins are increasingly thought to have significant effects on neuronal excitability and neurodegenerative processes (Andrews et al., 2005). UCP2 is up-regulated after seizures; and, when UCP2 is transgenically upregulated, there is reduced neuronal cell death associated with status epilepticus (Diano et al., 2003). After KD, UCPs are induced (Sullivan et al., 2004) and there are greater numbers of mitochondria in hippocampus (Bough et al., 2006). In mice, chronic treatment with a KD up-regulated the expression of UCPs (2, 4, and 5) and the increased abundance of UCP expression diminished the generation of ROS in juvenile mice (Sullivan et al., 2004). In rats, there was evidence for a 46% increase in the number of mitochondria after KD (Bough et al., 2006). Electron micrographic studies of hippocampal tissue showed that the number of mitochondrial profiles was increased after three weeks of diet treatment. Although there was no noted increase in the rate of TCA enzyme activities (Bough et al., 2006), energy reserves were elevated in rodents (DeVivo et al., 1978) and children (Pan et al., 1999) maintained on a KD. The ATP/ADP ratio levels were increased in mice (Nakazawa et al., 1983) and rats (DeVivo et al., 1978) after KD, and microarray studies show that diet treatment coordinately up-regulated 17 genes linked to oxidative phosphorylation (Bough et al., 2006) (Noh et al., 2004). These findings are also in line with work showing an increased metabolic efficiency (and decreased respiratory quotient) in rodents (Bough et al., 2000b) and the observation that the maximal mitochondrial respiratory rate was increased after consumption of a KD (Sullivan et al., 2004). These data collectively suggest that a dietary induction of UCPs and mitochondrial biogenesis may be a key part of a KD-induced diminution of neuronal hyperexcitability and, perhaps, neurodegeneration.

Anticonvulsant Actions of 'Optimized' Metabolism

The theory linking energy and seizure control is not new. It was theorized over 30 years ago that elevated energy reserves (in the form of an elevated ATP/ADP ratio and glycogen) would act to stabilize neurons and increase the resistance to seizures. What is novel is the elucidation of how specifically these changes might be occurring. Increasing evidence supports both the experimental (Kudin et al., 2002) and clinical (Antozzi et al., 1995; Kunz et al., 2000) view that impaired oxidative phosphorylation is likely to contribute appreciably to the epileptic phenotype. It follows that a KD-induced enhancement in cellular metabolism, via mitochondrial biogenesis and an increased expression of UCPs, are importantly linked to the limitation of neuronal hyperexcitability and the anticonvulsant nature of the diet.

It was theorized over 30 years ago that elevated energy reserves (in the form of an elevated ATP/ADP ratio and glycogen) would act to stabilize neurons and increase the resistance to seizures. In view of previous work showing impaired oxidative phosphorylation capacities in pilocarpine-treated rats (Kudin et al., 2002) and in patients with epilepsy (Antozzi et al., 1995; Kunz et al., 2000), a KD-induced increase in energy metabolism via mitochondrial biogenesis is likely to contribute appreciably to the anticonvulsant nature of the diet. But *how*?

Increased Na/K ATPase

One possibility could be through an enhanced (and/or prolonged) activation of the Na/K ATPase (Schwartzkroin, 1999). The Na/K ATPase is an electrogenic transporter that moves 3 Na^+ ions out for every two K^+ ions taken in; the net result is an outward flow of positive charge and a hyperpolarization of the cell's membrane potential. In neurons, increased activation of the Na/K ATPase might hyperpolarize the cell, reduce the resting membrane potential, and diminish firing probability. In glia, increased activation of the electrogenic Na/K ATPase might slow glial depolarization and allow for significantly lengthened periods of (depolarizing) K^+-uptake during periods of intense neuronal activity (e.g., high-frequency bursting). Either glial, neuronal, or both enhancements would be expected to limit hyperexcitability and increase the resistance to seizures as noted after treatment with KD.

In view of the high metabolic rate of brain tissue, PCr likely play a pivotal role in maintaining Na/K ATPase activity during periods of intense neuronal activation such as a seizure, in both glutamatergic and GABAergic neurons. GABAergic interneurons, which already rest at more depolarized potentials, must endure non-accommodating bursts of neuronal firing and must metabolically persist (Attwell and Laughlin, 2001), else network inhibition would become compromised. Indeed, there was a correlation between PCr/ATP ratio and the recovery of the membrane potential following a stimulus train in one study of human temporal lobe epilepsy (Williamson et al., 2005); this was inversely correlated with granule cell bursting. In view of the previous finding that creatine kinase was predominantly localized within GABAergic interneurons (Boero et al., 2003), these authors concluded that PCr and energy levels were especially critical in the ability to maintain GABAergic inhibitory output. In view of KD data showing an increase in the PCr/Cr ratio (acts to maintain ATP levels via the creatine kinase enzyme), enhanced energy reserves would be expected to maintain ATP levels at or near normal levels for prolonged periods of time and maintain synaptic function.

Toward this possibility, hippocampal slices taken from KD fed rats have recently been shown to be more metabolically resistant than is hippocampal tissue taken from control-fed animals (Bough et al., 2006). When challenged with a mild hypoglycemic stress, synaptic transmission within the dentate gyrus was maintained for approximately 60% longer in slices taken from KD-fed animals compared to controls. These data suggest that normal synaptic function (especially including activation of GABAergic inhibitory neurons) would be more metabolically resistant to metabolic stressors (e.g., a seizure) and may work to stabilize neuronal synaptic function (both excitatory and inhibitory) for prolonged periods of time.

Closure of K_{ATP} Channels Enhances Inhibitory Output

Another potential link between enhanced cellular metabolism, ATP production, and reduced neuronal excitability may be through modulation of the K_{ATP}-channel. There is an important role for K_{ATP}-channels in epilepsy. Genetic deletion of the Kir3.2 (*Kcnj6*) gene (a subtype of the K_{ATP}-channel) results in spontaneous seizures in mice (Signorini et al., 1997). K_{ATP}-channels, however, are somewhat 'misnamed';it is ADP, not ATP, opens these channels. Once activated, K_{ATP}-channels hyperpolarize the cell membrane of both neurons and glia (Zawar and Neumcke, 2000). ATP, conversely, keeps these channels closed. Thus, it is not immediately clear how enhanced energy reserves and higher levels of ATP might lead to diminished neuronal excitability. K_{ATP}-channels exhibit greater current density in inhibitory interneurons than in excitatory (CA1) pyramidal cells (Zawar and Neumcke, 2000) (Figure 3). This result suggests, perhaps, a selective role for K_{ATP}-channels in hippocampal inhibition. In this instance, a diet-induced elevation in ATP could *inhibit* K_{ATP}-channel opening and *depolarize* these inhibitory cells preferentially, resulting in a net-increase in inhibition and diminished hippocampal hyperexcitability, a possibility in accordance with the noted increase in GABAergic inhibition described above. Although many questions remain, these results support the notion that KD differentially inhibits (pyramidal cells) or activates (GABAergic interneurons) K_{ATP} channels. Collectively, this would be expected to enhance inhibitory output, limit network hyperexcitability, and increase the resistance to seizures.

Changes in Amino Acid Metabolism may further Enhance Inhibitory Output

Both ketone bodies (Erecinska et al., 1996; Yudkoff et al., 1997) and KD treatment (Yudkoff et al., 2001b) modify amino acid metabolism. Ketones, in particular acetoacetate, reduce the formation of aspartate via a reduction in the transamination of glutamate, the major excitatory amino acid in the brain (Yudkoff et al., 2001a). It has been theorized that a shift in metabolism including, in large part, the breakdown of ketone bodies as a primary energy source induced an increased synthesis of GABA, the major inhibitory neurotransmitter in the brain. This change is proposed to occur via an enhanced level of substrate availability (higher glutamate) for the glutamic acid decarboxylase (GAD) GABA synthetic enzyme and a reduction in the level of aspartate, an inhibitor of the GAD enzyme (Yudkoff et al., 2001a). Caloric restriction (as typically occurs during KD) enhanced brain GAD-65 and GAD-67 levels (Cheng et al., 2004). Although an increase in brain levels of GABA in either KD-fed mice (Yudkoff et al., 2001b) or rats (Al-Mudallal et al., 1996; DeVivo et al., 1978) has not been found, two recent studies in humans have reported increases in GABA levels after KD (Dahlin et al., 2005; Wang et al., 2003).

Excitation Leads to Inhibition

The aforementioned adaptive changes in metabolism – uncoupling of more abundant mitochondria – might be expected to *increase* excitation rather than decrease it. That is, UCPs would act to promote synaptic transmission (Andrews et al., 2005). Dissipation of the inner mitochcondrial membrane potential would decrease Ca^{2+} influx, increase local heat production (thermogenesis) – and coupled with more abundant mitochondria (no pun intended) – elevate ATP production, all key factors involved with processes of vesicle docking and neurotransmitter release. Greater ATP production, as discussed above, might act to (1) inhibit K_{ATP}-channel opening and *depolarize* inhibitory cells preferentially to increase inhibitory output and/or (2) allow for more rapid or sustained neuronal and/or glial membrane repolarization during periods of intense periods of neuronal activity.

Functional Inhibition in Vivo is Enhanced after KD

Functional inhibition is enhanced after CR or KD, and network excitability is reduced. Both CR and KD diet treatment groups showed significantly greater paired-pulse inhibition compared to controls at the 30ms interpulse interval (Bough et al., 2003). Greater stimulus intensities were also required to drive population spikes in CR- or KD-fed animals. When the field EPSP-slope (E-S) measures were compared, all were found to be similar; this indicated that the reduction in neuronal excitability may be attributed entirely to a reduction of the fEPSP slope and is consistent with a decreased probability of excitatory neurotransmitter release from presynaptic glutamatergic neurons (Bough et al., 2003). Collectively, these data were consistent with the notion that either CR or KD functionally enhance GABAergic inhibition, dampen network excitability within the hippocampus, and contribute to the anticonvulsant actions of the diet.

Taken together, these results suggest that a switch in cellular metabolism underlies the anticonvulsant actions of the KD. The KD 'optimizes' cellular metabolism by uncoupling mitochondria and inducing mitochondrial biogenesis. Enhanced inhibition as a result of diet seems likely to occur in at least three ways: elevated thermogenesis (increased expression of UCPs), increased ATP concentrations and energy reserves (i.e., PCr:Cr ratio), and diminished Ca^{2+} uptake into mitochondria. These energetic changes would inhibit K_{ATP}-channels and maintain Na/K ATPase activity for a faster membrane repolarization. Together with the potential metabolic increase in GABA production, enhanced metabolic output would lead to enhanced and/or prolonged activation of inhibitory interneurons, diminished network excitability throughout the brain, and increase in the resistance to a wide variety of seizure types.

DIETARY IMPLICATIONS FOR *PREVENTING* EPILEPSY

A Role for KD in Preventing Epilepsy

It has been noted anecdotally that some children maintained on a KD for two years or more can gradually be weaned off the KD and remain seizure free (Freeman et al., 2000). A role for diet in the prevention of epilepsy has been described in several experimental reports as well. In the kainate model of epilepsy, rats maintained on a KD exhibited fewer spontaneous seizures over an eight-week course of dietary treatment (Muller-Schwarze et al., 1999; Su et al., 2000). Further, there was reduced mossy fiber sprouting in KD-treated animals compared to controls, aberrant neuronal outgrowth often associated with developmental processes of limbic epilepsies. Similar results were observed in other models of epilepsy. In the maximal dentate activation (MDA)-model of epileptogenesis, the rate of increase in electrographic seizure duration was markedly reduced in KD animals compared to controls (Bough et al., 2003). In the kindling model, KD treatment delayed the progression focally-stimulated kindled seizures in rats (Hori et al., 1997), although it is interesting that these effects were only maintained transiently; after-discharge threshold was elevated for only two weeks after treatment onset. In a mouse model of epilepsy, treatment with a KD (Todorova et al., 2000) or CR (Greene et al., 2001) significantly slowed the development of epilepsy in 'epileptic' EL mice, further suggesting the KD can retard epileptogenesis (Todorova et al., 2000). Experimentally, these data indicate that chronic treatment with a KD, in addition to the anticonvulsant actions described above, slows the progression of the epilepsy.

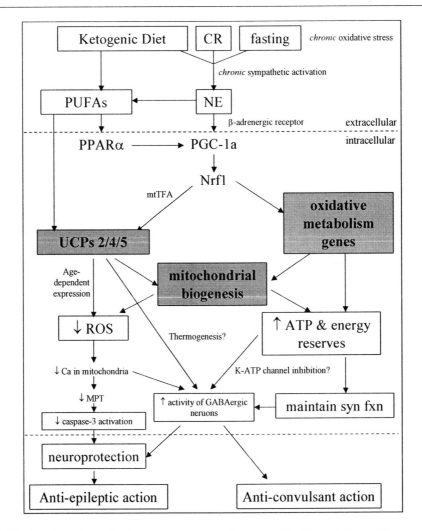

Figure 6. Working hypothesis for the anticonvulsant actions of a KD. Abbreviations: CR=calorie restricted; PUFAs=poly unsaturated fatty acids; PPARα=peroxisome proliferator activated receptor, alpha; UCP=uncoupling proteins; PGC-1a=PPAR, gamma cofactor-1 alpha; Nrf1=nuclear repiratory factor, 1; UCPs=uncoupling proteins; ROS=reactive oxygen species; MPT=mitochondrial permeability transition. See text for detailed descriptions of relationships.

Diminished Neurodegeneration after KD

One way that KD may slow the development of epilepsy is by limiting neuronal cell death. Non-necrotic cell death can be induced via a variety of mechanisms; KD is likely to diminish neuronal cell death by limiting the production of ROS. As discussed above, oxidative phosphorylation and electron transport are tightly coupled. Uncoupling proteins, in conjunction with PUFAs, allow for proton escape back into the mitochondrial matrix disassociating electron transport from ATP production, which, in turn, reduce ROS generation and increase local heat production (thermogenesis). Cellular metabolism and the production of ROS have been implicated in neuronal cell death and synaptic excitability (Mattson and Liu, 2002). These authors suggest that the high energy demands of the brain compared with other tissues, increase the generation of ROS within metabolically-active neurons and render them more susceptible to synaptic dysfunction and programmed cell death (Mattson and Liu, 2002).

By comparison, the KD reduces ROS generation and enhances cellular metabolism (Sullivan et al., 2004). It has been shown to limit neuronal degeneration in mice after kainate-induced status epilepticus (SE) (Noh et al., 2003). Although KD is not neuroprotective after pilocarpine-induced SE in rats (Muller-Schwarze et al., 1999; Su et al., 2000; Zhao et al., 2004), it has been shown to be neuroprotective in other, less severe models of neurotoxicity. For example, KD treatment reduced neuronal cell death induced by either controlled cortical injury (Prins et al., 2005) or by hypoglycemia (Yamada et al., 2005).

Modified Ca^{2+} Buffering after KD?

Another way that KD may slow the development of epilepsy is by modifying calcium homeostasis. There is an important role for Ca^{2+} homeostasis in neuronal cell death (Andrews et al., 2005) and diminished Ca^{2+} homeostasis in epilepsy (Raza et al., 2004). In epileptogenic tissue (i.e., tissue that is in the process of becoming ictogenic), calcium concentrations within neurons remained elevated, but were more rapidly sequestered in tissue from animals that did not go on to develop epilepsy (Raza et al., 2004). This was thought to occur through a diminution of the Ca^{2+}-binding calcium/calmodulin kinase II (CAMKII) enzyme (Churn et al., 2000a; Churn et al., 2000b) and/or a reduction in ATP-dependent Ca^{2+} reuptake back into the ER (i.e., SERCA pump activity) (Pal et al., 2000). After KD, microarray data showed that CAMKII and SERCA 2 were markedly upregulated (Bough et al., 2006). Together with an increase in ATP production capacity (i.e., an increased substrate for the SERCA pumps), these data suggest that KD may also act to enhance Ca^{2+} buffering within the cell and help curb potentially detrimental levels of calcium buildup.

DIETARY TREATMENT FOR OTHER NEUROLOGICAL DISORDERS

KD may also be effectively used to treat neurological conditions *other* than epilepsy. A clear indication for the KD is for patients with glucose transporter 1 (GLUT-1) and pyruvate dehydrogenase deficiency (Klepper et al., 2004; Wexler et al., 1997). In these conditions, glucose entry into the brain is significantly compromised, and energy supply is limited. In lieu of glucose, ketones become a major alternative source of energy. The KD increases the production of ketone bodies, enhances energy supply, and helps prevent associated sequale including seizures.

KD has also been suggested as a potential treatment for affective disorders. In 2001, KD was associated with an improvement in cognitive development, attention span, and social behavior (Pulsifer et al., 2001). Although this was the first prospective publication to specifically address the effects of KD on behavior, early investigations of the diet anecdotally reported improved behaviors after KD treatment, in often-dramatic fashion (Geyelin, 1921;

Peterman, 1924). Other reports followed in recent years, suggesting KD helped improved symptoms of depression, bipolar disorder, and the behavioral changes associated with Rett syndrome described (Liebhaber et al.,2003; Murphy et al., 2004; Yaroslavsky et al., 2002). A recent review stated, "trials of the KD in relapse prevention of bipolar mood episodes are warranted" (El-Mallakh and Paskitti, 2001). The diet has also been reported as effective for autism, as well, with 18 (60%) of 30 children improved (Evangeliou et al., 2003).

The KD has also been investigated as a potential treatment of migraine headaches. In the form of the Atkins diet, a KDhas been described anecdotally as potentially beneficial for migraine headaches (Atkins, 2002). Other than the temporary headaches, which can occur with induction of ketosis, the majority of children in ketosis do not have headaches. In a manner similar to anticonvulsant medications, dietary therapies may be helpful for headaches as well (Mauskop, 2005; Wiffen et al., 2005). A pilot study of the Atkins diet for adolescent chronic daily headache is underway. A single case report described the benefits of the diet for the myopathy glycogenosis type V (McArdle's Disease) (Busch et al., 2005). In addition, a low carbohydrate diet has been reported as effective for narcolepsy, diabetes, hyperinsulinemic hypoglycemia, and gastroesophageal reflux (Hosain et al., 2005; Plecko et al., 2002; Willi et al., 2004; Yancy et al., 2001).

The benefits of dietary therapies such as the KD might also be extended to the treatment and/or prevention of other neurodegenerative disorders including epilepsy, Alzheimer's and Parkinson's where neurodegeneration is thought to underlie disease progression. The infusion of the ketone body BHB in mice conferred partial protection from dopaminergic neurodegeneration and behavioral motor deficits induced by MPTP (Tieu et al., 2003). The KD has been shown to significantly reduce neuronal damage associated with head trauma and head injury protection (Prins et al., 2005). Interestingly, ketones protect neurons in models of Alzheimer's and Parkinson's disease (Kashiwaya et al., 2000), and from hypoxia (Masuda et al., 2005).

There may even be a role for KD in the treatment of certain cancers. As many tumors require large amounts of glucose for growth, it was hypothesized that a KD could limit tumor growth (Tisdale et al., 1987). In mice, KD limited tumor growth and reversed cancer-associated cachexia (Tisdale et al., 1987). Interestingly, only the MCT-based KD that produced chronic ketonemia reduced tumor size; a LCT-based diet that did not produce chronic ketonemia, did not reduce tumor size (Tisdale and Brennan, 1988). These findings were in accordance with findings that 40% calorie restriction and ketonemia after either KD or control diet limited tumor growth by approximately 80% (Seyfried et al., 2003). Although this has not been investigated clinically, at least one case report of two subjects exhibited reduced tumor glucose uptake, behavioral improvements and limited disease progression (in one patient) after 12 months (Nebeling et al., 1995).

CONCLUSION

After nearly 100 years of clinical use, the KD is known to be an effective treatment for many persons with pharmacologically refractory epilepsy. Relegation of the KD to "alternative" or secondary status denies its success, which is the equal of any of the current anti-epileptic drugs, lacking many of the undesirable side-effects and having comparatively few contraindications. Whether implemented as a very rigid and restrictive 4:1 ketogenic diet or as the more moderate Atkins diet, or as the even more moderate low-glycemic index diet, a therapeutically significant reduction of seizures is the norm. It is true that the mechanisms by which such diets produce their anti-ictal effects are unknown, but it is also true that the most effective drugs have multiple actions and that the identities of the actions that are therapeutic remain unclear. Good medical practice would dictate that the most effective treatment be used, ever mindful of the dictum to "first do no harm." The fact that a change in diet as simple as reduction of caloric intake can have therapeutic effects seems to proffer a "Rosetta Stone" for fundamental insights into interactions between diet, metabolism, and cognitive health.

All of the diets or diet strategies that have been used in the treatment of epilepsy have, in common, a reduction of calories provided by carbohydrates; the consistent physiological response is a reduction in circulating levels of glucose and insulin, along with a rise in free fatty acids, "ketone bodies" and glucagon. There are many other changes as well, but we have focused on those pertaining most directly to energy metabolism in this review.

The brain can use only two metabolic fuels: glucose and "ketone bodies" (including BHB, acetoacetate, and acetone). A central question is whether the reduction in calories provided to the brain as glucose is fully compensated by the calories provided as any, or all, of the "ketone bodies." Studies of humans and experimental animals are divided on this question, some indicating that BHB and acetoacetate are more efficient sources of energy than is glucose, metabolically (Veech et al., 2001), and that some indices of brain energetics show improvement on ketogenic diets (Pan et al., 1999), while others suggest that glucose restriction is key (Greene et al., 2003), noting that the brain can *never* live in the complete absence of glucose.

Current evidence suggests that the KD acts significantly to 'optimize' cellular metabolism. An endogenous dietary program – a switch in gene expression – produces mitochondrial proliferation within the brain to elevate energy reserves and reduce the production of ROS. This likely increases ionic homeostasis and normal membrane functioning, increases the stability of neurons, and, consequently reduces neuronal hyperexcitability and neurodegeneration. Seizures and perhaps the progression of epilepsy can be controlled.

Dietary treatment strategies – either primary or adjunctive – will be vitally important in future health and wellness. First, although strict and difficult to adhere to, treatments like the KD are likely to have fewer side effects and be more cost-effective than traditional pharmacological therapies when properly administered (Gilbert et al., 1999). Second, a frequent problem in the treatment of epilepsy, cancer, or disease in general – is pharmacoresistance. This may, in part, explain why the KD is effective in treating epilepsies where traditional medications fail. And, third, older individuals take on average four prescription and two over-the-counter drugs each day. This means that the incidence of epilepsy, Parkinson's, Alzheimer's and the like will only become more common with time. Indeed, the elderly represent one of the fastest growing segments of the population within the United States and the onset of epilepsy within this group is higher than for any other age group (Leppik, 2001); the prevalence of epilepsy in adults 65 and older is approximately

1.5%, twice that for younger adults. The elderly are also more than twice as susceptible to side effects of drugs as younger patients and side effects are also likely to be more severe, affecting quality of life and resulting in visits to the doctor and in hospitalization. Dietary approaches will allow practitioners the option of circumventing at least some of these issues.

Both clinical and scientific interest in KD has increased dramatically over the past decade (Kossoff and McGrogan, 2005). Diet is being used and studied *worldwide* at an increasingly rapid pace. Insights gleaned from the identification of key molecular and biochemical changes that underlie the actions of the KD will not only be expected to identify links between cellular metabolism and cognitive health, but may contribute to the development of novel treatment strategies for epilepsy and other neurodegenerative maladies such as Parkinson's, Alzheimer's, and/or stroke. By working together, both clinicians and researchers are finding clues to help each other address these issues and identify central aspects of diet that may contribute to improved health. Now that is some food for thought.

REFERENCES

Al-Mudallal, A. S., LaManna, J. C., Lust, W. D., and Harik, S. I. (1996). Diet-induced ketosis does not cause cerebral acidosis. *Epilepsia 37*, 258-261.

Andrews, Z. B., Diano, S., and Horvath, T. L. (2005). Mitochondrial uncoupling proteins in the CNS: in support of function and survival. *Nat Rev Neurosci 6*, 829-840.

Anson, R. M., Guo, Z., de Cabo, R., Iyun, T., Rios, M., Hagepanos, A., Ingram, D. K., Lane, M. A., and Mattson, M. P. (2003). Intermittent fasting dissociates beneficial effects of dietary restriction on glucose metabolism and neuronal resistance to injury from calorie intake. *Proc Natl Acad Sci U S A 100*, 6216-6220.

Antozzi, C., Franceschetti, S., Filippini, G., Barbiroli, B., Savoiardo, M., Fiacchino, F., Rimoldi, M., Lodi, R., Zaniol, P., and Zeviani, M. (1995). Epilepsia partialis continua associated with NADH-coenzyme Q reductase deficiency. *J Neurol Sci 129*, 152-161.

Appleton, D. B., and DeVivo, D. C. (1974). An animal model for the ketogenic diet. *Epilepsia 15*, 211-227.

Appleton, R. E., Peters, A. C., Mumford, J. P., and Shaw, D. E. (1999). Randomised, placebo-controlled study of vigabatrin as first-line treatment of infantile spasms. *Epilepsia 40*, 1627-1633.

Atkins, R. C. (2002). Dr. Atkins' New Diet Revolution (New York, Avon).

Attwell, D., and Laughlin, S. B. (2001). An energy budget for signaling in the grey matter of the brain. *J Cereb Blood Flow Metab 21*, 1133-1145.

Bahnsen, M., Burrin, J. M., Johnston, D. G., Pernet, A., Walker, M., and Alberti, K. G. (1984). Mechanisms of catecholamine effects on ketogenesis. *Am J Physiol 247*, E173-180.

Ballaban-Gil, K., Callahan, C., O'Dell, C., Pappo, M., Moshe, S., and Shinnar, S. (1998). Complications of the ketogenic diet. *Epilepsia 39*, 744-748.

Barborka, C. J. (1930). Epilepsy in adults: results of treatment by ketogenic diet in one hundred cases. Arch Neurol 6, 904-914.

Bergqvist, A. G., Chee, C. M., Lutchka, L., Rychik, J., and Stallings, V. A. (2003). Selenium deficiency associated with cardiomyopathy: a complication of the ketogenic diet. *Epilepsia 44*, 618-620.

Bergqvist, A. G., Schall, J. I., Gallagher, P. R., Cnaan, A., and Stallings, V. A. (2005). Fasting versus gradual initiation of the ketogenic diet: a prospective, randomized clinical trial of efficacy. *Epilepsia 46*, 1810-1819.

Berry-Kravis, E., Booth, G., Sanchez, A. C., and Woodbury-Kolb, J. (2001a). Carnitine levels and the ketogenic diet. *Epilepsia 42*, 1445-1451.

Berry-Kravis, E., Booth, G., Taylor, A., and Valentino, L. A. (2001b). Bruising and the ketogenic diet: evidence for diet-induced changes in platelet function. *Ann Neurol 49*, 98-103.

Best, T. H., Franz, D. N., Gilbert, D. L., Nelson, D. P., and Epstein, M. R. (2000). Cardiac complications in pediatric patients on the ketogenic diet. *Neurology 54*, 2328-2330.

Blondeau, N., Widmann, C., Lazdunski, M., and Heurteaux, C. (2002). Polyunsaturated fatty acids induce ischemic and epileptic tolerance. *Neuroscience 109*, 231-241.

Boero, J., Qin, W., Cheng, J., Woolsey, T. A., Strauss, A. W., and Khuchua, Z. (2003). Restricted neuronal expression of ubiquitous mitochondrial creatine kinase: changing patterns in development and with increased activity. *Mol Cell Biochem 244*, 69-76.

Bough, K. J., Chen, R. S., and Eagles, D. A. (1999). Path analysis shows that increasing ketogenic ratio, but not B-Hydroxybutarate, elevates seizure threshold in the rat., pp. 19.

Bough, K. J., Matthews, P. J., and Eagles, D. A. (2000a). A ketogenic diet has different effects upon seizures induced by maximal electroshock and by pentylenetetrazole infusion. *Epilepsy Res 38*, 105-114.

Bough, K. J., Schwartzkroin, P. A., and Rho, J. M. (2003). Calorie restriction and ketogenic diet diminish neuronal excitability in rat dentate gyrus in vivo. *Epilepsia 44*, 752-760.

Bough, K. J., Yao, S. G., and Eagles, D. A. (2000b). Higher ketogenic diet ratios confer protection from seizures without neurotoxicity. *Epilepsy Res 38*, 15-25.

Bough, K. J., Wetherington, J., Hassel, B., Pare, J. F., Gawryluk, J. W., Greene, J. G., Shaw, R., Smith, Y., Geiger, J. D., Dingledine, R. J. (2006). Mitochonridal biogenesis in the anticonvulsant mechanism of the ketogenic diet. *Ann Neurol 60*, 223.

Busch, V., Gempel, K., Hack, A., Muller, K., Vorgerd, M., Lochmuller, H., and Baumeister, F. A. (2005). Treatment of glycogenosis type V with ketogenic diet. *Ann Neurol 58*, 341.

Caraballo, R. H., Cersosimo, R. O., Sakr, D., Cresta, A., Escobal, N., and Fejerman, N. (2005). Ketogenic diet in patients with Dravet syndrome. *Epilepsia 46*, 1539-1544.

Cheng, C. M., Hicks, K., Wang, J., Eagles, D. A., and Bondy, C. A. (2004). Caloric restriction augments brain glutamic acid decarboxylase-65 and -67 expression. *J Neurosci Res 77*, 270-276.

Churn, S. B., Kochan, L. D., and DeLorenzo, R. J. (2000a). Chronic inhibition of Ca(2+)/calmodulin kinase II activity in the pilocarpine model of epilepsy. *Brain Res 875*, 66-77.

Churn, S. B., Sombati, S., Jakoi, E. R., Severt, L., and DeLorenzo, R. J. (2000b). Inhibition of calcium/calmodulin kinase II alpha subunit expression results in epileptiform activity in cultured hippocampal neurons. *Proc Natl Acad Sci U S A 97*, 5604-5609.

Conklin, H. W. (1922). Cause and treatment of epilepsy. J Am Osteopathic Assoc *22*, 11-14.

Coppola, G., Veggiotti, P., Cusmai, R., Bertoli, S., Cardinali, S., Dionisi-Vici, C., Elia, M., Lispi, M. L., Sarnelli, C., Tagliabue, A., *et al.* (2002). The ketogenic diet in children, adolescents and young adults with refractory epilepsy: an Italian multicentric experience. *Epilepsy Res 48*, 221-227.

Cullingford, T. E. (2004). The ketogenic diet; fatty acids, fatty acid-activated receptors and neurological disorders. *Prostaglandins Leukot Essent Fatty Acids 70*, 253-264.

Cunnane, S. C. (2004). Metabolism of polyunsaturated fatty acids and ketogenesis: an emerging connection. *Prostaglandins Leukot Essent Fatty Acids 70*, 237-241.

Cunnane, S. C. (2005). Origins and evolution of the Western diet: implications of iodine and seafood intakes for the human brain. *Am J Clin Nutr 82*, 483; author reply 483-484.

Dahlin, M., Elfving, A., Ungerstedt, U., and Amark, P. (2005). The ketogenic diet influences the levels of excitatory and inhibitory amino acids in the CSF in children with refractory epilepsy. *Epilepsy Res 64*, 115-125.

Dalsgaard, M. K., Ott, P., Dela, F., Juul, A., Pedersen, B. K., Warberg, J., Fahrenkrug, J., and Secher, N. H. (2004). The CSF and arterial to internal jugular venous hormonal differences during exercise in humans. *Exp Physiol 89*, 271-277.

Dekaban, A. S. (1966). Plasma lipids in epileptic children treated with the high fat diet. *Arch Neurol 15*, 177-184.

Dell, C. A., Likhodii, S. S., Musa, K., Ryan, M. A., Burnham, W. M., and Cunnane, S. C. (2001). Lipid and fatty acid profiles in rats consuming different high-fat ketogenic diets. *Lipids 36*, 373-378.

DeVivo, D. C., Leckie, M. P., Ferrendelli, J. S., and McDougal, D. B., Jr. (1978). Chronic ketosis and cerebral metabolism. *Ann Neurol 3*, 331-337.

DeVivo, D. C., Malas, K. L., and Leckie, M. P. (1975). Starvation and seizures. Observation on the electroconvulsive threshold and cerebral metabolism of the starved adult rat. *Arch Neurol 32*, 755-760.

Diano, S., Matthews, R. T., Patrylo, P., Yang, L., Beal, M. F., Barnstable, C. J., and Horvath, T. L. (2003). Uncoupling protein 2 prevents neuronal death including that occurring during seizures: a mechanism for preconditioning. *Endocrinology 144*, 5014-5021.

Eagles, D. A., Boyd, S. J., Kotak, A., and Allan, F. (2003). Calorie restriction of a high-carbohydrate diet elevates the threshold of PTZ-induced seizures to values equal to those seen with a ketogenic diet. *Epilepsy Res 54*, 41-52.

El-Mallakh, R. S., and Paskitti, M. E. (2001). The ketogenic diet may have mood-stabilizing properties. *Med Hypotheses 57*, 724-726.

Enyeart, J. A., Danthi, S. J., and Enyeart, J. J. (2004). TREK-1 K+ channels couple angiotensin II receptors to membrane depolarization and aldosterone secretion in bovine adrenal glomerulosa cells. *Am J Physiol Endocrinol Metab 287*, E1154-1165.

Erecinska, M., Nelson, D., Daikhin, Y., and Yudkoff, M. (1996). Regulation of GABA level in rat brain synaptosomes: fluxes through enzymes of the GABA shunt and effects of glutamate, calcium, and ketone bodies. *J Neurochem 67*, 2325-2334.

Erickson, J. C., Jabbari, B., and Difazio, M. P. (2003). Basal ganglia injury as a complication of the ketogenic diet. *Mov Disord 18*, 448-451.

Eun, S., Kang, H. C., Kim, D. W., Kim, H. D., and Kang, D. C. (2004). Efficacy and safety of the ketogenic diet for intractable infantile spasms. *Epilepsia 45*, 152-153.

Evangeliou, A., Vlachonikolis, I., Mihailidou, H., Spilioti, M., Skarpalezou, A., Makaronas, N., Prokopiou, A., Christodoulou, P., Liapi-Adamidou, G., Helidonis, E., *et al.* (2003). Application of a ketogenic diet in children with autistic behavior: pilot study. *J Child Neurol 18*, 113-118.

Farasat, S., Kossoff, E. H., Pillas, D. J., Rubenstein, J. E., Vining, E. P., and Freeman, J. M. (2006). The importance of parental expectations of cognitive improvement for their children with epilepsy prior to starting the ketogenic diet. *Epilepsy Behav 8*, 406-410.

Fink, M., Lesage, F., Duprat, F., Heurteaux, C., Reyes, R., Fosset, M., and Lazdunski, M. (1998). A neuronal two P domain K+ channel stimulated by arachidonic acid and polyunsaturated fatty acids. *Embo J 17*, 3297-3308.

Francois, L. L., Manel, V., Rousselle, C., and David, M. (2003). [Ketogenic regime as anti-epileptic treatment: its use in 29 epileptic children]. *Arch Pediatr 10*, 300-306.

Fraser, D. D., Hoehn, K., Weiss, S., and MacVicar, B. A. (1993). Arachidonic acid inhibits sodium currents and synaptic transmission in cultured striatal neurons. *Neuron 11*, 633-644.

Fraser, D. D., Whiting, S., Andrew, R. D., Macdonald, E. A., Musa-Veloso, K., and Cunnane, S. C. (2003). Elevated polyunsaturated fatty acids in blood serum obtained from children on the ketogenic diet. *Neurology 60*, 1026-1029.

Freeman, J. M., Kelley, M. T., and Freeman, J. B. (2000). *The Ketogenic Diet: A Treatment for Epilepsy*, 3rd edition. edn (New York, Demos).

Freeman, J. M., and Vining, E. P. (1998). Ketogenic diet: a time-tested, effective, and safe method for treatment of intractable childhood epilepsy [letter; comment]. *Epilepsia 39*, 450-451.

Freeman, J. M., and Vining, E. P. (1999). Seizures decrease rapidly after fasting: preliminary studies of the ketogenic diet. *Arch Pediatr Adolesc Med 153*, 946-949.

Freeman, J. M., Vining, E. P., Pillas, D. J., Pyzik, P. L., Casey, J. C., and Kelly, L. M. (1998). The efficacy of the ketogenic diet-1998: a prospective evaluation of intervention in 150 children. *Pediatrics 102*, 1358-1363.

Furth, S. L., Casey, J. C., Pyzik, P. L., Neu, A. M., Docimo, S. G., Vining, E. P., Freeman, J. M., and Fivush, B. A. (2000). Risk factors for urolithiasis in children on the ketogenic diet. *Pediatr Nephrol 15*, 125-128.

Garlid, K. D., Jaburek, M., and Jezek, P. (2001). Mechanism of uncoupling protein action. *Biochem Soc Trans 29*, 803-806.

Geyelin, H. (1921). Fasting as a method for treating epilepsy. Medical Record *99*, 1037-1039.

Gilbert, D. L., Pyzik, P. L., and Freeman, J. M. (2000). The ketogenic diet: seizure control correlates better with serum beta-hydroxybutyrate than with urine ketones. *J Child Neurol 15*, 787-790.

Gilbert, D. L., Pyzik, P. L., Vining, E. P., and Freeman, J. M. (1999). Medication cost reduction in children on the ketogenic diet: data from a prospective study. *J Child Neurol 14*, 469-471.

Giorgi, F. S., Pizzanelli, C., Biagioni, F., Murri, L., and Fornai, F. (2004). The role of norepinephrine in epilepsy: from the bench to the bedside. *Neurosci Biobehav Rev 28*, 507-524.

Greene, A. E., Todorova, M. T., McGowan, R., and Seyfried, T. N. (2001). Caloric restriction inhibits seizure susceptibility in epileptic EL mice by reducing blood glucose. *Epilepsia 42*, 1371-1378.

Greene, A. E., Todorova, M. T., and Seyfried, T. N. (2003). Perspectives on the metabolic management of epilepsy through dietary reduction of glucose and elevation of ketone bodies. *J Neurochem 86*, 529-537.

Hahn, T. J., Halstead, L. R., and DeVivo, D. C. (1979). Disordered mineral metabolism produced by ketogenic diet therapy. *Calcif Tissue Int 28*, 17-22.

Hamano, H., Nabekura, J., Nishikawa, M., and Ogawa, T. (1996). Docosahexaenoic acid reduces GABA response in substantia nigra neuron of rat. *J Neurophysiol 75*, 1264-1270.

Helmholz, H. F., and Keith, H. M. (1930). Eight years' experience with the ketogenic diet in the treatment of epilepsy. *JAMA 95*, 707-709.

Hemingway, C., Freeman, J. M., Pillas, D. J., and Pyzik, P. L. (2001). The ketogenic diet: a 3- to 6-year follow-up of 150 children enrolled prospectively. *Pediatrics 108*, 898-905.

Heurteaux, C., Guy, N., Laigle, C., Blondeau, N., Duprat, F., Mazzuca, M., Lang-Lazdunski, L., Widmann, C., Zanzouri, M., Romey, G., and Lazdunski, M. (2004). TREK-1, a K+ channel involved in neuroprotection and general anesthesia. *Embo J 23*, 2684-2695.

Hodgkin, A. L., and Huxley, A. F. (1952). Currents carried by sodium and potassium ions through the membrane of the giant axon of Loligo. *J Physiol 116*, 449-472.

Hopkins, I. J., and Lynch, B. C. (1970). Use of ketogenic diet in epilepsy in childhood. *Aust Paediatr J 6*, 25-29.

Hori, A., Tandon, P., Holmes, G. L., and Stafstrom, C. E. (1997). Ketogenic diet: effects on expression of kindled seizures and behavior in adult rats [see comments]. *Epilepsia 38*, 750-758.

Hosain, S. A., La Vega-Talbott, M., and Solomon, G. E. (2005). Ketogenic diet in pediatric epilepsy patients with gastrostomy feeding. *Pediatr Neurol 32*, 81-83.

Huttenlocher, P. R. (1976). Ketonemia and seizures: metabolic and anticonvulsant effects of two ketogenic diets in childhood epilepsy. *Pediatr Res 10*, 536-540.

Jaburek, M., Varecha, M., Gimeno, R. E., Dembski, M., Jezek, P., Zhang, M., Burn, P., Tartaglia, L. A., and Garlid, K. D. (1999). Transport function and regulation of mitochondrial uncoupling proteins 2 and 3. *J Biol Chem 274*, 26003-26007.

Kang, H. C., Chung da, E., Kim, D. W., and Kim, H. D. (2004). Early- and late-onset complications of the ketogenic diet for intractable epilepsy. *Epilepsia 45*, 1116-1123.

Kang, J. X., and Leaf, A. (1996). Evidence that free polyunsaturated fatty acids modify Na+ channels by directly binding to the channel proteins. *Proc Natl Acad Sci U S A 93*, 3542-3546.

Kang, J. X., Xiao, Y. F., and Leaf, A. (1995). Free, long-chain, polyunsaturated fatty acids reduce membrane electrical excitability in neonatal rat cardiac myocytes. *Proc Natl Acad Sci U S A 92*, 3997-4001.

Kann, O., Kovacs, R., Njunting, M., Behrens, C. J., Otahal, J., Lehmann, T. N., Gabriel, S., and Heinemann, U. (2005). Metabolic dysfunction during neuronal activation in the ex vivo hippocampus from chronic epileptic rats and humans. *Brain 128*, 2396-2407.

Karceski, S. (2001). The Expert Consensus Guideline Series: Treatment of Epilepsy. *2*, A1-A50.

Kashiwaya, Y., Takeshima, T., Mori, N., Nakashima, K., Clarke, K., and Veech, R. L. (2000). D-beta-hydroxybutyrate protects neurons in models of Alzheimer's and Parkinson's disease. *Proc Natl Acad Sci U S A 97*, 5440-5444.

Keith, H. M. (1933). Factors influencing experimentally produced convulsions. *Arch Neurol Psychiatr 29*, 148-154.

Kim, D. W., and Choi, J. H. (2000). Effects of age and dietary restriction on animal model SAMP8 mice with learning and memory impairments. *J Nutr Health Aging 4*, 233-238.

Kim, D. W., Kang, H. C., Park, J. C., and Kim, H. D. (2004). Benefits of the nonfasting ketogenic diet compared with the initial fasting ketogenic diet. *Pediatrics 114*, 1627-1630.

Kim, Y., Bang, H., Gnatenco, C., and Kim, D. (2001). Synergistic interaction and the role of C-terminus in the activation of TRAAK K+ channels by pressure, free fatty acids and alkali. *Pflugers Arch 442*, 64-72.

Kinsman, S. L., Vining, E. P., Quaskey, S. A., Mellits, D., and Freeman, J. M. (1992). Efficacy of the ketogenic diet for intractable seizure disorders: review of 58 cases. *Epilepsia 33*, 1132-1136.

Klepper, J., Diefenbach, S., Kohlschutter, A., and Voit, T. (2004). Effects of the ketogenic diet in the glucose transporter 1 deficiency syndrome. *Prostaglandins Leukot Essent Fatty Acids 70*, 321-327.

Klepper, J., Florcken, A., Fischbarg, J., and Voit, T. (2003). Effects of anticonvulsants on GLUT1-mediated glucose transport in GLUT1 deficiency syndrome in vitro. *Eur J Pediatr 162*, 84-89.

Klepper, J., Leiendecker, B., Bredahl, R., Athanassopoulos, S., Heinen, F., Gertsen, E., Florcken, A., Metz, A., and Voit, T. (2002). Introduction of a ketogenic diet in young infants. *J Inherit Metab Dis 25*, 449-460.

Kossoff, E. H. (2004). More fat and fewer seizures: dietary therapies for epilepsy. *Lancet Neurol 3*, 415-420.

Kossoff, E. H., Krauss, G. L., McGrogan, J. R., and Freeman, J. M. (2003). Efficacy of the Atkins diet as therapy for intractable epilepsy. *Neurology 61*, 1789-1791.

Kossoff, E. H., and McGrogan, J. R. (2005). Worldwide use of the ketogenic diet. *Epilepsia 46*, 280-289.

Kossoff, E. H., McGrogan, J. R., Bluml, R. M., Pillas, D. J., Rubenstein, J. E., and Vining, E. P. (2006). A modified atkins diet is effective for the treatment of intractable pediatric epilepsy. *Epilepsia 47*, 421-424.

Kossoff, E. H., McGrogan, J. R., and Freeman, J. M. (2004a). Benefits of an all-liquid ketogenic diet. *Epilepsia 45*, 1163.

Kossoff, E. H., Pyzik, P. L., Furth, S. L., Hladky, H. D., Freeman, J. M., and Vining, E. P. (2002a). Kidney stones, carbonic anhydrase inhibitors, and the ketogenic diet. *Epilepsia 43*, 1168-1171.

Kossoff, E. H., Pyzik, P. L., McGrogan, J. R., and Rubenstein, J. E. (2004b). The impact of early versus late anticonvulsant reduction after ketogenic diet initiation. *Epilepsy Behav 5*, 499-502.

Kossoff, E. H., Pyzik, P. L., McGrogan, J. R., Vining, E. P., and Freeman, J. M. (2002b). Efficacy of the ketogenic diet for infantile spasms. *Pediatrics 109*, 780-783.

Kossoff, E. H., Thiele, E. A., Pfeifer, H. H., McGrogan, J. R., and Freeman, J. M. (2005). Tuberous sclerosis complex and the ketogenic diet. *Epilepsia 46*, 1684-1686.

Kudin, A. P., Kudina, T. A., Seyfried, J., Vielhaber, S., Beck, H., Elger, C. E., and Kunz, W. S. (2002). Seizure-dependent modulation of mitochondrial oxidative phosphorylation in rat hippocampus. *Eur J Neurosci 15*, 1105-1114.

Kunz, W. S., Kudin, A. P., Vielhaber, S., Blumcke, I., Zuschratter, W., Schramm, J., Beck, H., and Elger, C. E. (2000). Mitochondrial complex I deficiency in the epileptic focus of patients with temporal lobe epilepsy. *Ann Neurol 48*, 766-773.

Kwiterovich, P. O., Jr., Vining, E. P., Pyzik, P., Skolasky, R., Jr., and Freeman, J. M. (2003). Effect of a high-fat ketogenic diet on plasma levels of lipids, lipoproteins, and apolipoproteins in children. *Jama 290*, 912-920.

Laux, L. C., Devonshire, K. A., Kelley, K. R., Goldstein, J., and Nordli, D. R. (2004). Efficacy of the ketogenic diet in myoclonic epilepsy of Doose. *Epilepsia 45*, 251.

Leaf, A., Kang, J. X., Xiao, Y. F., Billman, G. E., and Voskuyl, R. A. (1999). Functional and electrophysiologic effects of polyunsaturated fatty acids on exictable tissues: heart and brain. *Prostaglandins Leukot Essent Fatty Acids 60*, 307-312.

Lebel, D., Morin, C., Laberge, M., Achim, N., and Carmant, L. (2001). The carbohydrate and caloric content of concomitant medications for children with epilepsy on the ketogenic diet. *Can J Neurol Sci 28*, 322-340.

Lefevre, F., and Aronson, N. (2000). Ketogenic diet for the treatment of refractory epilepsy in children: A systematic review of efficacy. *Pediatrics 105*, E46.

Lennox, W. G., and Cobb, S. (1928). Studies in epilepsy. VIII. The clinical effect of fasting. *Arch Neurol Psychiatr 20*, 771-779.

Leppik, I. E. (2001). Epilepsy in the elderly. *Curr Neurol Neurosci Rep 1*, 396-402.

Levy, R., and Cooper, P. (2003). Ketogenic diet for epilepsy. *Cochrane Database Syst Rev*, CD001903.

Liebhaber, G. M., Riemann, E., and Baumeister, F. A. (2003). Ketogenic diet in Rett syndrome. *J Child Neurol 18*, 74-75.

Likhodii, S. S., Musa, K., Mendonca, A., Dell, C., Burnham, W. M., and Cunnane, S. C. (2000). Dietary fat, ketosis, and seizure resistance in rats on the ketogenic diet. *Epilepsia 41*, 1400-1410.

Likhodii, S. S., Serbanescu, I., Cortez, M. A., Murphy, P., Snead, O. C., 3rd, and Burnham, W. M. (2003). Anticonvulsant properties of acetone, a brain ketone elevated by the ketogenic diet. *Ann Neurol 54*, 219-226.

Liu, C., Au, J. D., Zou, H. L., Cotten, J. F., and Yost, C. S. (2004). Potent activation of the human tandem pore domain K channel TRESK with clinical concentrations of volatile anesthetics. *Anesth Analg 99*, 1715-1722, table of contents.

Liu, Y. M., Williams, S., Basualdo-Hammond, C., Stephens, D., and Curtis, R. (2003). A prospective study: growth and nutritional status of children treated with the ketogenic diet. *J Am Diet Assoc 103*, 707-712.

Lyczkowski, D. A., Pfeifer, H. H., Ghosh, S., and Thiele, E. A. (2005). Safety and tolerability of the ketogenic diet in pediatric epilepsy: effects of valproate combination therapy. *Epilepsia 46*, 1533-1538.

Mady, M. A., Kossoff, E. H., McGregor, A. L., Wheless, J. W., Pyzik, P. L., and Freeman, J. M. (2003). The ketogenic diet: adolescents can do it, too. *Epilepsia 44*, 847-851.

Martillotti, J., Weinshenker, D., Liles, L. C., and Eagles, D. A. (2005). A ketogenic diet and knockout of the norepinephrine transporter both reduce seizure severity in mice. *Epilepsy Res.*

Masuda, R., Monahan, J. W., and Kashiwaya, Y. (2005). D-beta-hydroxybutyrate is neuroprotective against hypoxia in serum-free hippocampal primary cultures. *J Neurosci Res 80*, 501-509.

Mattson, M. P., and Liu, D. (2002). Energetics and oxidative stress in synaptic plasticity and neurodegenerative disorders. *Neuromolecular Med 2*, 215-231.

Mauskop, A. (2005). Vagus nerve stimulation relieves chronic refractory migraine and cluster headaches. *Cephalalgia 25*, 82-86.

Maydell, B. V., Wyllie, E., Akhtar, N., Kotagal, P., Powaski, K., Cook, K., Weinstock, A., and Rothner, A. D. (2001). Efficacy of the ketogenic diet in focal versus generalized seizures. *Pediatr Neurol 25*, 208-212.

McGarry, J. D., and Foster, D. W. (1980). Regulation of hepatic fatty acid oxidation and ketone body production. *Annu Rev Biochem 49*, 395-420.

Merritt, H. H., and Putnam, T. J. (1938a). A new series of anticonvulsant drugs tested by experiments in animals. *Arch Neurol Psychiatr 39*, 1003-1015.

Merritt, H. H., and Putnam, T. J. (1938b). Sodium diphenyl hydantinoate in the treatment of convulsive disorders. *JAMA 111*, 1068-1073.

Miller, P., Peers, C., and Kemp, P. J. (2004). Polymodal regulation of hTREK1 by pH, arachidonic acid, and hypoxia: physiological impact in acidosis and alkalosis. *Am J Physiol Cell Physiol 286*, C272-282.

Muller-Schwarze, A. B., Tandon, P., Liu, Z., Yang, Y., Holmes, G. L., and Stafstrom, C. E. (1999). Ketogenic diet reduces spontaneous seizures and mossy fiber sprouting in the kainic acid model. *Neuroreport 10*, 1517-1522.

Murphy, P., Likhodii, S., Nylen, K., and Burnham, W. M. (2004). The antidepressant properties of the ketogenic diet. *Biol Psychiatry 56*, 981-983.

Musa-Veloso, K., Likhodii, S. S., Rarama, E., Benoit, S., Liu, Y. M., Chartrand, D., Curtis, R., Carmant, L., Lortie, A., Comeau, F. J., and Cunnane, S. C. (2006). Breath acetone predicts plasma ketone bodies in children with epilepsy on a ketogenic diet. *Nutrition 22*, 1-8.

Nakamura, M. T., Cheon, Y., Li, Y., and Nara, T. Y. (2004). Mechanisms of regulation of gene expression by fatty acids. *Lipids 39*, 1077-1083.

Nakazawa, M., Kodama, S., and Matsuo, T. (1983). Effects of ketogenic diet on electroconvulsive threshold and brain contents of adenosine nucleotides. *Brain Dev 5*, 375-380.

Nebeling, L. C., Miraldi, F., Shurin, S. B., and Lerner, E. (1995). Effects of a ketogenic diet on tumor metabolism and nutritional status in pediatric oncology patients: two case reports. *J Am Coll Nutr 14*, 202-208.

Nishikawa, M., Kimura, S., and Akaike, N. (1994). Facilitatory effect of docosahexaenoic acid on N-methyl-D-aspartate response in pyramidal neurones of rat cerebral cortex. *J Physiol 475*, 83-93.

Noh, H. S., Kim, Y. S., Lee, H. P., Chung, K. M., Kim, D. W., Kang, S. S., Cho, G. J., and Choi, W. S. (2003). The protective effect of a ketogenic diet on kainic acid-induced hippocampal cell death in the male ICR mice. *Epilepsy Res 53*, 119-128.

Noh, H. S., Lee, H. P., Kim, D. W., Kang, S. S., Cho, G. J., Rho, J. M., and Choi, W. S. (2004). A cDNA microarray analysis of gene expression profiles in rat hippocampus following a ketogenic diet. *Brain Res Mol Brain Res 129*, 80-87.

Nordli, D. R., Jr., and De Vivo, D. C. (1997). The ketogenic diet revisited: back to the future [editorial; comment] [see comments]. *Epilepsia 38*, 743-749.

Nordli, D. R., Jr., Kuroda, M. M., Carroll, J., Koenigsberger, D. Y., Hirsch, L. J., Bruner, H. J., Seidel, W. T., and De Vivo, D. C. (2001). Experience with the ketogenic diet in infants. *Pediatrics 108*, 129-133.

Paez, X., Stanley, B. G., and Leibowitz, S. F. (1993). Microdialysis analysis of norepinephrine levels in the paraventricular nucleus in association with food intake at dark onset. *Brain Res 606*, 167-170.

Pal, S., Limbrick, D. D., Jr., Rafiq, A., and DeLorenzo, R. J. (2000). Induction of spontaneous recurrent epileptiform discharges causes long-term changes in intracellular calcium homeostatic mechanisms. *Cell Calcium 28*, 181-193.

Pan, J. W., Bebin, E. M., Chu, W. J., and Hetherington, H. P. (1999). Ketosis and epilepsy: 31P spectroscopic imaging at 4.1 T. *Epilepsia 40*, 703-707.

Peterman, M. G. (1924). The ketogenic diet in the treatment of epilepsy: a preliminary report. *Am J Dis Child 28*, 28-33.

Peterson, S. J., Tangney, C. C., Pimentel-Zablah, E. M., Hjelmgren, B., Booth, G., and Berry-Kravis, E. (2005). Changes in growth and seizure reduction in children on the ketogenic diet as a treatment for intractable epilepsy. *J Am Diet Assoc 105*, 718-725.

Pfeifer, H. H., and Thiele, E. A. (2005). Low-glycemic-index treatment: a liberalized ketogenic diet for treatment of intractable epilepsy. *Neurology 65*, 1810-1812.

Plecko, B., Stoeckler-Ipsiroglu, S., Schober, E., Harrer, G., Mlynarik, V., Gruber, S., Moser, E., Moeslinger, D., Silgoner, H., and Ipsiroglu, O. (2002). Oral beta-hydroxybutyrate supplementation in two patients with hyperinsulinemic hypoglycemia: monitoring of beta-hydroxybutyrate levels in blood and cerebrospinal fluid, and in the brain by in vivo magnetic resonance spectroscopy. *Pediatr Res 52*, 301-306.

Prins, M. L., Fujima, L. S., and Hovda, D. A. (2005). Age-dependent reduction of cortical contusion volume by ketones after traumatic brain injury. *J Neurosci Res 82*, 413-420.

Pulsifer, M. B., Gordon, J. M., Brandt, J., Vining, E. P., and Freeman, J. M. (2001). Effects of ketogenic diet on development and behavior: preliminary report of a prospective study. Dev Med Child Neurol *43*, 301-306.

Rapoport, S. I. (2001). In vivo fatty acid incorporation into brain phosholipids in relation to plasma availability, signal transduction and membrane remodeling. *J Mol Neurosci 16*, 243-261; discussion 279-284.

Rapoport, S. I. (2003). In vivo approaches to quantifying and imaging brain arachidonic and docosahexaenoic acid metabolism. *J Pediatr 143*, S26-34.

Raza, M., Blair, R. E., Sombati, S., Carter, D. S., Deshpande, L. S., and DeLorenzo, R. J. (2004). Evidence that injury-induced changes in hippocampal neuronal calcium dynamics during epileptogenesis cause acquired epilepsy. *Proc Natl Acad Sci U S A 101*, 17522-17527.

Rho, J. M., Anderson, G. D., Donevan, S. D., and White, H. S. (2002). Acetoacetate, acetone, and dibenzylamine (a contaminant in l-(+)-beta-hydroxybutyrate) exhibit direct anticonvulsant actions in vivo. *Epilepsia 43*, 358-361.

Rubenstein, J. E., Kossoff, E. H., Pyzik, P. L., Vining, E. P., McGrogan, J. R., and Freeman, J. M. (2005). Experience in the use of the ketogenic diet as early therapy. *J Child Neurol 20*, 31-34.

Sampath, H., and Ntambi, J. M. (2004). Polyunsaturated fatty acid regulation of gene expression. *Nutr Rev 62*, 333-339.

Sampath, H., and Ntambi, J. M. (2005). Polyunsaturated fatty acid regulation of genes of lipid metabolism. *Annu Rev Nutr 25*, 317-340.

Schlanger, S., Shinitzky, M., and Yam, D. (2002). Diet enriched with omega-3 fatty acids alleviates convulsion symptoms in epilepsy patients. *Epilepsia 43*, 103-104.

Schwartz, R. H., Eaton, J., Bower, B. D., and Aynsley-Green, A. (1989a). Ketogenic diets in the treatment of epilepsy: short-term clinical effects. *Dev Med Child Neurol 31*, 145-151.

Schwartz, R. M., Boyes, S., and Aynsley-Green, A. (1989b). Metabolic effects of three ketogenic diets in the treatment of severe epilepsy. *Dev Med Child Neurol 31*, 152-160.

Schwartzkroin, P. A. (1999). Mechanisms underlying the anti-epileptic efficacy of the ketogenic diet. *Epilepsy Res 37*, 171-180.

Seyfried, T. N., Sanderson, T. M., El-Abbadi, M. M., McGowan, R., and Mukherjee, P. (2003). Role of glucose and ketone bodies in the metabolic control of experimental brain cancer. *Br J Cancer 89*, 1375-1382.

Shulman, R. G., Rothman, D. L., Behar, K. L., and Hyder, F. (2004). Energetic basis of brain activity: implications for neuroimaging. *Trends Neurosci 27*, 489-495.

Signorini, S., Liao, Y. J., Duncan, S. A., Jan, L. Y., and Stoffel, M. (1997). Normal cerebellar development but susceptibility to seizures in mice lacking G protein-coupled, inwardly rectifying K+ channel GIRK2. *Proc Natl Acad Sci U S A 94*, 923-927.

Sirven, J., Whedon, B., Caplan, D., Liporace, J., Glosser, D., O'Dwyer, J., and Sperling, M. R. (1999). The ketogenic diet for intractable epilepsy in adults: preliminary results. *Epilepsia 40*, 1721-1726.

Stafstrom, C. E., and Rho, J. M., eds. (2004). *Epilepsy and the Ketogenic Diet* (Totowa, New Jersey, Humana Press).

Stewart, W. A., Gordon, K., and Camfield, P. (2001). Acute pancreatitis causing death in a child on the ketogenic diet. *J Child Neurol 16*, 682.

Su, S. W., Cilio, M. R., Sogawa, Y., Silveira, D. C., Holmes, G. L., and Stafstrom, C. E. (2000). Timing of ketogenic diet initiation in an experimental epilepsy model. *Brain Res Dev Brain Res 125*, 131-138.

Sullivan, P. G., Rippy, N. A., Dorenbos, K., Concepcion, R. C., Agarwal, A. K., and Rho, J. M. (2004). The ketogenic diet increases mitochondrial uncoupling protein levels and activity. *Ann Neurol 55*, 576-580.

Szot, P., Weinshenker, D., Rho, J. M., Storey, T. W., and Schwartzkroin, P. A. (2001). Norepinephrine is required for the anticonvulsant effect of the ketogenic diet. *Brain Res Dev Brain Res 129*, 211-214.

Tabb, K., Szot, P., White, S. S., Liles, L. C., and Weinshenker, D. (2004). The ketogenic diet does not alter brain expression of orexigenic neuropeptides. *Epilepsy Res 62*, 35-39.

Taha, A. Y., Ryan, M. A., and Cunnane, S. C. (2005). Despite transient ketosis, the classic high-fat ketogenic diet induces marked changes in fatty acid metabolism in rats. *Metabolism 54*, 1127-1132.

Takeoka, M., Riviello, J. J., Jr., Pfeifer, H., and Thiele, E. A. (2002). Concomitant treatment with topiramate and ketogenic diet in pediatric epilepsy. *Epilepsia 43*, 1072-1075.

Talbot, F. B., Metcalf, K. M., and Moriarty, M. E. (1927). Epilepsy: chemical investigations of rational treatment by production of ketosis. *Am J Dis Child 33*, 218-225.

Tan, J. H., Liu, W., and Saint, D. A. (2004). Differential expression of the mechanosensitive potassium channel TREK-1 in epicardial and endocardial myocytes in rat ventricle. *Exp Physiol 89*, 237-242.

Tempel, D. L., and Leibowitz, S. F. (1993). Glucocorticoid receptors in PVN: interactions with NE, NPY, and Gal in relation to feeding. *Am J Physiol 265*, E794-800.

Than, K. D., Kossoff, E. H., Rubenstein, J. E., Pyzik, P. L., McGrogan, J. R., and Vining, E. P. (2005). Can you predict an immediate, complete, and sustained response to the ketogenic diet? *Epilepsia 46*, 580-582.

Thavendiranathan, P., Mendonca, A., Dell, C., Likhodii, S. S., Musa, K., Iracleous, C., Cunnane, S. C., and Burnham, W. M. (2000). The MCT ketogenic diet: effects on animal seizure models. *Exp Neurol 161*, 696-703.

Theda, C., Woody, R. C., Naidu, S., Moser, A. B., and Moser, H. W. (1993). Increased very long chain fatty acids in patients on a ketogenic diet: a cause of diagnostic confusion. *J Pediatr 122*, 724-726.

Thio, L. L., Wong, M., and Yamada, K. A. (2000). Ketone bodies do not directly alter excitatory or inhibitory hippocampal synaptic transmission. *Neurology 54*, 325-331.

Tieu, K., Ischiropoulos, H., and Przedborski, S. (2003). Nitric oxide and reactive oxygen species in Parkinson's disease. *IUBMB Life 55*, 329-335.

Tisdale, M. J., and Brennan, R. A. (1988). A comparison of long-chain triglycerides and medium-chain triglycerides on weight loss and tumour size in a cachexia model. *Br J Cancer 58*, 580-583.

Tisdale, M. J., Brennan, R. A., and Fearon, K. C. (1987). Reduction of weight loss and tumour size in a cachexia model by a high fat diet. *Br J Cancer 56*, 39-43.

Todorova, M. T., Tandon, P., Madore, R. A., Stafstrom, C. E., and Seyfried, T. N. (2000). The ketogenic diet inhibits epileptogenesis in EL mice: a genetic model for idiopathic epilepsy. *Epilepsia 41*, 933-940.

Uauy, R., Hoffman, D. R., Mena, P., Llanos, A., and Birch, E. E. (2003). Term infant studies of DHA and ARA supplementation on neurodevelopment: results of randomized controlled trials. *J Pediatr 143*, S17-25.

Vaisleib, II, Buchhalter, J. R., and Zupanc, M. L. (2004). Ketogenic diet: outpatient initiation, without fluid, or caloric restrictions. *Pediatr Neurol 31*, 198-202.

Vamecq, J., Vallee, L., Lesage, F., Gressens, P., and Stables, J. P. (2005). Antiepileptic popular ketogenic diet: emerging twists in an ancient story. *Prog Neurobiol 75*, 1-28.

Veech, R. L. (2004). The therapeutic implications of ketone bodies: the effects of ketone bodies in pathological conditions: ketosis, ketogenic diet, redox states, insulin resistance, and mitochondrial metabolism. *Prostaglandins Leukot Essent Fatty Acids 70*, 309-319.

Veech, R. L., Chance, B., Kashiwaya, Y., Lardy, H. A., and Cahill, G. F., Jr. (2001). Ketone bodies, potential therapeutic uses. *IUBMB Life 51*, 241-247.

Vigevano, F., and Cilio, M. R. (1997). Vigabatrin versus ACTH as first-line treatment for infantile spasms: a randomized, prospective study. *Epilepsia 38*, 1270-1274.

Vining, E. P., Freeman, J. M., Ballaban-Gil, K., Camfield, C. S., Camfield, P. R., Holmes, G. L., Shinnar, S., Shuman, R., Trevathan, E., and Wheless, J. W. (1998). A multicenter study of the efficacy of the ketogenic diet [see comments]. *Arch Neurol 55*, 1433-1437.

Vining, E. P., Pyzik, P., McGrogan, J., Hladky, H., Anand, A., Kriegler, S., and Freeman, J. M. (2002). Growth of children on the ketogenic diet. *Dev Med Child Neurol 44*, 796-802.

Voskuyl, R. A., Vreugdenhil, M., Kang, J. X., and Leaf, A. (1998). Anticonvulsant effect of polyunsaturated fatty acids in rats, using the cortical stimulation model. *Eur J Pharmacol 341*, 145-152.

Vreugdenhil, M., Bruehl, C., Voskuyl, R. A., Kang, J. X., Leaf, A., and Wadman, W. J. (1996). Polyunsaturated fatty acids modulate sodium and calcium currents in CA1 neurons. *Proc Natl Acad Sci U S A 93*, 12559-12563.

Wang, Z. J., Bergqvist, C., Hunter, J. V., Jin, D., Wang, D. J., Wehrli, S., and Zimmerman, R. A. (2003). In vivo measurement of brain metabolites using two-dimensional double-quantum MR spectroscopy--exploration of GABA levels in a ketogenic diet. *Magn Reson Med 49*, 615-619.

Weeks, D. F., Renner, D. S., Allen, F. M., and Wishart, M. B. (1923). Observations on fasting and diets in the treatment of epilepsy. *J Metab Res 3*, 317-364.

Wexler, I. D., Hemalatha, S. G., McConnell, J., Buist, N. R., Dahl, H. H., Berry, S. A., Cederbaum, S. D., Patel, M. S., and Kerr, D. S. (1997). Outcome of pyruvate dehydrogenase deficiency treated with ketogenic diets. Studies in patients with identical mutations. *Neurology 49*, 1655-1661.

Wheless, J. W. (2001). The ketogenic diet: an effective medical therapy with side effects. *J Child Neurol 16*, 633-635.

Wiffen, P., Collins, S., McQuay, H., Carroll, D., Jadad, A., and Moore, A. (2005). Anticonvulsant drugs for acute and chronic pain. *Cochrane Database Syst Rev*, CD001133.

Wilder, R. M. (1921). The effect of ketonemia on the course of epilepsy. *Mayo Clin Bulletin 2*, 307-308.

Willi, S. M., Martin, K., Datko, F. M., and Brant, B. P. (2004). Treatment of type 2 diabetes in childhood using a very-low-calorie diet. *Diabetes Care 27*, 348-353.

Williams, S., Basualdo-Hammond, C., Curtis, R., and Schuller, R. (2002). Growth retardation in children with epilepsy on the ketogenic diet: a retrospective chart review. *J Am Diet Assoc 102*, 405-407.

Williamson, A., Patrylo, P. R., Pan, J., Spencer, D. D., and Hetherington, H. (2005). Correlations between granule cell physiology and bioenergetics in human temporal lobe epilepsy. *Brain 128*, 1199-1208.

Wirrell, E. C., Darwish, H. Z., Williams-Dyjur, C., Blackman, M., and Lange, V. (2002). Is a fast necessary when initiating the ketogenic diet? *J Child Neurol 17*, 179-182.

Wu, B. J., Hulbert, A. J., Storlien, L. H., and Else, P. L. (2004). Membrane lipids and sodium pumps of cattle and crocodiles: an experimental test of the membrane pacemaker theory of metabolism. *Am J Physiol Regul Integr Comp Physiol 287*, R633-641.

Xiao, Y., and Li, X. (1999). Polyunsaturated fatty acids modify mouse hippocampal neuronal excitability during excitotoxic or convulsant stimulation. *Brain Res 846*, 112-121.

Yamada, K. A., Rensing, N., and Thio, L. L. (2005). Ketogenic diet reduces hypoglycemia-induced neuronal death in young rats. *Neurosci Lett 385*, 210-214.

Yancy, W. S., Jr., Provenzale, D., and Westman, E. C. (2001). Improvement of gastroesophageal reflux disease after initiation of a low-carbohydrate diet: five brief case reports. *Altern Ther Health Med 7*, 120, 116-129.

Yaroslavsky, Y., Stahl, Z., and Belmaker, R. H. (2002). Ketogenic diet in bipolar illness. *Bipolar Disord 4*, 75.

Yehuda, S., Carasso, R. L., and Mostofsky, D. I. (1994). Essential fatty acid preparation (SR-3) raises the seizure threshold in rats. *Eur J Pharmacol 254*, 193-198.

Young, C., Gean, P. W., Chiou, L. C., and Shen, Y. Z. (2000). Docosahexaenoic acid inhibits synaptic transmission and epileptiform activity in the rat hippocampus. *Synapse 37*, 90-94.

Yudkoff, M., Daikhin, Y., Nissim, I., and Grunstein, R. (1997). Effects of ketone bodies on astrocyte amino acid metabolism. *J Neurochem 69*, 682-692.

Yudkoff, M., Daikhin, Y., Nissim, I., and Lazarow, A. (2001a). Brain amino acid metabolism and ketosis. *J Neurosci Res 66*, 272-281.

Yudkoff, M., Daikhin, Y., Nissim, I., and Lazarow, A. (2001b). Ketogenic diet, amino acid metabolism, and seizure control. *J Neurosci Res 66*, 931-940.

Yuen, A. W., and Sander, J. W. (2004). Is omega-3 fatty acid deficiency a factor contributing to refractory seizures and SUDEP? A hypothesis. *Seizure 13*, 104-107.

Yuen, A. W., Sander, J. W., Fluegel, D., Patsalos, P. N., Bell, G. S., Johnson, T., and Koepp, M. J. (2005). Omega-3 fatty acid supplementation in patients with chronic epilepsy: a randomized trial. *Epilepsy Behav 7*, 253-258.

Zawar, C., and Neumcke, B. (2000). Differential activation of ATP-sensitive potassium channels during energy depletion in CA1 pyramidal cells and interneurones of rat hippocampus. *Pflugers Arch 439*, 256-262.

Zhao, Q., Stafstrom, C. E., Fu, D. D., Hu, Y., and Holmes, G. L. (2004). Detrimental effects of the ketogenic diet on cognitive function in rats. *Pediatr Res 55*, 498-506.

In: Nutrition Research Advances
Editor: Sarah V. Watkins, pp. 47-80

ISBN 1-60021-516-5
© 2007 Nova Science Publishers, Inc.

Chapter II

RELATIONSHIP BETWEEN DIET AND WERNICKE'S ENCEPHALOPATHY

GianPietro Sechi[1], Alessandro Serra[1], Maria I. Pirastru[1], Giulio Rosati[1], Luisanna Bosincu[2], Paolo Cossu Rocca[2] and Maurizio Conti[3]

[1]Institute of Clinical Neurology, University of Sassari, Sassari, Italy;
[2]Institute of Pathology, University of Sassari, Sassari, Italy;
[3]Institute of Radiological Science, University of Sassari, Sassari, Italy.

ABSTRACT

Wernicke's encephalopathy is an acute neuropsychiatric syndrome characterized in its classical form by paralysis of eye movements, stuggering gait and mental changes, a triad not frequently encountered in clinical practice. It results from a deficiency in vitamin B1, or thiamine, an essential coenzyme in intermediate carbohydrate metabolism. Thiamine requirements are directly related to total caloric intake and to the proportion of calories provided as carbohydrates. As a consequence, high caloric and high carbohydrate oral diets increase the demand for thiamine. Moreover, genetic factors may determine the response to diet and hence influence the susceptibility to Wernicke's encephalopathy. Additional, environmental factors that may modify thiamine requirements or usefulness include prolonged cooking of foods, ethanol ingestion (which impairs thiamine transport across intestinal mucosa), post-operative intravenous hyperalimentation, the consumption of foods containing thiaminases or antithiamine compounds (e.g., the use of some raw fish and certain teas), the use of some chemotherapy agents that may impair conversion of thiamine into its active metabolite thiamine pyrophosphate, and the occurrence of magnesium depletion which may induce a refractory response to thiamine. The recommended thiamine doses for healthy adults range between 0.5 and 0.66 mg per 1000 Kcal. These doses are likely higher in children, in critically ill conditions, during pregnancy and lactation. However, the precise amount of thiamine to be given in these cases remains an important unsettled issue. Wernicke's encephalopathy may occur in chronic alcoholism, when the dietary intake of thiamine is inadequate, and may complicate any condition in which there is poor nutrition. In particular, the conditions of poor nutrition associated with Wernicke's encephalopathy include persistent vomiting, anorexia nervosa, prolonged starvation for the treatment of obesity, prolonged fasting, and the use of dietary commercial formulae, with or without thiamine, in severely ill patients. An emerging, leading potential risk factor for Wernicke's encephalopathy in susceptible individuals is the use of prolonged, apparently balanced slimming diets. Usually, these diets contain thiamine in amounts that conform to standard nutritional recommendations. Thus, the occurrence of Wernicke's encephalopathy following a slimming diet, it is not something one would predict on general principles. Common, additional supplementations to these diets include herbal preparations and certain teas. These supplements may interfere with thiamine's intestinal absorption, or act as thiamine antagonists. Moreover, another important question is "do these diets actually contain the amount of thiamine reported on the label?". These products are not well monitored by the public health authorities, and quality control can be poor as recently demonstrated by tests on other dietary formulae (e.g., a soy-based formula for infants, defective in thiamine, identified in Israel in 2003). Even when suspected, thiamine deficiency is difficult to diagnose, since the available tests for measuring thiamine activity in blood or other tissues are usually not available routinely. Wernicke's encephalopathy remains a clinical diagnosis. It is very important to make a presumptive diagnosis of this encephalopathy and treat the patient as soon as possible. Prompt vitamin B1 replenishment in suspected cases is the safest approach to prevent neurological symptoms and may be a life-saving measure.

INTRODUCTION

Diet, from the Latin *diaeta*, way of living, is the food and drink regularly consumed by a person for nourishment. The usual food and drink consumed may be regulated in time for medical reasons, regional, philosophical or practical factors, and for cosmetic weight loss. To maintain a healthy condition, nutritionists usually recommend a diet that contains the proper proportions of carbohydrates, fats, proteins, vitamins, minerals, and water. This may be accomplished either by eating a wide variety of foods, or by a very limited diet. Vegetarians, for example, exclude meat from their diet, and therefore, to achieve the proper proportions of nutrients, need to eat a wide variety of plants whose nutrients complement each other, providing a balance of essential aminoacids and vitamins [1]. The most important factors in determining a balanced, healthy diet are the continous availability of food, the personal choice and the cross-cultural influences. An important factor in the near future should be an accurate nutritional information supplied by public health authorities.

Diets and the amount of calories assumed by a person vary greatly throughout the world. Unbalanced diets and an inadequate or excessive amount of calories assumed are unhealthy conditions and increase the risk of disease and mortality [2,3]. Whereas, an adequate caloric restriction seems to extend the lifespan of numerous species, from yeast to rodents, through specific biochemical mechanisms that maintain DNA stability [4]. Thus, the nutritional status of a person may influence all bodily systems, in particular brain functioning [5], and changes in diet are used in medicine to treat neurological disorders (e.g., the chetogenic diet to improve some epileptic syndromes) [6]. Conversely, unbalanced diets that do not provide all the necessary daily nutrients may induce severe neurological pathologies [7]. The evidence is now conclusive that a diet deficient in vitamin B_1, or thiamin, may lead, within a few weeks, mainly in susceptible individuals, to Wernicke's encephalopathy: an acute neuropsychiatric syndrome that, if untreated, causes severe and irreversible damage to the brain, leading to death [8]. It is the purpose of this chapter to review our present knowledge on the relationship between many kinds of diets and the risk of developing Wernicke's encephalopathy, and moreover, to discuss the diagnostic criteria, the pathophysiology, and the therapeutic measures of this disorder.

Wernicke's Encephalopathy

Carl Wernicke described this distinctive entity in 1881 as acute superior hemorrhagic polioencephalitis, in two alcoholic men and a young woman who developed persistent vomiting due to pyloric stenosis following the ingestion of sulphuric acid [9]. All of them died within 10-14 days from the onset of neurologic manifestations. The patients shared a clinical triad, nystagmus and ophthalmoplegia, mental status changes and unsteadiness of stance and gait. Pupillary function was spared. Fundoscopic changes, consisting of swelling of the optic discs and retinal hemorrhages were also observed [9]. Campbell and Russell in the 1940's stressed the nutritional aspect of the encephalopathy and suggested thiamin deficiency as a causative factor [10].

PATHOPHYSIOLOGY

Studies in experimental animals, such as monkeys and rats, and clinical studies have demonstrated that Wernicke's encephalopathy results from a deficiency in thiamin, a water-soluble vitamin of the B-group that, like all vitamins, cannot be synthesized by the human body and needs to be consumed in food as part of the diet on a regular basis [11]. The sequence of events that lead to brain lesions during thiamin deficiency is not completely understood. The vitamin is transported actively at the blood-brain barrier by two cationic transporters [12]. Into neuronal and glial cells thiamin is converted to its active form thiamin pyrophosphate (also called thiamin diphosphate, or cocarboxylase) which acts as a coenzyme in more than 24 enzymes involved in several biochemical pathways in the brain, such as the intermediate carbohydrate metabolism (for energy production by ATP synthesis), lipid metabolism for production and manteinance of myelin sheath), as well as the production of aminoacids and glucose-derived neurotransmitters (e.g, gamma-aminobutyric acid; glutamic acid) [13]. Other functions of thiamin include a putative role in axonal conduction and a role in synaptic transmission, mainly at acetylcholinergic and serotonergic synapses [14]. At the cellular level, the major thiamin-dependent enzymes involved are the pyruvate dehydrogenase complex (PHD) and the α-ketoglutarate dehydrogenase complex (alpha-KGDH) at tricarboxylic acid cycle, and transketolase (TK) at pentose-phosphate pathway [15]. Experimental findings in vivo and in vitro indicate that thiamine deficiency produces a diffuse decrease in the use of glucose in the brain [16], which leads to a severe impairment of energy metabolism both in neuronal and glial cells within a few days [17]. This is related to the limited body stores of thiamin which are only sufficient for 10-20 days [18]. In Wernicke's encephalopathy, the earliest brain biochemical alteration is the decrease in alpha-KGDH activity in astrocytes, which occurs after about 4 days of thiamine deficiency [19,20]. After 7-10 days of thiamine deficiency, a reduction in the activity of TK is also noticed, while no change in the activity of PDH is observed following thiamine deficiency treatment for up to 10 days [20]. The metabolic impairment at tricarboxylic acid cycle and pentose-phosphate pathway disrupts many astrocytic-related functions, such as the control of intracellular and extracellular glutamate concentrations, with consequent, probable occurrence of glutamate-mediated excitotoxicity; maintenance of ionic gradients across the cell membrane and blood-brain barrier permeability [21]. DNA fragmentation in neurons resulting in apopitotic cell death, restricted to the thalamus, appears, instead, from day 14 of Wernicke's encephalopathy [22]. Moreover, in Wernicke's encephalopathy at the symptomatic stage, an increased lactate production by both neurons and astrocytes has been pointed out, with intracellular accumulation of lactate, reductions in pH and focal acidosis, restricted to the selectively vulnerable regions of the Wernicke's encephalopathy brain [23]. Interestingly, lactate accumulation within brain structures is increased further after glucose loading and it seems parallel the worsening and progression of neurological symptoms in Wernicke's encephalopathy [23].

Other mechanisms involved in the pathogenesis of selective neuronal loss in Wernicke's encephalopathy may include a mitochondrial dysfunction and oxidative stress with early significant increases of expression of the brain endothelial isoform of nitric oxide synthase, production of free radicals and cytokines [24], resulting in an amplification of the previously discussed cell death mechanisms in thiamine deficiency [24]. The consequence of the cascade of metabolic alterations reported in Wernicke's encephalopathy is the loss of osmotic gradients across cell membranes, with the occurence of cytotoxic edema and a progressive cell volume increase firstly in astrocytes after about 4 days of thiamine deficiency [25]. Early occurence of cerebral edema, both in glia cells and neurons, with characteristic topographical distribution of lesions, has also been documented in humans with Wernicke's encephalopathy by magnetic resonance imaging (MRI) studies [26-30]. In the same restricted cerebral regions, after a few days of thiamine deficiency, both cytotoxic and vasogenic edema have been documented with breakdown of blood-brain barrier [29-32]. Importantly, various clinical studies have shown that a prompt and sufficient thiamin replacement therapy leads to the disappearance of the MRI abnormal signal intensities due to cerebral edema within 14 days [30-32]. Conversely, in Wernicke's encephalopathy, the lack or a delayed thiamin therapy may lead to structural, irreversible lesions in discrete regions of the brain with possible major, permanent neurological sequelae (e.g., Korsakoff psychosis) or a fatal outcome [18,33]. The probable, temporal sequence of metabolic and morphologic alterations that occurs at the cellular level in discrete regions of the brain during thiamin deficiency is synthesized in Table 1.

NEUROPATHOLOGY

Macroscopic examination of the brain of patients diagnosed with Wernicke's encephalopathy reveals gross neuropathological changes in only about fifty per cent of the cases [34,35]. These include symmetrical grayish discoloration, shrinkage, congestion, fresh pinpoint hemorrhages in some gray matter structures, including the periaqueductal gray matter, the mammillary bodies and medial thalamus [18]. Also, an increase in the size of the lateral and third ventricles is reported [18]. Gross hemorrhage is encountered in about 5 per cent of cases and is thought to be a late change in patients with rapid depletion of thiamin (e.g., patients on parenteral nutrition without vitamin supplements) [36]. Histopathological changes affect specific areas of the brain, mainly in periventricular regions of diencephalon, midbrain, brainstem and superior vermis of the cerebellum [18]. Why thiamin deficiency preferentially affects neurons in particular areas of the nervous system is unknown. Thiamin content and turnover is high in these areas, and these structures may have a high rate of oxidative metabolism which could make them more vulnerable [24]. Victor et. al. [18] reported observed microscopic involvement of the mammillary bodies and the thalamus, the most frequently affected region was the medial dorsal nucleus, in 100 per cent of the cases studied. Lesions of the cerebellum were reported in approximately one-third of the cases. Other areas affected include the periaqueductal region at the level of the third cranial nerve nuclei, the pontine tegmentum, the reticular formation of the midbrain, and the posterior corpora quadrigemina [18]. On histological examination, acute lesions display edema, swelling of astrocytes with decreases in myelinated fibres, minimal loss of neurons, patchy loss of nerve cells accompanied by activated microglia and reactive astrogliosis, moreover prominent vessels as a result of swelling and hyperplasia (Figure 1). Interestingly, in a study by Torvik [37], the nature of the neuropathological lesions in patients with Wernicke's encephalopathy was found to vary depending on the region of the brain. In particular, in the mammillary body and paraventricular structures neuropil destruction and preserved but small neurons have been shown, while in the thalamus and inferior olives a definite neuronal loss with preserved neuropil have been shown [37]. These findings are consistent with recent ultrastructural data on the content of the proteins complexin I and complexin II in neurons of the medial thalamus and inferior colliculus in rats with Wernicke's encephalopathy [38]. In this study, these proteins were decreased in the thalamus, at the symptomatic stage of Wernicke's encephalopathy, but were unchanged in inferior colliculus [38]. These data indicate the likelihood of more than one mechanism of brain cell damage in patients with Wernicke's encephalopathy [21].

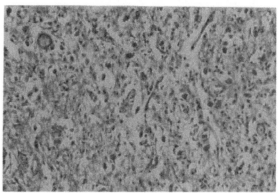

Figure 1. Hystological examination of the hypothalamic region in a patient with Wernicke's encephalopathy (haematoxylin and eosin, original magnification 10✕) shows characteristic loosening of the neuropil, marked small vessel proliferation, reactive astrocytes with plump cytoplasm, relative neuronal and axonal sparing.

Table 1. Proposed temporal sequence of metabolic and morphologic alterations that occurs at the cellular level in discrete regions of the brain during thiamin deficiency. From experimental findings in vivo and in vitro, and MRI studies in humans

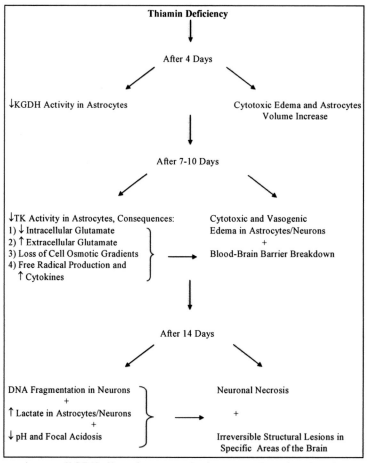

For references, see the text; KGDH=Ketoglutarate Dehydrogenase Complex; TK=Transketolase.

CLINICAL FEATURES

Early detection of subclinical thiamin deficiency poses considerable problems as symptoms, when present, are vague and aspecific (e.g., unusual fatigue, anorexia, irritability, abdominal discomfort, frequent headaches, some falling off in the growth rate of children, and slight, occasional weight loss in adults) [39]. Patients with clinical thiamin deficiency present with Wernicke's encephalopathy, a neuropsychiatric disorder of acute onset characterized, in its classic form, by ocular abnormalities, incoordination of gait and mental status changes, a triad encountered in clinical practice in only 16 per cent of the cases [40].

Ocular abnormalities are the most consistent clinical manifestation of Wernicke's encephalopathy and occur in about 96 per cent of patients. According to clinically based series [8]. These include nystagmus (mainly on horizontal plane, but also on vertical), palsy of both lateral recti and sometimes other ocular muscles, and conjugate-gaze palsies, reflecting lesions of the pontine tegmentum and of abducens and oculomotor nuclei [8]. Rarely, a sluggish reaction of the pupils to light, anisocoria and light near dissociation are seen [41]. Bilateral visual loss with optic disc edema, sometimes with retinal hemorrhages, and optic neuropathy may be present and should not prompt the clinician to exclude Wernicke's encephalopathy [42].

The loss of equilibrium with incoordination of gait and trunkal ataxia occurs in 87 per cent of patients and may result both from an involvement of the anterior and superior cerebellar vermis and from vestibular dysfunction [8,43]. In some cases the occurrence of polyneuropathy may be a contributing factor. Rarely, limb ataxia and dysartria may occur [8].

The mental status changes occur in about 90 per cent of patients and range from a global or partial confusional state to mental sluggishness, apathy, impaired awareness of the immediate situation, restlessness, inability to concentrate, and, if left untreated, patients may progress through stupor (i.e., the requirement of constant stimulation to be roused), coma (i.e., the patient is unarousable even with the most intense sensory stimuli) and death [8,44].

Noteworthy, about 19 per cent of patients showed none of the classic elements at the presentation of Wernicke's encephalopathy [35,40], although, usually, one or more symptoms of the classical triad appear later over the course of Wernicke's encephalopathy [45,46]. In unsuspected cases the presenting symptoms may be stupor or coma, mainly related to damage within the thalami; hypotension and tachycardia, due either to a defect in efferent sympathetic outflow and decreased peripheral resistance, or to a coexistent cardiovascular-wet beriberi; hypothermia, due to involvement of the posterior hypothalamic regions (when the more anterior hypothalamic regions are spared); and bilateral visual loss with papilledema, likely due to the loss of cellular osmotic gradients in the optic discs and retinas.

Wernicke's encephalopathy is an acute, rapidly progressive disease which can evolve over several days, if left untreated. However, little is known about the temporal progression of neurological signs in humans. In rhesus monkeys, the number of cerebral structures affected tends to increase with increasing periods of thiamin deficiency [47]. In our experience, over the course of the disease, mainly in a late stage (i.e., about one or two weeks after the beginning of the symptoms), other neurological signs may be noticed including epileptic seizures, until status epilepticus, due to excessive glutamatergic activity, hyperthermia, unresponsive to antipyretics, due to involvement of anterior hypothalamic regions, increased motor tone with nuchal and lower spine rigidity, and intermittent choreic dyskinesias of hands and feet due to damage to structures or fiber systems at mesopontine tegmental areas [45,46]. In rare instances, in a late stage of Wernicke's encephalopathy, the contemporary occurrence of stupor, ophthalmoplegia, hyperthermia, and severe nuchal and lower spine rigidity may mimic a skull basal meningitis [45]. Obviously, the knowledge of how Wernicke's encephalopathy progresses is of direct clinical relevance and may be essential in the diagnosis and treatment of this reversible, but potentially fatal condition. From our experience and based on literature data, the clinical features of Wernicke's encephalopathy may be categorized as symptoms common at presentation, symptoms uncommon at presentation, and late stage symptoms (Table 2). The relationship between neurological signs in Wernicke's encephalopathy and the cerebral structures affected are summarized in Table 3.

Table 2. Clinical features of Wernicke's encephalopathy at its presentation and at a late stage of the disease

Clinical Features of Wernicke's Encephalopathy
A) Common Symptoms at Presentation
- Ocular Abnormalities
- Mental Status Changes
- Incoordination of Gait and Trunkal Ataxia
B) Uncommon Symptoms at Presentation
- Stupor
- Hypotension / Tachycardia
- Hypothermia
- Bilateral Visual Loss / Papilledema
C) Late Stage Symptoms
- Epileptic Seizures / Status Epilepticus
- Coma
- Hyperthermia
- Increased Muscular Tone
- Choreic Dyskinesias
- Memory Deficits

In some patients with chronic, intermittent thiamin deficiency, peripheral neurological changes (dry beriberi[*]) may occur. The symptoms include the occurrence of bilateral and symmetric paresthesias involving predominantly the lower extremities, with a burning sensation in the feet (particularly severe at night), calf muscle cramps, and pains in the legs. Difficulty in rising from a squatting position, a diminution in the vibratory sensation in the toes, and plantar dysesthesia are all early signs. Ankle jerks are absent. Continued deficiency

---

[*] beriberi: the term beriberi is derived from the Sinhalese word meaning extreme weakness.

causes a loss of knee jerk, atrophy of the calf and thigh muscles, and finally foot and toe drop.

Table 3. Relationship between neurological signs in Wernicke's encephalopathy (WE) and cerebral structures affected

Neurological Signs in WE	Cerebral Structures Affected
Nystagmus / Palsy of Extraocular Muscles / Conjugate-Gaze Palsies	Pontine Tegmentum / Abducens and Oculomotor Nuclei
Incoordination of Gait / Trunkal Ataxia	Anterior / Superior Cerebellar Vermis; Vestibular Nuclei
Mental Status Changes	Thalami / Mammillary Bodies
Disturbances of Wakefulness	Reticular Formation of Midbrain / Thalami
Hypotension	Sympathetic System
Hypothermia	Posterior Hypothalamic Regions
Hyperthermia	Anterior Hypothalamic Regions
Increased Motor Tone	Mesopontine Tegmental Areas
Choreic Dyskineseas	Mesopontine Tegmental Areas
Memory Deficits	Mammillary Bodies
Bilateral Visual Loss	Optic Disks

In a few patients a cardiovascular (wet) beriberi may also occur. This takes 2 forms: a) a more common, high output state, characterized by early tachycardia, sweating, and warm skin. Following heart failure, orthopnea, pulmonary and peripheral edema, peripheral vasoconstriction causing cold and cyanosed extremities are evident; b) a rare, low output state (Shoshin disease*), characterized by severe hypotension, lactic acidosis and absence of edema.

A peculiar clinical form is the infantile beriberi, which occurs in infants breast-fed by thiamin-deficient mothers, or in infants fed with soy-based formula defective in thiamin [48], usually between the 2nd and 12th months of life. Cardiomyopathy, aphonia, absent deep tendon reflexes, vomiting, diarrhea, weight loss, lethargy, restlessness, nystagmus, ophthalmoplegia and respiratory symptoms may occur [48].

It is interesting that among humans, Asians and Europeans respond to thiamin deficiency differently: Asians tend to develop mainly a cardiovascular (wet) beriberi, whereas Europeans tend to develop a dry beri beri with polineuropathy and Wernicke's encephalopathy, with the late occurrence of severe memory defects (Korsakoff psychosis). Obviously, in an individual, thiamin deficiency may induce both neurological and cardiovascular disturbances to different degrees, according to the nature of thiamin deficiency (clinical setting, acute, subacute, or chronic-intermittent forms) and the peculiar genetic susceptibility.

CLINICAL SETTINGS

A continuously increasing number of clinical settings in which Wernicke's encephalopathy may be encountered has been focused on in recent years. These range from gastrointestinal surgery to patients with cancer, especially if treated with chemotherapy, and acquired immunodeficiency syndrome (AIDS). In the past, the most common conditions associated with a high incidence of thiamin deficiency were chronic alcholism in Western countries and the use of highly polished rice in Asian countries. The variety of clinical settings related to Wernicke's encephalopathy more commonly encountered in clinical practice has been summarized in Table 4, and will be discussed below:

1) *Alcohol Abuse and Malnutrition:* Studies in animals and humans have shown that chronic alcohol ingestion does not result in Wernicke's encephalopathy if the dietary intake of thiamin is adequate [49]. Ethanol is a rich source of non-nutritive calories and, usually, alcoholic beverages contain few vitamins and minerals. While the supply of vitamins is reduced, the metabolism of alcohol increases the demand beyond normal, so that alcoholics usually require amounts of vitamins that exceed the demand of healthy subjects [50]. In particular, for an individual, about 40 liters of beer or 200 liters of wine are needed to cover the daily requirements for B vitamins [50]. As a consequence, heavy drinking is often complicated by malnutrition and inadequate dietary intake of minerals and vitamins including thiamin [51]. Other contributing factors to the deficiency of thiamin in alcoholics are the alcohol-related, reduced transport of thiamin across intestinal mucosa, the reduced capacity of the liver to store the vitamin, and the impaired activation of thiamin pyrophosphate from thiamin [52,53]. Furthermore, since not every individual with a similar degree of malnutrition and abuse of alcohol develops Wernicke's encephalopathy or other neurologic complications, it has been suggested that both environmental and genetic factors contribute to disease expression. Blass and Gibson [54] found a variant form of transketolase having a decreased affinity for thiamin pyrophosphate in four cases of Wernicke's encephalopathy, with respect to controls. The abnormalities in this form of transketolase appeared to be genetic, and hence hereditary, rather than a consequence of Wernicke's encephalopathy, since they persisted in fibroblasts through more than 20 generations of culture medium containing thiamin and not ethanol [54]. This trait may be more common in certain individuals, leaving them more susceptible when on a diet marginal or deficient in thiamin, especially if challenged with a large carbohydrate load. However, sequencing of the transketolase's coding region failed to demonstrate a specific variation which may account for an altered enzyme activity, [55], thus further studies are needed to define the nature of the altered transketolase activity in Wernicke's encephalopathy. Chronic alcohol misuse and malnutrition may also lead to a significant magnesium depletion [56]. This finding may be relevant for alcoholics prone to Wernicke's encephalopathy, since this divalent cation acts as a co-factor for

---

* Shoshin disease: shoshin is the Japanese word for damage to the heart.

many enzymes, including transketolase, in the pentose phosphate pathway and magnesium is thought to have a crucial role in a proper catalytical action of these enzymes [57]. Consequently, patients with Wernicke's encephalopathy may be unresponsive to parenteral thiamin in the presence of hypomagnesiemia [58] and, as indicated by clinical studies, this refractoriness may reverse with magnesium replenishment [58]. Thus, the risk for Wernicke's encephalopathy in alcoholics is high and, in the United States, this encephalopathy is most commonly associated with chronic alcohol abuse [33]. Fortification of alcoholic beverages with thiamin has been proposed to reduce the incidence of Wernicke's encephalopathy [59]. In Australia, the enrichment of bread flour with thiamin has caused a 40 per cent reduction of the incidence of acute Wernicke's encephalopathy and Korsakoff psychosis [60]. Since this disease complex has, however, not been eliminated, the opportunity of adding thiamin to beer or wine is presently being studied [61].

2) *Polished Rice and Thiamin Deficiency:* For many countries, about two-thirds of the world population, where rice is the main part of the diet, a major cause of thiamin deficiency remains a staple diet of milled or polished rice. Milling removes the husk, which contains most of the thiamin, but boiling before husking disperses the vitamin throughout the grain, thus preventing its loss. In these countries beriberi, and not Wernicke's encephalopathy, has been endemic until that most of the population used polished rice rather than the traditional brown rice, because the consumption of brown rice was considered inferior and status lowering. As all countries in the world started to use thiamin-enriched food, the incidence of beriberi decreased dramatically. However, thiamin deficiency due to polished rice remains an important health care issue in particular populations, mainly in Asia, such as the displaced persons in refugee camps [62,63]. In these populations, the clinical presentation of thiamin deficiency is mainly as polineuropathy or infantile Beriberi rather than Wernicke's encephalopathy [62,63]. The reasons for this peculiar clinical presentation are still unknown. Perhaps, in these populations, the combined use of foods that have a considerable amount of thiaminase may play a role [64].

3) *Gastrointestinal Surgery:* Many gastrointestinal surgery procedures for a variety of disorders (e.g., peptic ulcer disease, colonic carcinoma, severe obesity with a body mass index greater than 40 kg/m^2), which lead to exclusion of portions of the gastrointestinal tract, are predisposing risk factors for the development of Wernicke's encephalopathy, polyneuropathy, and, rarely, wet beriberi with cardiac failure [65-67]. In most of these patients, thiamin deficiency is frequently associated with low levels of other nutrients (e.g., niacin, pyridoxin, vitamin B_{12}, iron), leading to the clinical condition of a multi-vitamin deficiency [68]. The surgical procedures implicated range from gastrectomy or gastrojejunostomy to partial colectomy, to gastroplasty/gastric bypass surgery, and to therapy with an intragastric balloon [66-69]. Wernicke's encephalopathy occurs most commonly between the second and the eighth month after surgery and with weight loss of 13 to 45 kg. Sometimes, it occurs 20-30 days after surgery, if intravenous hyperalimentation without vitamin supplementation is given [69]. Patients usually give a history of nonremitting nausea and persistent vomiting, with difficulty drinking or eating [68,69]. Rarely, Wernicke-

Korsakoff syndrome may occur after a long latent interval following gastectomy (2 to 20 years) [70]. In these patients with a long-standing latent deficiency in thiamin levels, minor changes in dietary habit may lead to the development of Wernicke's encephalopathy [70]. The mechanisms responsible for Wernicke's encephalopathy after gastrointestinal surgery are numerous. These include the limited amount of food ingested, the poor compliance with an adeguate dietary intake, the maldigestion of food with consequent malabsorption, and the reduced area of the gastric and jejunal mucosa useful for absorbing thiamin mainly by active transport [71,72]. In all patients, an important role seems to be played by the occurrence of persistent vomiting.

4) *Recurrent Vomiting, Diarrhea and Hyperemesis Gravidarum:* Recurrent vominting, sometimes with associated diarrhea, in a variety of clinical settings may result in Wernicke's encephalopathy. Rarely, severe malabsorption related to persistent diarrhea as a unique symptom may also lead to Wernicke's encephalopathy (e.g., lithium-induced diarrhea) [73]. More common clinical settings include patients with gastrointestinal disorders (e.g., pyloric stenosis and peptic ulcer; drugs-induced gastritis; vomiting due to biliary colics; Crohn's disease; obstruction; perforation) [74-78]. Moreover, the profuse vomiting during migraine attacks [79], the self-induced vomiting in anorexia nervosa [80], the vomiting associated with possibile diarrhea and malnutrition sometimes with signs of multi-organ failure, in the setting of a delayed (about 2 weeks) encephalopathy complicating an acute pancreatitis [81,82], and the persistent and severe nausea and vomiting in pregnancy that can progress to hyperemesis gravidarum [83,84]. The latter is a rare condition that, if inadequately or inappropriately treated (e.g., intravenous glucose supplementation without thiamin), it may cause Wernicke's encephalopathy, central pontine myelinolisis and death [84-86]. Thiamin deficiency is common in pregnancy [85,87], mainly if the woman is suffering from gestational diabetes, even when on standard prenatal thiamin supplementation [86,88]. Thus, the management of patients with hyperemesis gravidarum should always include thiamin supplementation, in combination with intravenous fluid and electrolyte replacement, use of conventional antiemetics and psychological support [89,90]. In these clinical settings, the long-standing poor oral intake due to recurrent vomiting and, sometimes, the concomitant malabsorption of vitamins, including thiamin, due to diarrhea, may easily explain the occurence of Wernicke's encephalopathy, although some Authors suggested the possibility that vomiting per se may in some cases constitute part of the syndrome of Wernicke's encephalopathy rather than represent its cause or precipitating event [79].

5) *Cancer and Medical Treatment:* The occurrence of thiamin deficiency with associated, severe, right-sided congestive heart failure (wet beriberi), or Wernicke's encephalopathy has been reported in oncological literature, both in early stages of cancer and in terminally ill cancer patients [91-93]. In addition, in a recent study, malignancy was the most common underlying disorder that preceded Wernicke's encephalopathy onset in a pediatric population [46]. Thiamin deficiency related to cancer was first reported in 1992 in a patient with acute myeloid leukemia with heart

failure that responded to treatment with thiamin [91,92]. Since leucocytes contain relatively high concentrations of thiamin-dependent enzymes, compared with erythrocites, and because no other cause could be found, it was postulated that consumption of thiamin by fast-growing blast cells was responsible for the deficiency [91,93]. Further reports of Wernicke's encephalopathy related to cancer and/or medical treatment, sometimes in combination with acute metabolic acidosis, include patients undergoing allogenic bone marrow transplantation, where thiamin deficiency was caused by a lack of vitamin supplementation during total parenteral nutrition administration [94], and patients with several kinds of cancer (e.g., inoperable gastric carcinoma, non-Hodgkin's lymphoma, myelomonocitic leukemia, large B-cell lymphoma) undergoing different chemotherapic treatments (e.g., 5-fluorouracil, cisplatin, ifosfamide, cytarabine, cyclophosphamide, doxorubicin, vincristine, rituximab, tolazamide and erbulozole) [95,96]. For erbulozole, in particular, a dose-limiting toxicity has been documented at respectively 100 mg/m^2 (one administration every three weeks) and 50 mg/m^2 (weekly administration). At this level, patients may display a dose-limiting Wernicke's encephalopathy-like syndrome [97]. Causes of thiamin deficiency in patients with cancer include the poor dietary intake related to inappetence and nausea, malabsorption, increased thiamin consumption and an elevated thiamin requirement [93]. In these settings, common precipitating events to Wernicke's encephalopaty may be the refeeding after starvation, and a carbohydrate loading without vitamin suplementation [94,96].

How medical treatment and chemotherapy in particular may lead to thiamin deficiency and Wernicke's encephalopathy is putzling but fascinating issue. Tolezamide can produce Wernicke's encephalopathy by lowering thiamin levels in susceptible individuals with borderline thiamin levels [96,98]. Moreover, many chemiotherapic agents are diluted in carbohydrate or alcoholic solutions that may act as a carbohydrate loading that facilitates Wernicke's encephalopathy. A direct metabolic effect of the diluent ethyl alcohol and propilene glycol on thiamin metabolism seems to be responsible for the occurence of Wernicke's encephalopathy after the intravenous infusion of high-dose nitroglycerine [99]. The chemiotherapic agent erbulozole is diluted in a solution of cyclodextrin, a hydrosoluble carbohydrate containing 6-12 glucose residues, thus both the drug and its solution may be responsible for Wernicke's encephalopathy-like neurotoxicity-induced by erbulozole. However, since no similar toxicity has been reported at low doses of the drug (less than 100 mg/m^2) administered in the same cyclodextrin solution, erbulozole rather than the cyclodextrin solution seems to be responsible for the encephalopathy [98,100]. Ifosfamide, another chemiotherapic agent extensively used in cancer therapy, may induce a Wernicke's encephalopathy-like syndrome that may be reversed by the administration of thiamin [101]. Since in patients with cancer, on therapy with erbulozole or ifosfamide, the thiamin levels in whole blood did not change after the administration of the drugs, it has been hypothesyzed that these chemiotherapic agents and/or their metabolites may interfere with thiamin function, or with the enzymes of the intermediate carbohydrate metabolism [100,101]. In particular, for both drugs a direct interference with the activation of thiamin pyrophosphate from thiamin seems likely [100,101]. Recognition of cancer and chemotherapy-associated Wernicke's encephalopathy is important, since thiamin administration and dose reduction, or discontinuation of chemotherapy most of the times results in the resolution of clinical symptoms and neuroimaging abnormalities.

6) *Systemic Illness and Drugs*: Many systemic diseases that affect thiamin uptake and metabolism may predispose to the development of Wernicke's encephalopathy. These include patients with end-stage renal disease undergoing regular dialysis [102], patients with AIDS [103], with thyrotoxicosis [104], with prolonged infectious-febrile conditions [8], and with magnesium depletion due to long-term diuretic use, or other causes [105].

   a] Renal Diseases

   In renal diseases, both patients on peritoneal dialysis and hemodialysis may rarely develop Wernicke's encephalopathy [106]. The main causes are the low intake of thiamin due to anorexia and vomiting, and the accelerated loss of the vitamin during dialysis [107,108]. Other factors altering thiamin requirements in these patients may be the intravenous or intradialytic parenteral nutrition with a percentage of glucose without thiamin addition, or infections [107]. An additional factor, in patients with uremic encephalopathy may be the increased brain content of guanidosuccinic acid [102]. This compound possibly inhibits transketolase, a thiamin-dependent enzyme that seems to play a key role in the pathophysiology of Wernicke's encephalopathy [21]. In patients with renal failure, encephalopathy is a common problem that may be caused by uremia, thiamin deficiency, dialysis, transplant rejection, hypertension, fluid and electrolyte disturbances or drug toxicity [102]. Clinically, it may be difficult to differentiate Wernicke's encephalopathy from other neurological complications that may occur in patients with renal failure [109]. In regular dialysis patients, it may be a good medical practice to treat with parenteral thiamin any patient with encephalopathy and unexplained neurological pictures. Since in some patients thiamin can be reduced during hemodialysis, thiamin supplementation may be required even after normalized food intake [107]. However, no consensus has been reached on the most appropriate dose of thiamin for the secondary prevention of Wernicke's encephalopathy in dialysis patients [107].

   b] AIDS

   The occurence of Wernicke's encephalopathy in a patient with AIDS treated with zidovudine was first reported in 1987 [110]. The patient had none of the known risk factors for Wernicke's encephalopathy and the diagnosis was not ascertained before death. The Authors suggested that zidovudine, by impairment of DNA synthesis, might increase the likelihood of Wernicke's encephalopathy in susceptible patients with AIDS [110]. Butterworth in 1991, reported biochemical evidence of thiamin deficiency in 23 per cent of patients with AIDS or AIDS-related complex, without clinical signs of Wernicke's encephalopathy [103]. Main suggested causes were the cachexia and the catabolic state characteristic of AIDS [103]. Recent reports confirm that Wernicke's encephalopathy may play a role in the morbidity and mortality associated with

AIDS [111,112]. According to other Authors [103,112], we believe that thiamin supplementation should be considered in all patients with AIDS, especially where access to antiretroviral therapy is limited.

c] *Chronic Infectious/Febrile Conditions*

The possibile occurrence of Wernicke's encephalopathy after prolonged infectious-febrile conditions (e.g., bronchopneumonia of undetermined nature) [113] is mentioned by several Authors [18,29,46]. Prolonged fever may induce thiamin deficiency secondary to increased requirement of the vitamin, often associated to deficient oral intake. However, documented reports on this topic in literature are scanty and the reliability of clinical data quite uncertain [113].

d] *Thyrotoxicosis*

Very few reports are available on Wernicke's encehalopathy related to severe hyperthyroid Grave's disease [114]. Relatively more common are the reports of hyperthyroidism due to gestational thyrotoxicosis associated with Wernicke's encephalopathy [104]. In the latter event, usually the thyroid gland is only slightly palpable, bruits are not audible, and exophtalmos is not present [104]. Main causes of thiamin deficiency are the hypermetabolic state characteristic of thyrotoxicosis and eventually, the occurrence of intermittent vomiting and diarrhea. To improve the prognosis, the proper therapy for hyperthyroidism and the administration of parenteral thiamin should be started as soon as possibile.

e] *Magnesium Deficiency and Drugs*

Magnesium deficiency has been reported frequently in patients on long-term diuretic therapy (e.g., furosemide, ethacrynic acid, bumetanide) for heart failure [115,116], likely due to impaired reassorbtion of this divalent cation in the kidneys [105,117]. In addition, low whole blood levels of thiamin have been found in congestive heart failure patients who have been treated with loop diuretics [118]. Other systemic diseases that may have magnesium depletion include hyperemesis gravidurum [117], diarrhea due to Crohn's disease [117], and gluten enteropathy [117]. Since magnesium is an essential cofactor in the conversion of thiamin into active diphosphate and triphosphate esters [119,120], in patients with Wernicke's encephalopathy, its deficiency may lead to a refractory response to thiamin until magnesium is given [120].

Magnesium may be given orally even without regular control of serum levels, provided that renal function is unpaired. Dosage is 3x 100–150 mg per day before meals (daily magnesium requirement for adults is 400-600 mg). Parenteral administration of magnesium, balanced according to the deficit measured, may also be given.

Occasionally, a mild to moderate thiamin deficiency may also be found in individuals exposed to formaldheyde, and following long-term use of several prescription drugs such as phenytoin, penicillins, chephalosporins, aminoglycosides, tetracycline derivatives, fluoroquinolones, sulfamide derivatives, trimethoprim and other drugs [121]. However, the chemical relevance of this deficiency is uncertain.

7) *Unbalanced Nutrition:* In a normal, healthy individual, any condition of unbalanced nutrition lasting 2-3 weeks may lead to Wernicke's encephalopathy. This period is the time necessary to deplete the body reserves of thiamin that in physiological conditions are only sufficient for up to 18 days [122]. In individuals with marginal stores of thiamin, due to a myriad of causes (see, Table 4), Wernicke's encephalopathy may occur after a few days of unbalanced nutrition, mainly if the staple diet has been very rich in carbohydrates. Some reports indicate that genetic factors may predispose some individuals to Wernicke's encephalopathy [54] although, until now, genetic association studies have failed to identify genetic mutations or polymorphisms influencing the susceptibility to the encephalopathy [55].

Causes of thiamin deficiency due to unbalanced nutrition may be defined primary, when the deficiency arises from inadequate intake in people or populations because of economic, cultural, geographical, or political reasons. In this setting the clinical correlates of thiamin deficiency (wet beriberi, dry beriberi, or Wernicke's encephalopathy) occur usually in epidemic or endemic way. For example, people in Asia subsisting on high polished rice and victims of political trade embargoes in Cuba, during 1992 and 1993, which after a long period of dietary restrictions and excessive carbohydrate intake developed optic neuropathy, deafness, myelopathy, and sensory neuropathy responsive to B group vitamins [123]. Secondary, when the deficiency usually arises in a sporadic way, from 1) iatrogenic causes, as in patients who develop Wernicke's encephalopathy and sometimes lactic acidosis during total parenteral nutrition without proper replacement of thiamin [124-127]. The vitamin deficiency may also occur when the patients are receiving an oral dose of thiamin but, due to concurrent malabsorption, they may not absorb thiamin adequately [125]; or when the patients are on intravenous hyperalimentation with a high percentage of glucose not balanced with adequate doses of thiamin [125]; moreover, during the early postoperative oral food intake period following one-two weeks of intravenous nutrition without adequate vitamin supplements, a condition which may deplete body reserves of thiamin [refeeding syndrome] [128]; 2) a background of psychogenic food refusal, as in in patients with anorexia nervosa, major depressive illness, or schizoaffective psychosis, or in people after prolonged fasting for religious-philosophical reasons, during prolonged starvation for the treatment of obesity, and after a long-term hunger strike as it may occur in political prisoners [29,129-132]; 3) the use, in technological advanced societies, of dietary commercial formulae, with or without thiamin, in infants [48,133], and in severely ill patients [134]; moreover, from the use of prolonged, unbalanced, or apparently balanced slimming diets in obese women, or food faddism [79,135,136]. The use of slimming diets, in particular, is an emerging, leading, potential risk factor for Wernicke's encephalopathy in susceptible individuals [135]. Usually, these diets contain thiamin in amounts that conform to standard nutritional recommendations. Thus, the occurrence of Wernicke's encephalopathy following an apparently balanced slimming diet, is not something we would predict on general principles. Common, additional supplements to these diets include herbal preparations and certain teas.

These supplements may interfere with thiamin's intestinal absorption, or act as thiamin antagonists [64,135,137]. Moreover, another inportant question is, "Do these diets actually contain the amount of thiamin reported on the label?". These products are not well-monitored by the public health authorities and quality control can be poor as recently demonstrated by texts on other dietary formulae. For example, a soy-based formula for infants, defective in thiamin, identified in Israel in 2003 [48,133]. Following the extensive use of this formula, an outbreak of life-threatening thiamin deficiency in infants with consequent neurological and cardiological symptoms, has been reported [48]. The formula was tested by the Israeli public health authorities and the thiamin level was found to be undetectable (less than 0.5 µg/g) [48]. The cause for the low thiamin level in the formula was probably human error [138]. However, it is important to make a note of similar cases int the past, always infants or children receiving a soya bean product because of atopic and gastrointestinal allergy, in these cases also a Wernicke's encephalopathy-like sindrome was documented [139,140]. Given these findings, a controlled supplementation of thiamin for all the dietary commercial formulae containing soya products seems mandatory.

Within the developed nations, another nutrional factor that may lead to thiamin deficiency is the extensive use of chemical food additives useful in preserving them and for elimination or control of natural contaminants of food. Common food additives are sulphites, salt, or ester derived from sulphureous acid, which act as antioxidants and preservatives. Sulphites are found frequently in processed fruit and vegetables, fresh grapes, dried fruits, fermented sausage, vinegar, meat, wine and dessicated coconut. Thiamin is sensitive to degradation in the presence of critical concentrations of sulphite ions both in food and in parenteral nutrition solutions [141]. In particular, the ability of sulphites to destroy thiamin is dependent on the dose used. When multivitamins were added directly to aminoacids solutions containing 0.1% (9.6 mM) sulphite, significant degradation of thiamin occurred within 5 hours. Thiamin was stable for at least 22 hours when added to total parenteral nutrition solutions containing less than 0.05% (4.8 mM) sulphite [141]. It is relevant that diets high in simple carbohydrates consisting mainly of processed food (e.g., the average American diet in adolescents), it has been documented by plasma levels, red cell transketolase, or thiamin pyrophosphate percentage effect, are usually deficient in thiamin [142,143]. Interestingly, thiamin deficiency and the occurrence of a Wernicke's encephalopathy-like sindrome has recently been documented in dogs due to prolonged feeding with sulphite preserved meat [144]. However, to our knowledge, no cases of Wernicke's encephalopathy strictly related to processed food with sulphites have been reported until now in humans.

The websites devoted to promoting dietary advice, dietary supplements, or potential hazardous "very low caloric diets" are increasing in number and their relevance and quality of the sites vary enormously, and certain regimes are potentially dangerous [145]. As there is an increasing use of dietary commercial formulae, even in the medical framework, and the number of people on slimming diets for cosmetic weight loss continues to climb, and the popularity of various kinds of slimming diets increases, we are likely to experience a marked rise in the number of people at risk for Wernicke's encephalopathy. In our opinion, these people could be a new group of potential patients to watch for.

Table 4. Clinical Settings Related to Wernicke's Encephalopathy

1)   Alcohol Abuse and Malnutrition
2)   Polished Rice in Particular Populations
3)   Gastrointestinal Surgery
4)   Recurrent Vomiting, Diarrhea, and Hyperemesis Gravidarum
5)   Cancer and Medical Treatment
6)   Systemic Illness and Drugs
7)   Unbalanced Nutrition

DIET, THIAMIN REQUIREMENT, AND WERNICKE'S ENCEPHALOPATHY

Dietary requirements depend on age, sex, height, weight, activity (metabolic and physical), physiological state of individuals (i.e., growth rate, pregnancy, lactation), genetic make-up and general health condition. Chronic illness that increases metabolism and, hence, energy expenditure (i.e., infections, fever, trauma, hyperthyroidism, cancer, AIDS), or alters the digestion and absorption of food (i.e., gastrointestinal, hepatic and pancreatic diseases) strongly influences an individual's dietary requirements. The ideal diet, which provides all the nutrients necessary for life and health, is well-balanced, energy-appropriate for age, height and general health condition, and includes a variety of food, and possibly, micronutrient supplements (i.e., vitamins and minerals). Diets that are energy-restricted to less than 1200 kcal/d may not be adequate in one or more of the essential nutrients. Most nutritionists indicate that in a diet, the appropriate quantities of nutrients have to be balanced to maintain an acceptable body weight for height, a body mass index of approximately 19 to 25 kg/m^2.

Thiamin requirements, in particular, are directly related both to total caloric intake and to the proportion of calories provided as carbohydrates [146]. As a consequence, high caloric and high carbohydrate oral diets increase the demand for thiamin. Moreover, genetic factors may determine the response to diet and the requirement of thiamin, and therefore can influence the individual's susceptibility to Wernicke's encephalopathy [54]. Additional, environmental factors that could potentially modify thiamin requirements or usefulness include prolonged cooking of foods, that may destroy the vitamin, the regular use of alcohol and antacids that may interfere with the absorption of thiamin, and the consumption of foods containing thiaminases or antithiamin compounds. For example, certain raw fish and shellfish that contain in the viscera bacteria rich in thiaminases [137,147]. These enzymes split thiamin and render it inactive biologically. Also, drinking tea, coffee, decaffeinated coffee, and chewing betel nut, which contain antithiamin factors [137,147]. The most likely substance in tea that inactivates thiamin is tannic acid, by forming a tannin-thiamin adduct. Moreover, a variety of conditions and substances previously discussed in the Clinical Settings paragraph which may strongly alter the requirement of the vitamin.

Thiamin exists in nature in many chemical forms: thiamin hydrochloride, thiamin mononitrate, thiamin diphosphate, thiamin disulphite, thiamin triphosphate, O,S-dibenzoyl thiamin, and tetrahydrofurfuryldisulphide thiamin. All of these forms have now been synthesized, although, they occur in different amounts in animal tissues and vegetals. Thiamin hydrochloride and thiamin mononitrate are the forms of thiamin typically used in nutritional supplements and for food fortification. The major form of thiamin that occurs in food is thiamin hydrochloride. It is fine for vitamin supplements, but it cannot be used for food fortification because the cooking process destroys most of the thiamin hydrochloride. On the other hand, thiamin mononitrate, which is found primarily in plant leaves, is completely stable when exposed to heat and moisture. All thiamin-enriched products that must be cooked now contain thiamin as thiamin mononitrate. Breakfast cereals, however, still use thiamin hydrochloride because it is much cheaper than thiamin mononitrate. Other chemical forms of thiamin found in nature are thiamin diphosphate and triphosphate, found in animal tissues (mainly in the brain); thiamin disulphide, found in onions and garlic; O,S-dibenzoyl thiamin, and tetrahydrofurfuryldisulphide thiamin, found in broccoli.

The total metabolic pool of thiamin in the body is approximately 30 milligrams. This vitamin is mainly present in skeletal muscles (about 50% of the body's total thiamin), but it is also found in the heart, liver, kidneys, and brain. The predominant form of thiamin in the body is thiamin pyrophosphate. Other forms include thiamin triphosphate (about 10%), and thiamin monophosphate and free thiamin (about 10%). Approximately 80% of thiamin in blood is present in erythrocytes as thiamin pyrophosphate. Thiamin is absorbed from the lumen of the small intestine, mainly in the jejunum and ileum, by an active, carrier-mediated, rate-limited process that is energy-dependent as well as sodium-dependent. The enzymes involved require thiamin themselves for their own production. Interestingly, certain lipid-soluble thiamin derivatives, known as allithiamins (e.g., tetrahydrofurfuryldisulphide thiamin), do not appear to be subject to the rate-limiting transport mechanism [148].

In healthy subjects, the maximum amount of thiamin which can be absorbed from a single oral dose is ≈ 4.5 mg. Thus, a single oral dose of 30 mg or 100 mg of the vitamin will achieve the same figure [74]. A dose of 100 mg orally three times per day would allow ≈ 4.5mg x 3 = 13.5 mg to be absorbed daily [149]. This dose would be largely adequate for healthy subjects and, likely, in individuals with mild deficiency. In humans, the transport of thiamin across the blood-brain barrier, unlike the small intestine, occurs by both passive and active mechanisms [149]. This allows rapid correction of brain thiamin deficiency, mainly by passive diffusion, if a steep plasma-brain concentration gradient is established, as after intravenous or intramuscular administration of thiamin [149]. Thiamin and its metabolites are mainly excreted by the kidneys.

Prevention of Wernicke's encephalopathy is strictly dependent on adequate dietary thiamin supplementation. The recommended dose of thiamin for an average healthy adult is 1.4 mg per day, or 0.5 mg of thiamin per 1000 kcal consumed [33]. The vitamin may be assumed in one or two separate doses. In particular, Ziporin et al. [150] studied thiamin requirements in eight healthy adult individuals and found daily needs of 0.54 – 0.66 mg/1000 kcal. Samberlich et al. [146], evaluated thiamin requirements in adult humans, in terms of erythrocyte transketolase activity and urinary excretion of the vitamin. The results of the study established a defined relationship between the requirement and caloric intake and expenditure. When the calories utilized were derived mainly from carbohydrates, the minimum adult male requirement for thiamin appeared to be 0.30 mg per 1000 kcal. These results fit the recommended intake for the adult human of 0.40 mg of thiamin for 1000 kcal by Food and Agriculture Organization of the United Nations / World Health Organization of the United Nations (FAO / WHO), and the recommended allowance of 0.5 mg per 1000 kcal by the Food and Nutritional Board of the National Academy of Sciences-National Research Council of the United States (NAS / NRC) [146,151] (Table 5).

Table 5. NAS / NRC Recommended Dietary Intake of Thiamin

The Food and Nutrition Board of the Institute of Medicine of the National Academy of Sciences recommends the following dietary reference intakes (DRIs) for thiamin:	
Infants 0-6 months 7-12 months	**Adequate Intake (AI)** 0.2 mg/day　0.3 mg/kg 0.3 mg/day　0.3 mg/kg
Children 1-3 years 4-8 years	**Allowances (RDA)** 0.5 mg/day 0.6 mg/day
Boys 9-13 years 14-18 years	0.9 mg/day 1.2 mg/day
Girls 9-13 years 14-18 years	0.9 mg/day 1.0 mg/day
Men 19 years and older	1.2 mg/day
Women 19 years and older	1.1 mg/day
Pregnancy 14-50 years	1.4 mg/day
Lactation 14-50 years	1.4 mg/day

The U.S. RDA (Recommended Dietary Daily Allowance) for thiamin, which is used for determining per centage of daily values on nutritional supplement and food labels, is 1.5 milligrams.

These doses are likely higher in children, in critically ill conditions, during pregnancy and lactation [46,62], and in the other several clinical settings associated with Wernicke's encephalopathy previously discussed. For example, in chronic alcohol misusers, malnutrition and alcohol itself can reduce intestinal thiamin absorption by ≈ 70% [150]. Thus, three oral thiamin doses of 100 mg each would be reduced to one third of that in healthy subjects, that is≈5mg in 24h. This finding indicates that the prevention and therapy of Wernicke's encephalopathy in alcoholic subjects requires high blood thiamin concentrations which can only result from parenteral administration [149].

Since there is a scarcity of studies on thiamin requirements in these settings due to the difficulty performing studies in humans for ethical reasons, the precise amount of thiamin to be given in these cases (e.g., in alcoholics, in children, in cancer patients) remains an important unsettled issue [46]. To prevent Wernicke's encephalopathy in the clinical settings often associated with this encephalopathy, the following measures are mandatory: 1) educating individuals about proper dietary habits (natural sources of thiamin include whole-grain products, brown rice, meat products, especially pork liver, vegetables, fruits, legumes, and seafood), 2) supplementation of patients with thiamin by enteral or parenteral route when there is the doubt of a relative thiamin deficiency, especially if most of the calories are provided as carbohydrates, 3) treating, when possible, the underlying disorder.

DIAGNOSIS OF WERNICKE'S ENCEPHALOPATHY

Wernicke's encephalopathy is a relatively common, potentially fatal disease, greatly underdiagnosed in adults and in children [18,34,46]. In adults, autopsy studies have repeatedly revealed a higher incidence of Wernicke's encephalopathy-like lesions in general populations (0.8-2.8%) than is predicted by clinical studies (0.04-0.13%) [18,34]. Similar data have been reported in children [46]. In particular, in the adult studies, only 5-14% of patients with Wernicke's encephalopathy were diagnosed in life [18,34]. In children this figure is ≈ 58% [46]. The very high rate of incorrect diagnosis of Wernicke's encephalopathy, both in adults and children, may be due to either a relatively non-specific clinical presentation of the disease in some cases, or to not properly recognized clinical data and neurological signs.

Wernicke's encephalopathy remains a clinical diagnosis since there is no specific routine laboratory test available, and no specific diagnostic abnormalities have been revealed in cerebrospinal fluid, brain imaging, electroencephalogram (EEG), or evoked potentials [33,149]. In this regard, clinical suspicion is the best aid for a correct diagnosis. Accordingly, the clinician is obliged to consider Wernicke's encephalopathy in any patient with a clinical history revealing a possible poor nutritional state or a period of high metabolic demand, in the context of the clinical settings previously discussed, also when the patient presents only one component of the classical triad, paralysis of eye movements, staggering gait and mental status changes. The extent of thiamin deficiency in a patient with possible Wernicke's encephalopathy may be confirmed by the determination of blood thiamin levels or by checking the thiamin status, measuring the red blood cell transketolase activity [149]. These are useful tests to confirm the presumptive diagnosis of Wernicke's encephalopathy. However, these measurements are generally not routinely available and are limited by lack of specificity and technical difficulty [18,149].

Other paraclinical studies often performed in patients with Wernicke's encephalopathy include lumbar puncture, EEG, and neuroimaging studies. The cerebrospinal fluid examination is usually normal at an early stage of the disease, but may show a mildly elevated protein level in a late stage. The EEG is within normal limits at an early stage, but always shows diffuse, synchronous, bilateral slow waves consistent with a metabolic encephalopathy or with meningoencephalitis in a late stage (Figure 2). Among the neuroimaging studies, currently, magnetic resonance imaging (MRI) is considered the most valuable imaging technique to diagnose Wernicke's encephalopathy, since cranial computed tomography (CT) often fails to demonstrate density alterations and yields a definite diagnosis in only a few patients [29]. In particular, according to Antunez et al. [152], the sensitivity of CT to detect lesions characteristic of acute Wernicke's encephalopathy was low (13%), so it is not useful in the diagnosis of this disease, while MRI was useful in almost half of the patients (sensitivity 53% and specificity 93%). Typically in Wernicke's encephalopathy patients, MRI studies have demonstrated an increased T_2 signal, bilaterally symmetric, in the paraventricular regions of the thalamus, the hypothalamus, mammillary bodies, the periaqueductal region, the floor of the fourth ventricle, and midline cerebellum [26,27,32,153,154] (Figure 3). Disruption of the blood-brain barrier, indicated by contrast enhancement on T_1 weighted spino-echo sequences, after intravenous gadolinium administration, has been pointed out in the same regions in about half of the 12 patients studied [28]. Another study of 12 patients with Wernicke's encephalopathy showed that the MRI examinations revealed a typical pattern of lesions in only 58% of the cases [155]. Given the low sensitivity of MRI studies (53%) in the diagnosis of Wernicke's encephalopathy, it is obvious that normal MRI does not exclude the diagnosis, mainly in an early stage of the disease.

Promising, valuable adjunct for an early diagnosis of Wernicke's encephalopathy are the diffusion-weighted MRI and the proton MR spectroscopy [153,156,157]. These tools may also provide additional information on the pathophysiology of the disease both in acute and subacute/chronic phases. However, the signal characteristics and the site of the lesions documented on MRI are not specific for Wernicke's encephalopathy and may be due to a wide range of possible causes. Especially when the clinical history does not reveal a clinical setting not associated with a possible poor nutritional state or with a period of high metabolic demand, other conditions need to be differentiated. These include paramedian thalamic infarction due to occlusion of the posterior thalamoperforating arteries (top-of-the-basilar syndrome), cytomegalovirus ventriculoencephalitis, primary cerebral lymphoma, Behcet's disease, mitochondrial disorders such as Leigh's disease, variant Creutzefeldt-Jakob disease [pulvinar sign], paraneoplastic encephalitis, severe hypophosphatemia, and acute or chronic intoxication from methylbromide or bromvalerylurea [158-167] [Table 6]. However, it is important to emphasize that in most of these diseases [e.g., Behcet's disease, paraneoplastic encephalitis, primary cerebral lymphoma] the altered signal intensities on MRI have usually an asymmetrical distribution, while the brain lesions in Wernicke's encephalopathy are always symetrically distributed. Ultimately, a definite diagnosis of Wernicke's encephalopathy in a living patient is mainly supported by the dramatic response of neurological signs to the administration of thiamin; post-mortem, by autopsy study.

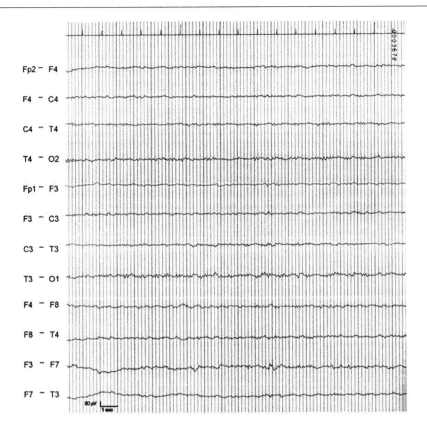

Figure 2. Patient with a late-stage Wernicke's encephalopathy, 16 days after the onset of diplopia and unsteadiness of the gait. The patient is now stuporous. EEG shows diffuse, bilateral, slow waves in the theta range.

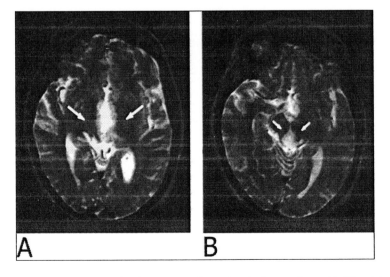

Figure 3. T2-W axial MR scans obtained at two contigous levels, in a patient with Wernicke's encephalopathy 16 days after onset of diplopia, and unsteadiness of gait. The patient is now stuporous. Symmetrical high intensity lesions in medial thalami (A), as well as in the periaqueductal gray matter of the midbrain (B), are evident.

Table 6. Differential Diagnosis of Wernicke's Encephalopathy at Brain MRI

1) Paramedian Thalamic Infarctions
2) Cytomegalovirus Ventriculoencephalitis
3) Primary Cerebral Limphoma
4) Behcet's Disease
5) Leigh's Disease
6) Variant Creutzfeldt-Jakob Disease
7) Paraneoplastic Encephalitis
8) Severe Hypophosphatemia
9) Acute Intoxication from Methyl Bromide
10) Chronic Intoxication from Bromvalerylurea

MANAGEMENT OF WERNICKE'S ENCEPHALOPATHY

Wernicke's encephalopathy is a medical emergency with a mortality rate estimated at 17 per cent [18]. In patients suspected of having Wernicke's encephalopathy, thiamin should be initiated immediately, either intravenously or intramuscularly, to ensure adequate absorption. Any therapeutic delay may result in permanent neurological damage and/or death. The thiamin hydrochloride solutions should be fresh, since old solutions that have been exposed to heat may be inactivated. At least 200 mg of parenteral thiamin per day, for at least five days, should be given. Since the intravenous administration of glucose can precipitate Wernicke's encephalopathy in thiamin-deficient patients, thiamin should always be given prior to any intravenous glucose administration to avoid this complication whenever the diagnosis is suspected.

Victor et al. [18], in a study on alcoholic patients, found that after thiamin administration, the recovery from the ophthalmoplegia was complete within hours after the administration, except for a residual, fine, horizontal nystagmus in 60% of the patients. Recovery from ataxia, usually occurred after a few days, although in some cases was incomplete. The mental signs tended to improve slowly, usually within 2 weeks of therapy. Deficiencies of other vitamins, especially niacin, and electrolytes, especially magnesium, should be corrected simultaneously. Because a higher enteral intake of thiamin is not toxic [168,169], in our opinion, oral thiamin supplementation should be continued for several months at a dose of 50 mg daily.

Considering that Wernicke's encephalopathy, in some cases, has a variable clinical and MRI presentation, it is a good clinical practice to treat with parenteral thiamin all patients presenting with coma, or a stuporous state, or hypothermia, or hyperthermia of unknown origin, or tachycardia and intractable hypotension of unknown cause, regardless of the symptoms, especially if a known clinical setting associated with Wernicke's encephalopathy has been pointed out [170]. In these cases a prompt therapy with thiamin is the safest approach to avoid neurological damage and may be a life-saving measure.

REFERENCES

[1]   The Columbia Electronic Encyclopedia, Sixth Edition Copyright 2003. Columbia University Press. www.cc.columbia.edu/cu/cup

[2]   Koletzko, B. Early nutrition and its later consequences: new opportunities. *Adv Exp Med Biol*, 2005 569, 1-12.

[3]   Flegal, KM; Graubard, BI; Williamson, DF; Gail MH. Excess deaths associated with underweight, overweight, and obesity. *Obstet Gynecol Surv*, 2005 60, 593-595.

[4]   Lamming, DW; Latorre-Esteves, M; Medvedik, O; Wong, SN; Tsang, FA; Wang, C; Lin, SJ; Sinclair, DA. HST2 mediates SIR2-independent life-span extension by calorie restriction. *Science*, 2005 309, 1861-1864.

[5]   Lutz, M. Diet as determinant of central nervous system development: role of essential fatty acids. *Arch Latinoam Nutr*, 1998 48, 29-34.

[6]   Sheth, RD; Stafstrom, CE; Hsu, D. Nonpharmacological treatment options for epilepsy. *Semin Pediatr Neurol*, 2005 12, 106-113.

[7]   Tarnopolsky, MA; Saris, W. Nutrition and neurological disorders: in the absence of cure, what can we offer? *Curr Opin Clin Nutr Metab Care*, 2002 5, 597-599.

[8]   Victor, M. The Wernicke-Korsakoff syndrome. *Handbook of Clinical Neurology*. PJ Vinken, GW Bruyn. Vol 28-Part II. Amsterdam: North-Holland Pushing Company; 1976; 243-270.

[9]   Wernicke, C. Die akute haemorrhagiscke poliencephalitis superior. In: Fisher Verlag, Kassel. *Lekrbuch der Gehirnkrankheiten, für Aertze und Studirende Vol II*. 1881, 229-242.

[10] Campbell, ACP; Russel, WR. Wernicke's encephalopathy. *Quart J Med*, 1941 10, 41.

[11] Mc Ilwain, HI; Bachelard, HS. *Biochemistry and the central nervous system*. 4th edn. Churchill-Livingstone. Edinburgh and London; 1971.

[12] Lockman, PR; McAfee, JH; Geldenhuys, WJ; Allen, DD. Cation transport specificity at the blood-brain barrier. *Neurochem Res*, 2000 29, 2245-2250.

[13] Neal, RA; Sauberlich, HE. Thiamin. In: Goodhart RS, Shils ME, editors. *Modern nutrition in health and disease. 6th ed.* Philadelphia: Lea & Febiger; 1980; 191-197.

[14] Iwata, H. Possible role of thiamine in the nervous system. *TIPS*, 1982 4, 171-173.

[15] Mc Candless, DW; Schenicer, S; Cook, M. Encephalopathy of thiamine deficiency: studies of intracerebral mechanisms. *J Clin Invest*, 1968 47, 2268-2280.

[16] Hakim, AH; Pappius, HM. Sequence of metabolic, clinical, and histological events in experimental thiamine deficiency. *Ann Neurol*, 1983 13, 365-375.

[17] Schenker, S; Henderson, GI; Hoyumpa, AM jr; Mc Candless, DW. Hepatic and Wernicke's encephalopathy: current concepts of pathogenesis. *Am J Clin Nutr*, 1980 22, 2719-2726.

[18] Victor, M; Adams, RD; Collins, GH. The Wernicke-Korsakoff syndrome. A clinical and pathological study of 245 patients, 82 with post-mortem examinations. *Contemp Neurol Ser*, 1971 7, 1-206.

[19] Butterworth RF. Cerebral thiamine dependent enzyme changes in experimental Wernicke's encephalopathy. *Metab Brain Dis*, 1986 1, 165-175.

[20] Hazell, AS; Pannunzio, P; Raok, VR; Pow, DV; Rambaldi, A. Thiamine deficiency results in downregulation of the GLAST glutamate transporter in cultured astrocytes. *Glia,* 2003 43, 175-184.

[21] Hazell, AS; Todd, KG; Butterworth, RF. Mechanisms of neuronal cell death in Wernicke's encephalopathy. *Metab Brain Dis*, 1998 13, 97-122.

[22] Matsushima, K; MacManus, JP; Hakim, AM. Apoptosi is restricted to the thalamus in thiamine-deficient rats. *Neuroreport,*1997 8, 867-870.

[23] Navarro, D; Zwinghann, C; Hazell, AS; Butterworth, RF. Brain lactate synthesis in thiamine deficiency: a re-evaluation using ^{1}H-^{13}C nuclear magnetic spectroscopy. *J Neurosci Res*, 2005 79, 33-41.

[24] Desjardins, P; Butterworth, RF. Role of mitochondrial dysfunction and oxidative stress in the pathogenesis of selective neuronal loss in Wernicke's encephalopathy. *Mol Neurobiol*, 2005 31, 17-25.

[25] Chan, F; Butterworth, RF; Hazell, AS. Primary cultures of rat astrocytes respond to thiamine deficiency-induced swelling by downregulating aquaparin-4 levels. *Neurosci Lett*, 2004 366, 231-234.

[26] Gallucci, M; Bozzao, A; Splendihni, A; Masciocchi, C; Passariello, R. Wernicke's encephalopathy: MR findings in five patients. *AJNR Am J Neuroradiol*, 1990 11, 887-892.

[27] Victor, M. MR in the diagnosis of Wernicke-Korsakoff syndrome. *AJR Am Roentgenol*, 1990 155, 1415-1416.

[28] Mascalchi, M; Simonelli, P; Tessa, C; Giancaspero, F; Petruzzi, P; Bosincu, L; Conti, M; Sechi, GP; Salvi, F. Do acute lesions of Wernicke's encephalopathy show contrast enhancement? Report of three cases and review of literature. *Neuroradiology*, 1999 41, 249-254.

[29] Unlu, E; Cakir, B; Astl, T. MRI findings of Wernicke's encephalopathy revisited due to hunger stroke. *Eur J Radiol*, 2005 (In Press).

[30] Bergui, M; Bradac, GB; Zhong, JJ; Barbero, PA; Durelli, L. Diffusion-weighted MR in reversible Wernicke encephalopathy. *Neuroradiology*, 2001 43, 969-972.

[31] Niclot, P; Gutchard, JP; Djomby, R; Sellier, P; Bousser, MG; Chabriat, H. Transient decrease of water diffusion in Wernicke's encephalopathy. *Neuroradiology*, 2002 44, 305-307.

[32] Chu, K; Kang, DW; Kim, HJ; Lee, YS; Park, SH. Diffusion-weighted imaging abnormalities in Wernicke's encephalopathy: reversible cytotoxic edema? *Arch Neurol*, 2002 59, 123-127.

[33] Reuler, JB; Girard, DE; Cooney, TG. Wernicke's encephalopathy. *N Engl J Med*, 1985 312, 1035-1039.

[34] Harper, C. Wernicke's encephalopathy: a more common disease than realised; a neuropathological study of 51 cases. *J Neurol Neurosurg Psychiatry*, 1979 42, 226-231.

[35] Torvik, A; Linboe, CF; Rodge, S. Brain lesions in alcoholics: a neuropathological study with clinical correlations. *J Neurol Sci*, 1982 56, 233-248.

[36] Vortmeyer, AO; Hagel, C; Laas, R. Haemorragic thiamine deficient encephalopathy following prolonged parenteral nutrition. *J Neurol Neurosurg Psychiatry*, 1992 55, 826-829.

[37] Torvik, A. Two types of brain lesions in Wernicke's encephalopathy. *Neuropath Appl Neurobiol*, 1985 11, 179-190.

[38] Hazell, A; Wang, G. Downregulation of complexin I and complexin II in the medial thalamus is blocked by N-acetylcisteine in experimental Wernicke's encephalopathy. *J Neurosci Res*, 2005 79, 200-207.

[39] Krill, JJ. Neuropathology of thiamine deficiency disorders. *Metab Brain Dis*, 1996 11, 9-17.

[40] Harper, CG; Giles, M; Finlay-Jones, R. Clinical signs in the Wernicke-Korsakoff complex: a retrospective analysis of 131 cases diagnosed at necropsy. *J Neurol Neurosurg Psychiatry*,1986 49, 341-345.

[41] Kulkarni, S; Lee, AG; Holstein, SA; Warner, JEA. You are what you eat. *Surv Ophthalmol*,2005 50, 389-393.

[42] Mumford, CJ. Papilloedema delaying diagnosis of Wernicke's encephalopathy in a comatose patient. *Postgrad Med J*, 1989 65, 371-373.

[43] Ghez, C. Vestibular paresis: a clinical feature of Wernicke's disease. *J Neurol Neurosurg Psychiatry*, 1969 32, 134-139.

[44] Wallis, WE; Willoughby, E; Baker, P. Coma in Wernicke-Korsakoff syndrome, *Lancet*, 1978 2, 400-401.

[45] Sechi, GP; Bosincu, L; Cossu Rocca, P; Deiana, GA; Correddu, P; Murrighile, RM. Hyperthermia, choreic dyskinesias and increased motor tone in Wernicke's encephalopathy. *Eur J Neurology*, 1996 3 suppl 5, 133.

[46] Vasconcelos, MM; Silva, KP; Vidal, G; Silva, AF; Domingues, RC; Berditchevsky CR. Early diagnosis of pediatric Wernicke's encephalopathy. *Pediatr Neurol*, 1999 20, 289-294.

[47] Witt, ED; Goldman-Rakic; PS. Intermittent thiamine deficiency in rhesus monkey. Progression of neurological signs and neuroanatomical lesions. *Ann Neurol*, 1983 13, 376-395.

[48] Fattal-Valevski, A; Kesler, A; Sela, B-A; Nitzan-Keloski, D; Rotsein, M; Mesterman, R; Toledano-Alhadef, H; Stolovitch, C; Hoffman, C; Globus, O; Eshel G. Outbreak of life-threatening thiamine deficiency in infants in Israel caused by a defective soy-based formula, *Pediatrics*, 2005 115, 233-238.

[49] Shaw, S; Gorkin, BD; Lieber, CS. Effects of chronic alcohol feeding on thiamine status: biochemical and neurological correlates. *Am J Clin Nutr*, 1981 34, 856-860.

[50] Thier, P. Acute and chronic alcohol related disorders. In: *Neurological Disorders. Course and Treatment.* Brandt T, Caplan LR, Dichgans J, Diever HC, Kennard C, editors. London: Academic Press; 1998; 677-693.

[51] Thompson, AD; Ryle, PR; Shaw, GK. Ethanol, thiamine, and brain damage. *Alcohol Alcohol*, 1983 18, 27-43.

[52] Tomasulo, PA; Kater, RMH, Iber, FL. Impairment of thiamine absorption in alcoholism. *Am J Clin Nutr*, 1968 21, 1341-1344.

[53] Camilo, ME; Morgan, MY; Sherlock, S. Erytrocyte transketolase activity in alcoholic liver disease. *Scand J Gastroenterol*, 1981 16, 273-279.

[54] Blass, JP; Gibson, GE. Abnormality of thiamine requiring enzyme in patients with Wernicke-Korsakoff Syndrome. *N Engl J Med*, 1977 297, 1367-1370.

[55] Mc Cool, BA; Plonk, Sg; Martin, PR; Singleton, CK. Cloning of human transketolase cDNAs and comparison of the nucleotide sequence of the coding region in Wernicke-Korsakoff and non- Wernicke-Korsakoff individuals. *J Biol Chem*, 1993 268, 1397-1404.

[56] Flink, EB. Magnesium deficiency in alcoholism, *Alcoholism: Clinical and Experimental Research*, 1986 10, 590-594.

[57] Shils, ME. Magnesium. In: *Present knowledge in nutrition*. Ziegler EE, Filer LJ, editors. Washington, DC: ILSI Press; 1996; 334-343.

[58] Traviesa, DC. Magnesium deficiency: a possible cause of thiamine refractoriness in Wernicke-Korsakoff encephalopathy. *J Neurol Neurosurg Psychiatry*, 1974 37, 959-962.

[59] Centerwall, BS; Criqui, MH. Prevention of the Wernicke-Korsakoff syndrome: a cost-benefit analysis. *N Engl J Med*, 1978 299, 285-289.

[60] Rolland, S; Truswell, AS. Wernicke-Korsakoff syndrome in Sydney hospitals after 6 years of thiamine enrichment of bread. *Public Health Nutr*, 1998 1, 117-122.

[61] Harper, GC; Sheedy, DL; Lama, AI; Garrick, TM; Hilton, JM, Raisanen; J. Prevalence of Wernicke-Korsakoff syndrome in Australia: has thiamine fortification made a difference? *Med J Aust*, 1998 168, 542-545.

[62] McGready, R; Simpson, JA; Cho, T; Dubowitz, L; Changbumrung, S; Bohm, V; Munger, RG; Sauberlich, HE; White, NJ; Nosten, F. Postpartum thiamine deficiency in a Karen displaced population. *Am J Clin Nutr*, 2001 74, 808-813.

[63] Luxemburger, L; White, NJ; Kuile, F; Singh, HM; Allier-Frachon, I; Ohn, M; Chongsuphajaisiddhi, T; Nosten, F. Beri-beri: the major cause of infant mortality in Karen refugees. *Trans R Soc Trop Med Hyg*, 2003 97, 251-255.

[64] Butterworth, F. Maternal thiamine deficiency: still a problem in some world countries. *Am J Clin Nutr*, 2001 24, 712-713.

[65] Haid, RW; Gutmann, L; Crosby, TW. Wernicke-Korsakoff encephalopathy after gastric plication. *JAMA*, 1982 247, 2566-2567.

[66] Chaves, LC; Faintuch, J; Kahwage, S; Alencar Fde, A. A cluster of polyneuropathy and Wernicke-Korsakoff syndrome in a bariatric unit. *Obes Surg*, 2002 12, 328-334.

[67] Bell, D; Robertson, CE; Muir, AL. Carbonated drinks, thiamine deficiency and right ventricular failure. *Scott Med J*, 1987 32, 137-138.

[68] Shuster, MH; Vazquez, JA. Nutritional concerns related to ranx-en-Y gastric bypass: what every clinician needs to know. *CCNUU*, 2005 28, 227-260.

[69] Shikata, E; Mizutani, T; Kokubun, Y; Takasu, T. "Iatrogenic" Wernicke's encephalopathy in Japan. *Eur Neurol*, 2000 44, 156-161.

[70] Shimoura, T; Mori, E; Hirono, N; Imamura, T; Yamashita, H. Development of Wernicke-Korsakoff syndrome after long-intervals following gastrectomy. *Arch Neurol*, 1998 55, 1242-1245.

[71] Thomson, AD. Mechanisms of vitamin deficiency in chronic alcohol misusers and the development of Wernicke-Korsakoff syndrome. *Alcohol and Alcoholism*, 2000 35 Suppl 1, 2-7.

[72] Yoshioka, H; Nishino, H; Usui, T; Sung, M; Ohshio, G; Sugiyama, T; Kita, T. Immunohistochemical demonstration of a new thiamine diphosphate-binding protein in the rat digestive tract. *Hystochemistry*, 1992 97, 121-124.

[73] Epstein, RS. Wernicke's encephalopathy following lithium-induced diarrhea. *Am J Psychiatry*, 1989 146, 806-807.

[74] Sakuma, A; Kato, I; Ogino, S; Okada, T; Takeyama, I. Primary position upbeat nystagmus with special reference to alteration to downbeat nystagmus. *Acta Otolaryngol*, 1996 Suppl 522, 43-46.

[75] Bataller, R; Salmeron, JM; Munoz, JE; Obach, V; Elizalde, JI; Mas, A; Tolosa, E; Teres, J. Pyloric stenosis complicated by Wernicke-Korsakoff syndrome. *Gastroenterol Hepatol*, 1997 20, 131-133.

[76] Larnaout, A; El-Euch, G; Kchir, N; Filali, A; Ben Amida, M; Hentati, F. Wernicke's encephalopathy in a patient with Chron's disease. A pahological study. *J Neurol*, 2001 248, 57-60.

[77] Eggspuhler, AW; Bauerfeind, P; Dorn, T; Siegel, AM. Wernicke's encephalopathy- a severe neurological complication in a clinically inactive disease. *Eur Neurol*, 2003 50, 184-185.

[78] Michowitz, Y; Copel, L; Shiloach, E; Litovchik, I; Rapaport, MJ. Non-alcoholic Wernicke's encephalopathy-unusual cliical findings. *Eur J Intern Med*, 2005 16, 443-444.

[79] Merkin-Zaborsky, H; Ifergane, G ; Frisher, S; Valdman, S; Herishanu, Y; Wirguin, I. Thiamine-responsive acute neurological disorders in nonalcoholic patients. *Eur Neurol*, 2001 45, 34-37.

[80] Hander, CE; Perkins, GD. Anorexia nervosa and Wernicke's encephalopathy: an underdiagnosed association. *Lancet*, 1982 2, 771-772.

[81] Wislet, MC; Donovon, IA; Aitchison, F. Wernicke's encephalopathy in association with complicated acute pancreatitis and morbid obesity. *Br J Clin Pract*, 1990 44, 771-773.

[82] Chen, L; Zhang, X. Pancreatic encephalopathy and Wernicke's encephalopathy. *Zhonghua Neike Za Zhi*, 2002 41, 94-97.

[83] Nightingale, S; Bates, D; Heath, PD; Barron, SL. Wernicke's encephalopathy in hyperemesis gravidarum. *Postgrad Med J*, 1982 58, 558-559.

[84] Lavin, PJM; Smith, D; Kori, SH; Ellemberger, C Jr. Wernicke's encephalopathy: a predictable complication of hyperemesis gravidarum. *Obstet Gynecol*, 1983 62 Suppl 3, 13-15.

[85] Chung, TI; Kim, JS; Park, SK; Kim, BS; Ahn, KJ; Yang, DW. Diffusion weighted MR imaging of acute Wernicke's encephalopathy. *Eur J Radiol*, 2003 45, 256-258.

[86] Wood, P; Murray, A; Sinha, B; Godley, M; Goldsmith, HJ. Wernicke's encephalopathy induced by hyperemesis gravidarum: case reports. *Br J Obstet Gynecol*, 1983 90, 583-586.

[87] Heller, S; Salked, RM; Korner, WE. Vitamin B1 status in pregnancy. *Am J Clin Nutr*, 1974 27, 1221-1224.

[88] Baker, H; Hocketein, S; De Angelis, B; Holland, BK. Thiamin status of gravidas treated for gestational diabetes mellitus compared to their neonates at parturition. *Int J Vit Nutr Res*, 2000 70, 317-320.

[89] Nelson-Piercy, C. Treatment of nausea and vomiting in pregnancy. When should it be treated and what can be safely taken? *Drug Saf,* 1998 19, 155-164.

[90] Indraccolo, U; Gentile, G; Pomili, G; Luzi, G; Villani, C. Thiamine deficiency and beriberi features in a patient with hyperemesis gravidarum. *Nutrition,* 2005 21, 967-968.

[91] Van Zaanen, HC; Van Der Lelie, J. Thiamine deficiency in hematological malignant tumors. *Cancer*, 1992 69, 1710-1713.

[92] Turner, JE; Alley, JG; Sharpless, NE. Wernicke's encephalopathy: an unusual acute neurological complication of linphoma and its therapy. *J Clin Oncology*, 2004 22, 4020-4022.

[93] Onishi, H; Kawanishi, C; Onose, M; Yamada, T; Saito, H; Yoshida, A; Noda, K. Succesful treatment of Wernicke's encephalopathy in terminally ill cancer patients: report of 3 cases and review of the literature. *Support Care Cancer*, 2004 12, 604-608.

[94] Bleggi-Torres, LF; De Medeiros, BC; Ogasawara, VS; Loddo, G; Zanis Neto, J; Pasquini, R; De Medeiros, CR. Iatrogenic Wernicke's encephalopathy in allogenic bone transplantation: a study of eight cases. *Bone Marrow Transplant*, 1997 20, 391-395.

[95] Kondo, K; Fujiwara, M; Murase, M; Kodera, Y; Akiyama, S; Ito, K; Takagi, H. Severe acute metabolic acidosis and Wernicke's encephalopathy following chemotherapy with 5-fluorouracil and cisplatin: case report and review of the literature. *Jpn J Clin Oncol*, 1996 26, 234-236.

[96] Vanhulle, C; Dacher, JN; Delangre, T; Garraud, V; Vannier, JP; Tron, P. Chimiotherapie anticancereuse at encephalopathie de Gayet-wernicke. *Arch Pediatr*, 1997 4, 243-246.

[97] Van Belle, SJ; Distelmans, W; Vandebroeck, J; Bruynscel, J; Van Ginckel, R; Storme, GA. Phase I trial of erbulozole (R55104). *Anticancer Res*, 1993 13, 2389-2391.

[98] Kwee, IL; Nakada, T. Wernicke's encephalopathy induced by talozamole. *N Engl J Med*, 1983 309, 599-600.

[99] Shorey, J; Bhardway, N; Loscalzo, J. Acute Wernicke's encephalopathy after intravenous infusion of high-dose nitroglycerin [Abstract]. *Ann Intern Med*, 1984 101, 500.

[100] De Klippel, N; De Keyser, J; De Greve, J; Van Belle, S. A Wernicke's encephalopathy-like neurotoxicity induced by erbulozole. *Neurology*, 1991 41, 762-763.

[101] Buesa, JM; Garcia-Tejdo, P; Losa, R; Fra, J. Treatment of ifosfamide encephalopathy with intravenous thiamin. *Clin Cancer Res*, 2003 9, 4636-4637.

[102] Brouns, R; De Deyn, PP. Neurological complications in renal failure: a review. *Clin Neurol Neurosurg*, 2004 107, 1-16.

[103] Butterworth, RF; Gaudreau, F; Vincelette, J; Bourgault, AM; Lamothe, F; Nutini, AM. Thiamine deficiency and Wernicke's encephalopathy in AIDS. *Metab Brain Dis*, 1991 6, 207-212.

[104] Ohmori, N; Tushima, T; Sekine, Y; Sato, K; Shibagaki, Y; Ijuchi, S; Akano, K. Gestational thyrotoxicosis with acute Wernicke's encephalopathy: a case report. *Endocr J*, 1999 46, 787-793.

[105] Mc Lean, J; Manchip, S. Wernicke's encephalopathy induced by magnesium depletion. *Lancet*, 1999 353, 1768.

[106] Hung, SC; Hung, SH; Tarng, DC; Yang, WC; Chen, TW; Huang, TP. Thiamine deficiency and unexplained encephalopathy in hemodialysis and peritoneal dialysis patients. *Am J Kidney Dis*, 2001 38, 941-947.

[107] Ihara, M; Ito, T; Yanagihara, C; Nishimura, Y. Wernicke's encephalopathy associated with hemodialysis: report of two cases and review of the literature. *Clin Neurol Neurosurg*, 1999 101, 118-121.

[108] Ookawara, S; Suzuki, M; Saitou, M. Acute encephalopathy due to thiamine deficiency with hyperamoniemia in a chronic hemodialysis patient: a case report. *Nippon Jinzo Gakkai Shi*, 2003 45, 393-397.

[109] Jagadha, V; Deck, JH; Halliday, WC; Smyth, HS. Wernicke's encephalopathy in patients on peritoneal dialysis or hemodialysis. *Ann Neurol*, 1987 21, 78-84.

[110] Davtyan, DG; Vinters, HV. Wernicke's encephalopathy in AIDS patient treated with zidovudine. *Lancet*, 1987 1, 919-920.

[111] Schwenk, J; Gosztonyi, G; Thierauf, P; Iglesias, J; Langer, E. Wernicke's encephalopathy in two patients with acquired immunodeficiency syndrome. *J Neurol*, 1990 237, 445-447.

[112] Alcaide, ML; Jayaweera, D; Espinoza, L; Kolber, M. Wernicke's encephalopathy in AIDS: a preventable case of fatal neurological deficit. *Int J STD AIDS*, 2003 14, 712-713.

[113] Lindboe, CF; Løberg, EM. Wernicke's encephalopathy in non-alcoholics. An autopsy study . *J Neurol Sci*, 1989 90, 125-129.

[114] Enoch, BA; Williams, DM. An association between Wernicke's encephalopathy and thyrotoxicosis. *Postgrad Med J*, 1968 4, 923-924.

[115] Lim, P; Jacob, E. Magnesium deficiency in patients on long-term diuretic therapy for heart failure. *BMJ*, 1972 3, 620.

[116] Ryan, MP. Magnesium and potassium-sparing effects of amiloride. Review and recent findings. *Magnesium*, 1984 3, 274-88.

[117] Durlach, J. *Magnesium in clinical practice*. London: John Libbey and Co Ltd; 1998.

[118] Brady, JA; Roch, CL; Horneffer, MR. Thiamine status, diuretic medications and the management of congestive heart failure. *J Am Diet Assoc*, 1995 95, 541-544.

[119] Zieve, I. Influence of magnesium deficiency on the utilization of thiamine. *Ann NY Acad Sci*, 1969 162, 732-743.

[120] Dyckner, T; Ek, B; Nybrin, H; Wester, Po. Aggravation of thiamine deficiency by magnesium depletion. *Acta Med Scand*, 1985 218, 129-131.

[121] Pelton, R; La Valle, JB; Hawkins, E; Krinsky, DL, eds. *Drugs-induced nutrient depletion handbook*. Hudson, Oil: Lexi-Comp; :1999; 258.

[122] Tanphaichtr, V. Thiamin. In: Skill ME, Olson JA, Shike M. *Modern nutrition in health and disease*. Philadelphia: Lea & Febiger; 1994; 359-364.

[123] Roman, GC. On politics and health: an epidemic of neurologic disease in Cuba. *Ann Intern Med*, 1995 122, 530-533.

[124] Nadel, M; Burger, PC. Wernicke's encephalopathy following prolonged intravenosu therapy. *JAMA*, 1976 235, 2403-2405.

[125] Hahn, JS; Berquist, W; Allorn, DM; Chamberlain, L; Bass, D. Wernicke's encephalopathy and beriberi during total parenteral nutrition attributable to multivitamin infusion shortage. *Pediatrics*, 1998 101, 10-14.

[126] D'Aprile, P; Tarantino, A; Santoro, N; Garella, A. Wernicke's encephalopathy induced by total parenteral nutrition in patient with acute leukaemia: unusual involvment of caudate nuclei and cerebral cortex on MRI. *Neuroradiology*, 2000 42, 781-783.

[127] Kuhn, J; Friedel, V; Knitelius, HO; Bewermeyer, H. Iatrogenic Wernicke-Korsakoff syndrome with unusual neurological deficits and MRI lesions. *Nervenarzt*, 2004 74, 795-780.

[128] Shiozawa, T; Shiota, H; Shikata, E; Kamei, S; Mizutani, T. Development of Wernicke's encephalopathy during the period of oral food intake after a subtotal colectomy for ulcerative colitis. *Rimsho Shinkeigaku*, 1995 35, 169-174.

[129] Drenik, EJ; Joven, CB; Swendseid, ME. Occurrence of Wernicke's encephalopathy during prolonged starvation for the treatment of obesity. *N Engl J Med*, 1966 274, 937-939.

[130] Doraiswamy, PM; Massey, EW; Enright, K; Palese, VJ; Lamonica, D; Boyko, O. Wernicke-Korsakoff syndrome caused by psychogenic food refusal: MR findings. *AJNR Am J Neuroradiol*, 1994 15, 594-596.

[131] Sharma, S; Sumich, PM; Francis, IC; Kiernan, MC; Spira, PJ. Wernicke's encephalopathy presenting with upbeating nystagmus. *J Clin Neurosci*, 2002 9, 476-478.

[132] Devathasan, G; Koh, C. Wernicke's encephalopathy in prolonged fasting. *Lancet*, 1982 2, 1108-1109.

[133] Prensky, AL. Wernicke's encephalopathy in infants. *J Neuro-Ophthalmol*, 2005 25, 167-168.

[134] Seear, MD; Norman, MG. Two cases of Wernicke's encephalopathy in children: an underdiagnosed complication of poor nutrition. *Ann Neurol*, 1988 24, 85-87.

[135] Sechi, GP; Serra, A; Pirastru, MI; Sotgiu, S; Rosati, G. Wernicke's encephalopathy in a woman on slimming diet. *Neurology*, 2002 58, 1697-1698.

[136] Arockie, D; Don, M; Romanoswki, CAJ. Wernicke's encephalopathy: unusual findings in nonalcoholic patients. *J Comput Assist Tomogr*, 2003 27, 235-240.

[137] Vimokesant, SL; Hilker, DM; Nakornchai, S; Rungruangsak, K; Dhanamitta, S. Effects of betel nut and fermented fish on thiamine status of northeastern thais. *Am J Clin Nutr*, 1975 28, 1458-1463.

[138] Kesler, A; Stolovitch, C; Hoffmann, C; Avni, I; Morad, Y. Acute ophthalmoplegia and nystagmus in infants fed a thiamine-deficient formula: an epidemic of Wernicke's encephalopathy. *J Neuro-Ophthalmol*, 2005 25, 169-172.

[139] Davis, RA; Wolf, A. Infantile beriberi associated with Wernicke's encephalopathy. *Pediatrics*, 1958 21, 409-410.

[140] Cochrane, WA; Collins-Williams, C; Donohue, WL. Superior hemorrhagic poliencephalitis (Wernicke's disease) occurring in an infant-probably due to thiamine deficiency from use of a soya bean product. *Pediatrics*, 1961 11, 771-777.

[141] Bowman, BB; Ngoyen, P. Stability of thiamine in parenteral nutrition solutions. *J Pen J Parenteral Enteral Nutr*, 1983 7, 567-568.

[142] Londsdale, D. *The nutritionist's giude to the clinical use of vitamin B1*. Tacoma, Wa: Life Sciences Press, 44-77.

[143] Londsdale, D; Schamberger, RJ. Red cell transketolase as indicator of nutritional deficiency. *Am J Clin Nutr*, 1980 33, 205-211.

[144] Singh, M; Thompson, M; Sullivan, N; Child, G. Thiamine deficiency in dogs due to feeding of sulphite preserved meat. *Aust Vet J*, 2005 83, 412-417.

[145] Miles, J; Petrie, C; Steel, M. Slimming on the internet. *J R Soc Med*, 2000 93, 254-257.

[146] Sauberlich, He; Herman YF; Stevens CO; Herman RM. Thiamine requirement of the adult human. *Am J Clin Nutr*, 1979 32, 2237-2248.

[147] Naing, KM; Uo, TT; Thein, K. Antithiamin activity in Burnase fish. *Union of Burma J Life Sci*, 1969 2, 63-66.

[148] Tanphaichitr, V. Thiamin. In: Shils ME. Olson JA, Shike M, Ross AC, eds. *Modern Nutrition in Health and Disease. 9th ed.* Baltimore, MD: Williams and Wilkins; 1999; 381-389.

[149] Thomson, AD; Cook, CCH; Touquet, R; Henry, JA. The royal college of physicians report on alcohol: guidelines for managing Wernicke's encephalopathy in the accident and emergency department. *Alcohol & Alcoholism*, 2002 37, 513-521.

[150] Ziporin, ZZ; Nuntes, WT; Powell, RC; Waring, PP; Sauberlich, CR. Thiamine requirement in the adult human as measured by urinary excretion of thiamine metabolites. *J Nutr*, 1965 85, 297-304.

[151] Dietary Reference Intakes For Thiamin, Riboflavin , Niacin, Vitamin B6, Folate, Vitamin B12, *Pantotenic Acid, Biotin and Choline*. Washington, DC: National Academic Press; 1998.

[152] Antunez, E; Estruch, R; Cardenal, C; Nicolas, JM; Fernandez-Sola, J; Urbano-Marquez, A. Usefulness of CT and MR imaging in the diagnosis of acute Wernicke's encephalopathy. *AJR Am J Roentgenol*, 1998 171, 1131-1137.

[153] Doherty, MJ; Watson, F; Uchino, K; Hallam, DK; Cramer, SC. Diffusion abnormalities in patients with Wernicke's encephalopathy. *Neurology*, 2002 58, 655-657.

[154] Chung, TI; Kim, JS; Park, SK; Kim, BS; Ahn, KJ; Yang, DW. Diffusion weighted MR imaging of acute Wernicke's encephalopathy. *Eur J Radiol*, 2003 45, 256-258.

[155] Weidauer, S; Nichtweiss, M; Lanfermann, H; Zanella, FE. Wernicke's encephalopathy: MR findings and clinical presentation. *Eur Radiol*, 2003 13, 1001-1009.

[156] Mascalchi, M; Belli G; Guerrini, L; Nistri, M; Del Seppia, I; Villari, N. Proton MR spectroscopy of Wernicke's encephalopathy. *AJNR Am J Neuroradiol*, 2002 23, 1803-1806.

[157] Rugilo, CA; Uribe Rocca, MC; Zurru, MC; Capizzano, AA; Pontello, GA; Gatto, EM. Proton MR spectroscopy in Wernicke's encephalopathy. *AJNR Am J Neuroradiol*, 2003 24, 952-955.

[158] Bogousslavsky, J; Regli, F; Uske, A. Thalamic infarcts: clinical syndromes, etiology and prognosis. *Neurology*, 1988 38, 837-848.

[159] Torgovnik, J; Arsura, EL; Lala, D. Cytomegalovirus ventriculoencephalitis presenting as Wernicke's encephalopathy. *Neurology*, 2000 55, 1910-1913.

[160] Brechtelsbauer, DL; Urbach, H; Sommer, T; Blumcke, I; Woitas, R; Solymosi, L. Cytomegalovirus encephalitis and primary cerebral limphoma mimicking Wernicke's encephalopathy. *Neuroradiology*. 1997 39, 19-22.

[161] Bae, SJ; Lee, HK; Lee, JH; Choi, CG; Suh, DC. Wernicke's encephalopathy: atypical manifestations at MR imaging. *AJNR Am J Neuroradiol*, 2001 22, 1480-1482.

[162] Harper, C; Butterworth, RF. Nutritional and metabolic disorders. In: Graham DI, Lantos PL. *Greenfield's Neuropathology Vol I*, 6th edn. London: Arnold, 1997; 601-652.

[163] Zeidler, M; Sellar, RJ; Collie, DA; Knight, R; Stewart, G; Hacleod, MA; Ironside, JW; Cousens, S; Coichester, AC; Hadley, DM; Will, RG; Colchester, AF. The pulvinar sign and magnetic resonance imaging in variant Creutzfeldt-Jakob disease. *Lancet*, 2000 355, 1412-1418.

[164] Dalmau, J; Graus, F; Vilarejo, A; Posner, JB; Blumenthal. D; Thiesse, B; Saiz, A; Meneses, P; Rosenfeld, MR. Clinical analysis of anti-Ma2-associated encephalitis. *Brain*, 2004 127, 1831-1844.

[165] Zurkirchen, MA; Mistel, M; Conten, D. Reversable neurological complications in chronic alcohol abuse with hypophosphatemia. *Schweiz Med Wochenschr*, 1994 124, 1807-1812.

[166] Squier, MV; Thompson, J; Rajgopalan, B. Case report: neuropathology of methyl bromite intoxication. *Neuropathol Appl Neurobiol*, 1992 6, 579-584.

[167] Fukazawa, T; Sasaki, H; Ito-Owada, Y; Hamada, T; Tashiro, K. A case of chronic bromvalerylurea intoxication with episodic neurological manifestations such as optic neuropathy, ophthalmoplegia and ataxia. *Rinsho Shinkeigaku*. 1996 6, 790-792.

[168] Seear, M; Lockitch, G; Jacobson, B; Quigley, G; MacNab, A. Thiamine, riboflavin, and pyridoxine deficiencies in a population of critically children. *J Pediatr*, 1992 121, 533-538.

[169] Hope, LC, Cook, C CH; Thomson, AD. A survey of the current clinical practice in the UK concerning vitamin supplementation for chronic alcohol misusers. *Alcohol & Alcoholism*, 1999 34, 862-867.

[170] Sechi, GP, Serra A. Wernicke's encephalopathy: new clinical settings and recent advances in diagnosis and management. *Lancet Neurol*, 2007 6, (in press).

In: Nutrition Research Advances
Editor: Sarah V. Watkins, pp. 81-101

ISBN 1-60021-516-5
© 2007 Nova Science Publishers, Inc.

Chapter III

MALNUTRITION, BRAIN DYSFUNCTION AND ANTISOCIAL CRIMINAL BEHAVIOR

Jianghong Liu[1], Adrian Raine[2], Peter Venables[1,3] and Sarnoff A. Mednick[1]

[1]Social Science Research Institute, University of Southern California, Los Angeles, CA 90089-0375, USA;
[2]Department of Psychology, University of Southern California, Los Angeles, CA 90089-1061, USA;
[3]Department of Psychology, University of York, Heslington, York, England.

INTRODUCTION

For decades, research intended to reduce the incidence of criminal violence has been largely unsuccessful. Such efforts include psychoanalytic approaches, behavior modification techniques, and experimental drug therapies. One of the possible reasons for the failure is that designs do not consider biological factors such as malnutrition in the development of antisocial, violent and criminal behavior (Raine, 2002a). Although the role of malnutrition in the development of antisocial behavior has gained some attention, research has still placed little weight on this topic (Fishbein, 2001, Rutter et al, 1998). This is despite decades of the dictum "you are what you eat" which emphasized the importance of nutritional factors impacting on human being behavior. The purpose of this chapter is to provide an overview of malnutrition as a risk factor for antisocial behavior, and to identify possible brain mechanisms which may account for the malnutrition – antisocial behavior link. To better illustrate the interplay among risk factors, mechanisms and behavioral outcome, a hypothetical malnutrition–psychopathology model will be outlined to provide a conceptual framework. Using this framework, we will first review empirical research on nutrition and antisocial behavior. Three key areas of brain dysfunction due to malnutrition will then be explored. Following this, our recent findings from Mauritius on malnutrition and externalizing behavior will be briefly presented. Finally, the current limitations of nutritional research on antisocial behavior and future research direction are outlined.

OVERVIEW OF THE MODEL

Figure 1 outlines the conceptual model for understanding psychopathy – nutrition relationships. This heuristic yet complex model indicates the relationships among risk factors (left), mechanisms (middle) and outcomes (right). Malnutrition caused either by environmental or genetic risk factors during the prenatal and postnatal periods are viewed in this model as risk factors of the outcome, i.e., psychopathology. Insufficient food supply or malabsorption of nutrients are fundamental risk factors for malnutrition. The types of malnutrition, macro-malnutrition or micro-malnutrition, rely on the individual bioavailability of utilizing nutrients. Such malnutrition can predispose to psychopathology through the possible mechanism of brain dysfunction / impairment caused by three independent yet related routes: reducing brain cell development, alteration of biochemical processes, and increasing neurotoxicity. Brain damage/dysfunction is ultimately viewed as being responsible for predisposing to psychopathology. The behavioral outcomes in this model include both antisocial behavior and schizophrenia-spectrum disorders, and we suggest that they both share the common risk factor of malnutrition and the similar mechanism of brain dysfunction. However, this chapter focuses on antisocial behavior as schizophrenia is covered elsewhere (Venables et al., 2006).

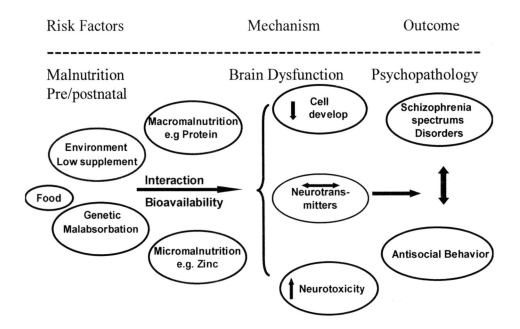

Figure 1. Malnutrition as risk factors for both schizophrenia spectrum disorder and antisocial behavior.

MALNUTRITION AS A RISK FACTOR
FOR ANTISOCIAL BEHAVIOR

Although diet and nutrition have theoretical and clinical implications for understanding antisocial behavior (Raine et al 2003, Rutter et al., 1998), research in this area is only beginning to receive attention. While most studies on diet, nutrition, and behavior have focused on hyperactivity, deficiency in nutrition has itself been rarely studied in relation to aggression, violence, and criminal behavior. Several studies have, however, demonstrated the general effects of related processes on human aggressive behavior, including food additives, hypoglycemia, and more recently cholesterol (Breakey, 1997; Fishbein et al., 1994; Fishbein, 2001; Raine, 1993). Epidemiological studies have shown associations between over-aggressive behaviors and deficiencies of several essential nutrients (Breakey, 1997; Werbach, 1992). However, findings are conflicting and controversial (Rutter et al., 1998). This section will outline recent empirical findings that support the view that malnutrition is a risk factor for the development of aggressive, violent, and criminal behavior. For the purpose of discussion, this section is divided into the following four topics to elucidate the four lines of research supporting the view of malnutrition as a risk factor for antisocial behavior.

Macro-Malnutrition vs. Micro-Malnutrition

Nutrients are normally divided into two categories, macronutrients, and micronutrients (Beers, and Berkow, 1999). While macro-nutrients often refer to protein, carbohydrates, fats, macro minerals, and water, micro-nutrients include vitamins and trace minerals. The amounts needed are small - micrograms or milligrams a day – so they are called "micro" nutrients. They are necessary for regulatory systems in the body, for efficient energy metabolism, and for other functions. Malnutrition can be either at the macro level or the micro level, and most cases may involve a mixture of both. The World Health Organization (WHO) defines malnutrition as "the cellular imbalance between the supply of nutrients and energy and the body's demand for them to ensure growth, maintenance, and specific functions" (WHO, 2000). Although either type of nutritional deficiency may take place alone, it is more common for several nutrition deficiencies to coexist. It is estimated that up to half of all of the children in the world are deficient in iron and/or zinc (WHO, 2001). Studies have indicated that both types of malnutrition are associated with increased behavioral problems (Liu et al., 2004a). Finally, bioavailability is viewed as the proportion of an ingested nutrient or drug that is truly absorbed into the bloodstream (Shargel and Yu, 1999). Bioavailability of nutritients is greatly influenced by both genetics factors (e.g. poor absorption from the gastrointestinal tract) and environmental factors (e.g. food inhibitors and enhancers (Hallberg et al, 1989).

Macro-Malnutrition

Protein-energy malnutrition (PEM), or protein-calorie malnutrition, is a deficiency syndrome caused by the inadequate intake of macronutrients and is characterized by an energy deficit due to a reduction in all macronutrients. Protein malnutrition is a global problem, affecting many young children in developing countries. In animals, male rats fed a low-protein diet in early postnatal life have been reported to show increased aggressive behavior in pair interactions (Tikal et al., 1976). Recent studies of humans support these findings. The male offspring of pregnant women starved during the German blockade of food to Holland at the end of World War II had 2.5 times the rates of antisocial personality disorder in adulthood compared to controls. Effects were found for severe malnutrition during the first and second trimesters of pregnancy, but not the third trimester (Neugerbauer et al., 1999), suggesting that good nutrition is particularly crucial when the fetal brain is developing rapidly in the second trimester.

Amino acids, the biochemical building blocks of protein, have been also implicated in aggressive and violent behavior. Both monkeys and rats fed diets depleted in the amino acid tryptophan become more aggressive than controls, while high-tryptophan food reduces aggressive behavior (Bjork et al., 1999). Because tryptophan is the dietary building block of serotonin, diets low in tryptophan could contribute to the low levels of serotonin found in impulsive violent offenders (Volavka, et al 1990; Virkkunen et al., 1995; Werbach, 1995).

Micro-Malnutrition

The influence of micronutrition such as zinc or iron, or of vitamins on brain function and behavior problems has been evidenced only recently (Rosen et al., 1985; Tu, 1994; Sever et al., 1997). Several studies reported iron deficiency in aggressive and conduct disordered children (Rosen et al., 1985; Werbach, 1995). Rosen et al. (1985) found iron deficiency in a third of juvenile delinquents. Furthermore, in a clinical trail, Sever et al. (1997) found that non-iron deficient children with attention deficit hyperactivity disorder showed both cognitive and behavioral improvement after iron supplementation treatment.

Researches have also implicated zinc deficiency in aggression and violence (Watts, 1990). In animals, the offspring of rats zinc-deprived during pregnancy have been found to be significantly more aggressive than controls (Halas et al., 1977). In humans, zinc deficiency in pregnancy was found to be associated with hyperactivity in the offspring (Brophy, 1986).

In addition to mineral deficiency, research is beginning to implicate micronutrition deficiency in interacting with heavy metals in predisposing to antisocial behavior. Importantly, studies indicate that mineral deficits alone may not produce behavior problems, but that instead low mineral levels exacerbate the effects of toxic metals (Walsh et al., 1997). For example, adding calcium to the diet can decrease the toxic effects produced by lead exposure (Bogden et al., 1997).

More recently, research has implicated docosahexaenoic acid (DHA) in relation to human behavior. It has been reported that behavior problems in boys such as temper tantrums occur more often in subjects with lower total fatty acid concentrations in the plasma phospholipids fraction (Stevens et al, 1996). Fish oil supplements have also been found to reduce impulsivity in girls compared with a control group (Itomura et al, 2005). Some studies have also failed to demonstrate the effectiveness of DHA supplement on reducing externalizing behavior. Voigt et al. (2001) reported that although a 4-month period of DHA supplementation (345 mg/day) increased plasma phospholipid DHA concentrations 2.6-fold compared with a placebo group, it did not improve any objective or subjective measure of symptoms related to attention deficit hyperactivity disorder (ADHD). Although research in this area is mixed, the potential implications of DHA on behavior problems is worth further investigation.

Environmental Influence vs. Genetic Predisposition

If nutrition factors are possible risk factors for antisocial and criminal behavior, an important question concerns whether individual malnutrition is the result of a genetic predisposition or is alternatively caused by the environment. At a general level, malnutrition may be due to inadequate food intake (deficiency in food consumption), or alternatively due to inadequate food utilization (malabsorption of food). While there is no clear understanding of the fundamental causes of malnutrition, it could be caused by the interaction of both environmental and genetic factors.

More specifically, from an environmental perspective, if food supply fails to provide adequate amounts of nutrients to meet human needs, malnutrition will occur. From a genetic perspective, if an individual genetically lacks internal biochemical elements such as the enzymes to absorb, metabolize, and utilize nutrients, malnutrition can develop. This later view of genetic influences on antisocial behavior is supported by twin studies (Rowe, 1983) and adoption / cross fostering studies (Hutchings and Mednick, 1975) which have shown that antisocial and criminal behavior are partly genetically determined. In their adoptee study, Mednick et al. (1984) assessed court convictions of 14,427 adoptees whose biological and adoptive parents were themselves either criminal or noncriminal. Results showed a significant relationship between biological parents' criminal convictions and criminal convictions in their adopted-away children. That is, those whose biological parents were criminal were more likely to commit crime themselves as adults. In addition, the more crimes the biological parent had committed, the higher the rate of criminality in the adopted-away offspring. In the context of a genetic predisposition to malnutrition, it could be that there are genetically-determined individual differences in metabolism that in turn alters brain biochemistry which in turn impacts on antisocial behavior. Furthermore, a genetic predisposition for malnutrition could also be explained by the fact that antisocial parents are not good care-givers and consequently have children who are under-nourished. Nevertheless, gene-environment interactions perhaps may best explain the development of antisocial behavior. One of the fundamental causes of violent crime could be a biochemical predisposition triggered by environmental stress.

Prenatal Period vs. Postnatal Stage

Both animal and human studies have illustrated that prenatal as well as postnatal malnutrition can impact both aggressive behavior and brain development (Neugebauer et al., 1999, Liu et al., 2004a). Malnutrition limited to the prenatal period is not only sufficient to produce permanent alterations in brain structure, but can also cause enduring changes in behavior that are at least as powerful as those produced by postnatal malnutrition (Smart, 1986). Furthermore, animal intervention studies have showed that prenatal vitamin B supplementation in rats advances their hippocampal development (Mellott et al, 2004). A reduction in the area of the hippocampus has been found to be linked to aggression in male mice (Sluyter et al., 1994). On the other hand, Granados-Rojas et al. (2004) found that the mossy fiber system of the hippocampal formation in rats is decreased by chronic postnatal but not prenatal protein malnutrition. Although data on the effects of prenatal vs. postnatal malnutrition on brain development and its impact on behavior remain conflicting, it is generally believed that the brain is most vulnerable and sensitive to insults when it is growing most rapidly. This argument receives some support by Neugebauer et al. (1999), who showed that the male offspring of nutritionally deprived pregnant women were found to have 2.5 times the normal rate of antisocial personality disorder in adulthood when severe malnutrition occurred during the first and second trimesters of pregnancy (when the brain is developing rapidly), but not during the third trimester.

Permanent Consequences vs. Temporary Effects

There continues to be ambiguity in the field of nutrition research as to whether the effect of malnutrition on brain and behavior is permanent or revisable. In the past, it was generally accepted that early malnutrition permanently decreases brain size and cell numbers, resulting in irreversible cognitive impairment. Reductions in cognitive ability have been observed to account for the relationship between malnutrition and antisocial behavior in children (Liu et al, 2004a).

However, more recent views suggest that while some parts of brain (such as the cerebellum) are indeed impacted by malnutrition, such effects appear to be reversible with nutritional rehabilitation. We recently demonstrated that a multi-modal postnatal enrichment that included better nutrition significantly reduced conduct disorder at age 17 and criminal behavior at age 23, and furthermore that these beneficial effects on conduct disorder were potentiated in children with signs of malnutrition at entry into the prevention program (Raine et al, 2003). This finding and recent work on the effects of nutritional supplements in reducing antisocial / aggressive behavior in prisoners are not consistent with the traditional view that the negative effects of early malnutrition are permanent (Gesch et al, 2002). Instead, it is suggested that whether prenatal or postnatal, the deleterious effects of early malnutrition can be addressed.

BRAIN DYSFUNCTION AS A MEDIATOR

From the above section, it is clear that malnutrition, either due to macro or micro malnutrition, may play a role in the development of antisocial and violent behavior. The causes of malnutrition could be both genetic and environmental. The effect of malnutrition on behavior could be both prenatal and postnatal. Long term effects of malnutrition on behavior could be reversible.

The important question that follows concerns the mechanism by which the risk factor of malnutrition predisposes to psychopathology. This section suggests that brain dysfunction may be a key consequence of malnutrition, and it explores the possibility that alterations in brain functioning account for the relationship between malnutrition and antisocial, criminal behavior. Although the precise mechanisms by which food and nutrients influence different aspects of brain functioning are not fully known, there is increasing understanding of how specific nutrients can operate both on brain and behavior. For example, while there is speculation that proteins and minerals play a direct role in brain cell growth and development, they may affect brain functioning by regulating neurotransmitters or hormones, or else by exacerbating neurotoxins, and in doing so predispose to aggressive and violent behavior (Coccaro, 1996, Liu, 2004b).

Decreasing Brain Cell Growth / Development

Investigations in animals have provided evidence that malnutrition during early life not only reduces the growth of the brain but also makes it permanently smaller in size and cellular content (Sara et al., 1976). Early in the study of malnutrition and the brain, the cerebellum was recognized as an area that is particularly sensitive to the effects of early malnutrition. Various cognitive-behavioral consequences are related to the effects of malnutrition on the brain, such as memory disturbance, learning impairments, and behavioral impairment. Studies have shown that following dietary protein restriction during pregnancy, the offspring of rats exhibit significantly smaller fetal body weight and alteration of brain cortical areas compared to controls (Gressens, 1997). The protein content of the diet is believed to play an important role on antioxidant mechanisms. Recent animal experimental studies have observed the effects of protein malnutrition on oxidation-reduction in the rat hippocampus. It has also been found that a deficiency in both the content of protein in the diet and in the essential amino acid methionine alters the antioxidant system and the oxidation-reduction state of the brain of rat (Bonatto, 2005).

It is increasingly recognized that micronutrients such as zinc and iron are essential elements in maintaining normal structure and function of the central nervous system (Liu et al., 2003). Thus, deficiency in iron or zinc can lead to alterations in brain growth and development. Recent studies on rats have indicated that supplementation of both zinc and iron help accelerate recovery of hippocampal functioning following iron deficiency (Shoham, and Youdim, 2002).

We now know from biochemical evidence that docosahexaenoic acid (DHA) deficiency and omega-3 long chain essential fatty acid (EFA) deficiency may exist in protein-energy malnutrition (PEM), and micronutrient deficiencies may contribute to impaired EFA bioavailability and metabolism (Smit et al, 2004). It is known that the brain is 60% fat, and DHA is the most rich fatty acid in the brain. DHA serves as the primary building block for the gray matter of the brain and the retina of the eye (Innis, 2004). Thus, DHA has a critical role in the brain development of the fetus, especially during the first few months of life when there is rapid cerebral cell membrane synthesis. In addition, EFA's are important components of nerve cell walls and are involved in the regulation of neurotransmitter release (Alessandri et al, 2004). There is increasing data to show that low levels of polyunsaturated fatty acids play a role in the pathophysiology of aggressive disorders. Buydens-Branchey et al (2003) in a sample of cocaine addict patients found that aggressive patients had significantly lower levels of DHA than patients without aggressive histories.

Furthermore, studies in human show that violent offenders display reduced glucose metabolism in the prefrontal region of the brain even after controlling for handedness, sex, ethnicity, and the presence/absence of head injury (Raine et al, 1997; Soderstrom et al., 2000). More recently, one study has shown that even slight, visually imperceptible reductions in prefrontal gray matter are significantly associated with antisocial personality disorder (Raine et al., 2000). Brain-imaging research is confirming that there are both structural and functional brain deficits in relation to violence. Malnutrition may directly cause this brain dysfunction by reducing brain cell growth and development and thus producing brain deficits that predispose to violent and criminal behavior (Liu, 2004b). Nevertheless, research in this area is limited.

Alternation in Neurochemistry

It is generally reported that neurochemical functioning in the brain is fundamentally related to the metabolism of nutrients (Wurtman et al, 1990). More specifically, neurotransmitter metabolism involves a chain of biochemical reactions that largely rely on vitamins and minerals which function as co-enzymes. Specific nutrients plays a role in neurotransmission functions such as production, release, inhibition, transmission, and receptor formation. Consequently, when the bioavailability of food / nutrients is impaired due to either environmental or genetic factors, alteration in neurotransmitters may occur. The neurotransmitter impairments implicated in impulsive and aggressive behavior include serotonin and dopamine.

For example, tryptophan is an essential amino acid. It is the precursor of the neurotransmitter serotonin. Its administration increases brain levels of tryptophan and may increase brain serotonin levels (Morand et al, 1983; Volavka, 1990). Considerable evidence from both animal and human studies indicate that alterations in brain tryptophan levels cause changes in brain neurotransmitters such as serotonin synthesis (Young, 2002). Serotonin (5-hydroxytryptamine; 5-HT) has been implicated in impulsiveness and aggression (Volavka et al, 1990). A recent study has shown that subjects who experience acute tryptophan depletion (by ingestion of a mixture of amino acids devoid of tryptophan) experience a decline in brain serotonin (Young, 2002). Furthermore, one new functional MRI study in humans reveals that tryptophan depletion produced by a dietary challenge reduces right inferior prefrontal activation during a response inhibition task (Rubia, et al. 2005).

Similarly, the bioavailability of iron in the brain has been shown to affect neurotransmitter production and function, mainly in the dopamine-opiate systems. Iron is an essential element in maintaining normal structure and function of the central nervous system. In the brain, zinc is with iron the most concentrated metal. The highest levels of zinc are found in the hippocampus in synaptic vesicles, and mossy fibers (Pfeiffer and Braverman, 1982). Furthermore, animal studies indicate that iron deficiency may alter behavior by reducing dopamine transmission (Weiser, 1994). It is also believed that zinc is a key co-factor for building up neurotransmitters and fatty acids, and indirectly involves metabolism of dopamine and fatty acids, which consequently effects on behavior (Arnold et al., 2000).

Moreover, animal studies have indicated that protein deficiency during pregnancy can induce a significant decrease in the activity of brain monoamine oxidase compare to controls. Low MAO-B activity has been reported to be linked to some personality traits, such as aggressiveness, impulsiveness and sensation-seeking behavior (Schalling et al., 1987; Stalenheim et al., 1997). Furthermore, recent animal studies have shown that there is a relationship between aggressiveness and MAO-A activity (Shih and Chen, 1999). MAO-A gene knock-out mice showed elevated brain levels of serotonin, norepinephrine and dopamine, and manifested aggressive behavior (Shih and Chen, 1999). Similarly, although the mechanisms linking cholesterol and antisocial/violent behavior are unknown, it has been suggested that low cholesterol influences 5-HT (serotonin) function. Monkeys fed a low-cholesterol diet have lower CSF serotonin than monkeys fed a high-cholesterol diet (Kaplan et al., 1997).

The relationship between neurotransmitters and aggressive behavior is reasonably well-known. Aggressive offenders have repeatedly been found to have lower levels of the neurotransmitter serotonin (Virkkunen et al., 1995; Halperin et al., 1994). Similarly, aggressive monkeys have also been found to have low levels of serotonin (Kyes et al., 1995). Both animal and human research suggests that increasing serotonin can significantly reduce aggressive behavior (Moskowitz et al, 2003). Drug research also suggests that the relationship may be causal. Prozac, which increases serotonin, has been found to reduce aggression in humans (Coccaro et al., 1997). Therefore, low serotonin could well predispose subjects to mood and impulse control disorders. Higher levels of serotonin may help to promote more constructive social interactions by decreasing aggression and increasing dominance (Young, 2002), and such effects apply to women as well as to men (Bond, 2001). Consequently, nutritional deficiency may directly and indirectly cause brain dysfunction by alterations in brain neurochemistry which in turn predispose to the likelihood of disruptive behavior. On the other hand, the exact mechanisms involve in this neurochemical process is a complex issue and further research needs to be conducted both in animals and human.

Increase in Neurotoxic Effects

Research in the effects of nutrition and environmental toxicity on children's behavior is beginning to recognize the significant effect of malnutrition in facilitating neurobehavioral toxicity in animals and humans. Although exactly how malnutrition is involved in this process is not fully understood, studies and clinical observations are beginning to provide initial empirical evidence to support this effect.

Research on the effects of metal toxicity on behavior has gained increasing attention in recent years. For example, lead exposure has long been known to negatively impact cognitive functions (Needleman et al., 1996). More recently, both animal studies (Delville, 1999) and human studies (Needleman et al., 1996) have found that higher lead exposure measured in bone and blood is significantly related to aggressive and delinquent behavior. Recently, research has found that postnatal lead exposure can have significant deleterious effects on progenitor cell proliferation and consequently affect the structure and function of the hippocampus (Schneider, 2005). In addition, research on rats has found that microinjections of manganese chloride (McCl2) can cause neurodegenerative processes that further alter the animal's emotional behavior (Ponzoni et al., 2000). Excessive copper in the neonatal brain is associated with abnormal development of the hippocampus, a brain structure that plays a critical role in learning and which functions abnormally in murderers (Masters et al., 1999; Raine et al., 1997b).

Notably, studies have shown that the individual effects of some neurotoxins do not directly cause behavior problems, but instead involve the occurrence of nutritional deficits such as protein or calcium deficiency. Animal research has found that protein deficiency during early life makes animals more susceptible to the neurobehavioral toxicity of styrene during both gestation and the early infancy period (Khanna et al, 1991). Masters et al. (1998) have reported that feeding animals a diet high in manganese does not lead to high levels of blood manganese when diets contained normal levels of calcium. In contrast, manganese uptake became significantly higher when the diet was deficient in calcium.

Although the mechanisms by which the neurotoxic effects on aggressive and violent behavior takes place are not fully understood, research has revealed that neurotoxins involve neurotransmitters processes. Murphy et al. (1991) found that levels of dopamine, norepinephrine, and serotonin were lowered in manganese-intoxicated animals. Thus, excessive manganese is thought to reduce brain levels of neurotransmitters such as serotonin while increasing serotonin concentrations elsewhere in the body (Masters et al., 1999). Interestingly, Moffitt et al. (1998) found antisocial individuals in a community sample had higher blood serotonin levels, a view opposite to the usual findings for CSF serotonin, but consistent with the notion that manganese exposure produces low CSF serotonin but high blood serotonin. As outlines earlier, the effects of manganese may be potentiated by low calcium. Just as manganese inhibits neurotransmitters, a recent molecular study on lead-exposed rats indicates that lead inhibits the NMDA receptor, which in turn plays a critical role in learning and conditioning (Nihei et al., 2000). Nevertheless, despite these findings, the research literature on the interaction effect of malnutrition and neurotoxins on externalizing behavior problems remains both limited and controversial.

It is concluded from this section that the effects of malnutrition on the brain can be the basis for the development of adverse behavior. Both animal and human studies provide evidence that malnutrition has a profound effect on the central nervous system and affects not only gross brain weight and cell structure and function, but also neurobiochemical constitution and processes. Consequently, malnutrition can cause brain dysfunction, which in turn can predispose to psychopathological behavior such as aggression and crime.

MALNUTRITION, IQ AND EXTERNALIZING BEHAVIOR: THE MAURITIUS STUDY

From the above discussion, there is reason to believe that malnutrition in the early years is linked to later psychopathological behavior, and that this link is mediated by brain dysfunction. However to date there appear to have been few prospective longitudinal studies testing this hypothesis. In this section, we will briefly present recent findings from the Mauritius longitudinal study indicating that malnutrition in the first few years of life predisposes to antisocial and aggressive behavior throughout childhood and late adolescence (see Liu et al 2004a for details). This analysis is of particular relevant to the theme of this book as Mednick and Venables initiated this study more than 30 years ago.

The Study Design

Participants consisted of a birth cohort of 1,795 children from Mauritius and are described in detail by Venables (1978). Subjects included both males (51.4%) and females (48.6%) with ethnic distribution consisting of Indian 68.7%, Creoles (African origin) 25.7%, and others (Chinese, English, and French) 5.6%. Verbal informed consent was obtained from the mothers of the participants in the early phases, and from participants themselves in the age 17 phase. The following three hypotheses were tested in this study: 1) poor nutrition at age 3 years predisposes to antisocial behavior at ages 8, 11, and 17 years, 2) such relationships are independent of early psychosocial adversity, and 3) IQ mediates the nutrition-antisocial relationship.

We tested the first hypothesis that poor nutrition at age 3 years predisposes to antisocial behavior at ages 8, 11, and 17 years. Participants were defined as suffering from nutritional deficits if at least one of the following four indicators was present at age three (22.6%): angular stomatitis (7.0 %.), hair dyspigmentation: (6.8%), sparse, thin hair (5.8%), and anemia (17%). Participants with no indicator present were defined as having relatively normative nutrition (77.4%) (Liu et al, 2003). We were also interested in a possible dose response relationship, i.e., that that the more indicators of malnutrition that the child has, the greater the level of later externalizing behavior. Subjects on whom behavior data were available were categorized into one of four groups: no malnutrition (N = 766 at age 8, N= 807 at age 11, N = 422 at age 17), one indicator of malnutrition (N = 160 at age 8, N = 172 at age 11, N = 90 at age 17), two indicators (N = 45 at age 3, N = 50 at age 11, N= 25 at age 17), three indicators (N = 10 at age 3, N = 13 at age 11, N = 4 at age 17). Because only two individuals had all four nutrition indicators, this category could not be included in dose-response analyses.

Externalizing behavior was assessed at three points of time among the subjects. The Childrens' Behavior Questionnaire (CBQ – Rutter, 1967) was used at age 8 years, with complete data of 1,130 on the aggression measure, and 1,128 on the hyperactivity measure. The three externalizing subscales (aggression, delinquency, hyperactivity) of the Child Behavior Checklist (CBCL- Achenbach and Edelbrock, 1983) were used at age of 11 years old with completed data on 1,206. The Revised Behavior Problem Checklist (RBPC - Quay and Peterson, 1987) was used at age of 17 years, with completed data on 608.

The Effects of Cognitive Ability and Psychosocial Adversity

We tested the second hypothesis that the malnutrition – externalizing behavior relationship is independent of psychosocial adversity. Psychosocial adversity was assessed at two points in time. The age 3 index of psychosocial adversity (Raine et al, 2002b, Raine et al, 1998) was based on nine psychosocial variables collected by social workers who visited the homes of the children at age 3 years (see Raine et al, 1997 for full details). Complete data for this construct were available on 1,795. The age 11 psychosocial adversity index (Raine et al., 2002b, Liu et al., 2003) was based on 14 variables collected by social workers who visited the homes of the children at age 11 years. Complete data were available on 1,272.

We also tested the third hypothesis that IQ mediates the relationship between nutrition and externalizing behavior problems. Cognitive ability was tested at two points of time. At age 3, measures of cognitive ability were derived from six sub-tests of the Boehm Test of Basic Concepts-Preschool Version (Boehm, 1986, Raine et al, 2002b), which assesses basic verbal and visual-spatial concepts that are fundamental for early school achievement. Data were available on 1,260 subjects. At age 11 years, estimates of full-scale IQ were assessed by using 7 subtests of the WISC (Wechsler, 1967), with Similarities and Digit Span forming an estimate of verbal IQ, while Block Design, Object Assembly, Coding, Mazes, and Picture Completion formed an estimate of performance IQ. Data were available on 1,260 subjects for the above three measure.

MALNUTRITION - LOW IQ – EXTERNALIZING BEHAVIOR PROBLEMS

The three hypotheses proposed above were confirmed in this study. First, malnutrition at age three years was founded to be associated with increase scores on externalizing behavior problems at ages 8, 11 and 17 (see Figure 2). Second, the malnutrition-externalizing relationship was not found to be confounded by psychosocial adversity. Third, the relationship of malnutrition – externalizing behavior was founded to be mediated by cognitive ability, indicating that malnutrition predisposes to lower IQ which in turn predisposes to externalizing behavior problems. These results are also supported by the finding of dose-response relationships between degree of malnutrition and degree of externalizing behavior problems at ages 8 and 17 (see Figure 3), relationships that were again found to be mediated by low IQ. We believe these are the first findings to show prospectively that malnutrition assessed in the early postnatal years is associated with externalizing behavior problems from childhood to late adolescence, and also to show the mediating effects of cognitive ability. These findings in turn have potential implications for public health attempts to prevent the occurrence of child and adolescent externalizing behavior problems.

Findings from the present study provide empirical support for the conceptual framework outlined at the beginning of this chapter. Findings suggest that early malnutrition could predispose to externalizing behavior problems by impairing brain mechanisms (such as the prefrontal cortex) which are thought to regulate emotion and inhibit impulsive aggressive behavior (e.g. Raine et al., 2000). Malnutrition could also predispose to externalizing behavior problems more indirectly by impacting cognitive functioning which in turn predisposes to externalizing behavior problems. Indicators of malnutrition in this study reflect deficits in protein (red hair, sparse/thin hair), iron (low hemoglobin), and zinc (red hair, sparse/thin hair). As we discussed above, there is extensive experimental evidence in animals both that zinc and protein deficiency impairs brain development (Bennis-Taleb, 1999, Halas, 1977, Oteiza et al., 1990), and also that protein, iron and zinc deficiency predisposes to aggression (Halas, 1977, Munro, 1987, and Tikal, 1976). Poor cognitive functioning (indirectly reflecting brain dysfunction) was recognized as a mediator for the malnutrition – externalizing relationship at ages 8 and 11 years in that controlling for the effect of IQ on externalizing behavior abolished the malnutrition – externalizing relationship. Poor cognitive ability has been found to be a consistent predisposition to externalizing behavior problems (Donnellan, 2000). Consequently, this study supports the conceptual framework outlined above which suggests that poor nutrition affects brain dysfunction which in turn predisposes to externalizing behavior.

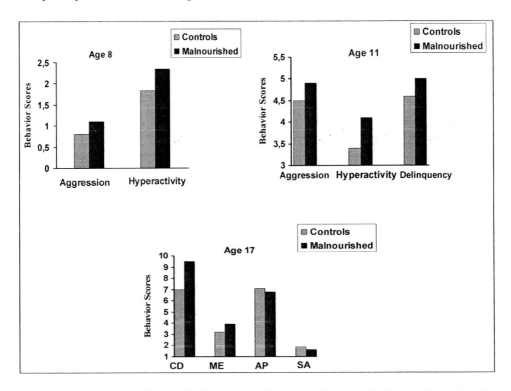

Figure 2. Scores for Externalizing Behaviors at Ages 8, 11, and 17 among Children in Mauritius Who Were or Were Not Malnourished at Age 3. CD: conduct disorder, SA: socialized aggression, ME: motor excess, and AP: attention problems.

Findings may have public health implications. Findings from Mauritius may provide a good model for understanding cognitive deficits in underserved sub-populations of U.S. society, particularly because up to 25% of adolescent girls in the U.S. are iron deficient (Bruner, 1996), because food insufficiency is relatively common in poor rural areas of the U.S. such as the Mississippi delta region (Smith et al, 1999), and because malnutrition is associated with poor behavioral functioning in low-income children in American inner-cities

(Murphy et al 1998, Smith et al 1999). Consequently, findings suggest that better attention to nutrition could have significant implications for brain development in children and adolescents and further decreased the likelihood of behavior problems (Liu, 2004a).

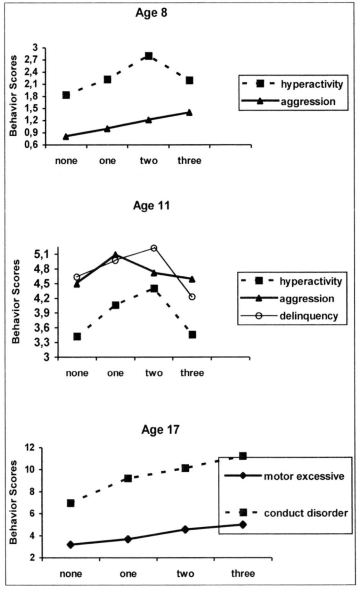

Figure 3. Dose-Response Relationships Between Number of Malnutrition Indicators at Age 3 and Externalizing Behaviors at Ages 8, 11, and 17 Among Children in Mauritius[a]. [a]Four indicators of malnutrition were assessed: angular stomatitis, hair dyspigmentation, sparse/thin hair, and anemia.

LIMITATIONS OF RESEARCH IN THIS FIELD AND FUTURE RESEARCH DIRECTIONS

Despite the potential significance of malnutrition in predisposing to violence, this research area has four important limitations. First, there are simply very few studies of this potential relationship. Second, little research has investigated prospectively the effects of early malnutrition on later violent behavior. Third, findings have not always been consistent. Fourth, few if any studies have tested for interactions with other risk factors.

Future research needs to place emphasis on investigating specific macro/micro-nutrition deficiency in relationship to the development of antisocial behavior, and experiments with animals can also establish *causal* relationships between early malnutrition, alterations in brain structures/function, and resulting psychopathology. Furthermore, the importance of early nutritional intervention on behavioral problems cannot be over-emphasized, although practical implications must be treated with caution.

ACKNOWLEDGEMENTS

This paper was written with the support of a NRSA fellowship (F32 NR-08661-2) from the National Institute of Health to the first author.

REFERENCES

Alessandri, JM., Guesnet, P., Vancassel, S, Astorg, P., Deni, I., Langelier, B., Aid, S., Poumes-Ballihaut, C., Champeil-Potokar, G., and Lavialle, M (2004). Polyunsaturated fatty acids in the central nervous system: evolution of concepts and nutritional implications throughout life. *Reprod Nutr 44*, 509-538.

Achenbach, TM., and Edelbrock, CS. (1983). *Manual for the Child Behavior Checklist and Revised Child Behavior Profile.* Burlington: University of Vermont Department of Psychiatry

Arnold, L.E., Pinkham, S.M., and Votolato, N. (2000). Does zinc moderate essential fatty acid and amphetamine treatment of attention-deficit/hyperactivity disorder? *Journal of Child and Adolescent Psycho pharmacology 10*, 111–117.

Beers, MH., and Berkow, R (1999). *The Merck Manual of Diagnosis and Therapy.* 17th Edition, Merck Research Laboratories.

Bennis-Taleb, N., Remacle, C., Hoet, JJ. and Reusens, B. (1999). A low-protein isocaloric diet during gestation affects brain development and alters permanently cerebral cortex blood vessels in rat offspring. *Journal of Nutrition. 129*, 1613-1619

Breakey, J. (1997). Journal of Pediatric Child Health. *The role of diet and behavior in childhood. 33*:190-194

Bjork, J. M., Dougherty, D. M., Moeller, F. G., Cherek, D. R., and Swann, A. C. (1999). The effects of tryptophan depletion and loading on laboratory aggression in men: Time course and a food-restricted control. *Psychopharmacology, 142,* 24-30.

Bogden, JD., Oleske, JM., and Louria, DB. (1997). Lead poisoning--one approach to a problem that won't go away. *Environ Health Perspect.105 (12):*1284-1287.

Bonatto, F., Polydoro, M., Andrades, ME., Frota, ML., Dal-Pizzol, F., Rotta, LN., Souza, DO., Perry, ML., and Moreira, JC. (2005). Effect of protein malnutrition on redox state of the hippocampus of rat. *Brain Res. 25,* 17-22.

Boehm, A. (1986). *Boehm Test of Basic Concepts - Preschool Version.* Psychological Corporation.

Bond, AJ., Wingrove, J., and Critchlow, DG. (2001). Tryptophan depletion increases aggression in women during the premenstrual phase. *Psychopharmacology. 156,* 477-480.

Brophy, M. H. (1986). Zinc and childhood hyperactivity. *Biological Psychiatry, 21,* 704-705.

Bruner, AB, Joffe, A., Duggan, AK., Casella, JF., Brandt, J (1996). Randomised study of cognitive effects of iron supplementation in non-anaemic iron-deficient adolescent girls. *Lancet. 348,* 992-996.

Buydens-Branchey, L., Branchey, M., McMakin, D., and Hibbeln, JR. (2003), Polyunsaturated fatty acid status and aggression in cocaine addicts *Drug and Alcohol Dependence 71*: 319-323

Coccaro, E. F., Kavoussi, R. J., and Hauger, R. L. (1997). Serotonin function and antiaggressive response to fluoxetine: a pilot study. *Biological Psychiatry, 42,* 546-552.

Delville, Y (1999). Exposure to lead during development alters aggressive behavior in golden hamsters. *Neurotoxicology and Teratology, 21,* 445-449.

Donnellan, MB., Ge, X., and Wenk, E. (2000). Cognitive abilities in adolescent-limited and life-course-persistent criminal offenders. *J Abnorm Psychol, 109,* 396-402

Fishbein, DH., Pease, SE. (1994). Diet, nutrition, and aggression. *Journal of Offender Rehabilitation 21,* 117-144

Fishbein, D., (2001). *Biobehavioral Perspectives in Criminology.* Wadsworth/Thomson Learning, Belmont, CA.

Gesch, C. B., Hammond, S M, Hampson, S E, Eves, A, and Crowder, M J. (2002). Influence of supplementary vitamins, minerals and essential fatty acids on the antisocial behaviour of young adult prisoners: Randomised, placebo- controlled trial. *British Journal of Psychiatry, 181,* 22-28.

Granados-Rojas, L., Aguilar, A., and Diaz-Cintra, S. (2004).The mossy fiber system of the hippocampal formation is decreased by chronic and postnatal but not by prenatal protein malnutrition in rats. *Nutr Neurosci. 7,* 301-308.

Gressens, P., Muaku, SM., Besse, L., Nsegbe, E., Gallego, J., Delpech, B., Gaultier, C., Evrard P, Ketelslegers, JM., and Maiter, D. (1997). Maternal protein restriction early in rat pregnancy alters brain development in the progeny. *Brain Res Dev Brain Res. 103,* 21-35.

Halas, E. S., Reynolds, G. M., and Sandstead, H. H. (1977). Intra-uterine nutrition and its effects on aggression. *Physiology and Behavior, 19,* 653-661.

Hallberg, L., Brune, M., Rossander, L (1989). Iron absorption in man: ascorbic acid and dose- dependent inhibition by phytate. *Am J Clin Nutr. 49*, 140-144

Halperin, JM., Sharma, V., Siever, L. J., Schwartz, S. T., Matier, K., Wornell, G. and others. (1994). Serotonergic function in aggressive and nonaggressive boys with ADHD. *American Journal of Psychiatry, 151*, 243-248.

Hutchings, B., and Mednick, S.A. (1975). Registered criminality in the adoptive and biological parents of registered male criminal adoptees. In S.A. Mednick, F. Schulsinger, J. Higgins, and B. Bell (Eds.), *Genetics, environment, and psychopathology* (pp. 215.227). Amsterdam: New Holland.

Innis, SM. (2004). Polyunsaturated fatty acids in human milk: an essential role in infant development. *Adv Exp Med Biol. 554*, 27-43.

Itomura, M., Hamazaki, K., Sawazaki S, Kobayashi, M., Terasawa, K., Watanabe, S, Hamazaki, T. (2005). The effect of fish oil on physical aggression in schoolchildren--a randomized, double-blind, placebo-controlled trial. *J NutrBiochem. 16,* 163-171. Khanna, VK., Husain, R, Hanig, JP., and Seth, PK. (1991). Increased neurobehavioral toxicity of styrene in protein-malnourished rats. *Neurotoxicol Teratol. 13*,153-159.

Kyes, R. C., Botchin, M. B., Kaplan, J. R., Manuck, S. B., and others. (1995). Aggression and brain serotonergic responsivity: response to slides in male macaques. *Physiol.and Beha. 5*, 205-208.

Lister, JP., Blatt, GJ., Debassio, WA., Kemper, TL., Tonkiss, J, Galler, JR., and Rosene, DL.(2005). Effect of prenatal protein malnutrition on numbers of neurons in the principal cell layers of the adult rat hippocampal formation. *Hippocampus.15*, 393-403.

Liu, J, Raine, A., Venables, P., and Mednick, S.A (2004a). Malnutrition at age 3 years predisposes to externalizing behavior problems at ages 8, 11 and 17 years. *American Journal of Psychiatry, 161, 2005-2013*

Liu, J (2004b). Concept Analysis: Aggression. *Issue in Mental Health Nursing 25, 693-714*

Liu, J, Raine, A, Venable, P, Dalais, C, and Mednick SA (2003) Malnutrition at age 3 years and lower cognitive ability at age 11 years: independence from psychosocial adversity. *Arch Pediatr Adolesc Med, 157, 593-600*

Masters, R.D, Hone, B., and Doshi. (1998). Environmental pollution, neurotoxicity, and criminal violence in J. Rose (Ed). *Environmental Toxicology* (pp. 13-48). London: Gordon and Breach. Masters, R. D., Coplan, M. (1999). A dynamic, multifactorial model of alcohol, drug abuse, and crime: linking neuroscience and behavior to toxicology. *Social Science Information*, 591-624. London: Sage.

Mednick, S. A., W. F. Gabrielli Jr., and B. Hutchings (1984) Genetic influences in criminal convictions: Evidence from an adoption cohort *Science 224*, 891-94

Mellott, TJ., Williams, CL., Meck, WH., Blusztajn, JK (2004). Prenatal choline supplementation advances hippocampal development and enhances MAPK and CREB activation. *FASEB J. 18*, 545-547.

Moffitt, T. E., Brammer, G. L., Caspi, A., Fawcett, J. P., Raleigh, M., Yuwiler, A. et al. (1998). Whole blood serotonin relates to violence in an epidemiological study. *Biological Psychiatry, 43,* 446-457

Morand, C., Young, SN., and Ervin FR (1983). Clinical response of aggressive schizophrenics to oral tryptophan. *Biol Psychiatry. 18*, 575-8.

Moskowitz, DS., Pinard, G., Zuroff, DC., Annable, L., and Young, SN.(2003) Tryptophan, serotonin and human social behavior. *Adv Exp Med Biol.527*:215-224.

Munro, N. (1987). A three year study of iron deficiency and behavior in rhesus monkeys. *International Journal of Biosocial Research, 9*, 35-62

Murphy, V., Rosenberg, J., Smith, Q., and Stanley, R. (1991). Elevation of brain manganese in calcium-deficient rats. *Neurotoxicology, 12*, 255-263.

Murphy JM, Wehler CA, Pagano ME, Little M, Kleinman RE, Jellinek MS (1998). Relationship between hunger and psychosocial functioning in low-income American children. *Journal of the American Academy of Child and Adolescent Psychiatry. 37*, 163-170.

Needleman, H. L., Riess, J. A., Tobin, M. J., Biesecker, G. E., and Greenhouse, J. B.(1996), Bone Lead Levels and Delinquent Behavior; *JAMA, 275* 363-369

Neugebauer, R., Hoek, HW., and Susser, E. (1999). Prenatal exposure to wartime famine and development of antisocial personality disorder in early adulthood. *JAMA 4*, 479–481

Nihei, MK., Desmond, NL., McGlothan, JL., Kuhlmann, AC., and Guilarte, TR. (2000). N-methyl-D-aspartate receptor subunit changes are associated with lead-induced deficits of long-term potentiation and spatial learning. *Neuroscience. 99(2)*:233-42.

Oteiza, PI. Hurley, L., Lonnerdal, B., Keen, C. (1990). Effects of marginal zinc deficiency on microtubule polymerization in the developing rat brain. *Biological Trace Element Research. 123*,13-23

Pfeiffer, C. C. and Braverman, E. R. (1982). Zinc, the brain and behavior. *Biol Psychiatry, 17*, 513-532.

Ponzoni, S., Guimaraes, F. S., Del Bel, E. A., and Garcia-Cairasco, N. (2000). Behavioral effects of intra-nigral microinjections of manganese chloride: Interaction with nitric oxide. *Progress in Neuro-Psychopharmacology and Biological Psychiatry, 24*, 307-325.

Quay, HC, Peterson, D. (1987). *Manual for the Revised Behavior Problem Checklist.* Coral Gables, FL, Department of Psychology, University of Miami.

Raine, A., Lencz, T., Bihrle, S., LaCasse, L., and Colletti, P. (2000). Reduced prefrontal gray matter volume and reduced autonomic activity in antisocial personality disorder. *Archives of General Psychiatry, 57,* 119-127.

Raine, A., (2002a). Biosocial studies of antisocial and violent behavior in children and adults: a review. *Journal of Abnormal Child Psychology, 30*, 311–326.

Raine, A., Yaralian, P., Reynolds, C., Venables, PH., and Mednick, SA (2002b). Spatial but not verbal cognitive deficits at age 3 years in persistently antisocial individuals. *Development and Psychopathology, 14*:25-44

Raine, A., Mellingen, K, Liu, J H, Venables, P H, and Mednick, S A. (2003). Effects of environmental enrichment at 3-5 years on schizotypal personality and antisocial behavior at ages 17 and 23 years. *American Journal of Psychiatry, 160*, 1627-1635.

Raine, A, Reynolds, C, Venables, PH, Mednick, SA, Farrington, DP. (1998). Fearlessness, stimulation-seeking, and large body size at age 3 years as early predispositions to childhood aggression at age 11 years . *Arch Gen Psychiatry, 55*, 745-751

Raine, A., Venables, PH., Mednick, SA. (1997). Low resting heart rate at age 3 years predisposes to aggression at age 11 years: Evidence from the Mauritius Child Health

Project. *Journal of the American Academy of Child and Adolescent Psychiatry, 36*,1457-1464

Raine, A., Buchsbaum, M., and LaCasse, L. (1997a). Brain abnormalities in murderers indicated by positron emission tomography. *Biological Psychiatry, 42,* 495-508.

Raine, A., Brennan, P., Farrington D., and Mednick, S. A. (1997b). *Biosocial basis of violence.* New York: Plenum Press.

Rosen, GM, Deinard, AS, Schwartz, S, Smith, C, Stephenson, B, and Grabenstein, B. (1985): Iron deficiency among incarcerated juvenile delinquents .*J.of Adol. Health Care, 6*, 419-423

Rowe, D.C. (1983). Biometrical genetic models of self-reported delinquent behavior: A twin study. *Behavior Genetics, 13*, 473.489.

Rubia, K., Lee, F., Cleare, AJ., Tunstall, N., Fu, CH., Brammer, M., McGuire, P. (2005) Tryptophan depletion reduces right inferior prefrontal activation during response inhibition in fast, event-related fMRI. *Psychopharmacology (Berl).* 26

Rutter, M., Giller, H., Hagell, A. (1998). *Antisocial behavior by young people.* New York, NY, Cambridge University Press

Rutter, M (1967). A children's behaviour questionnaire for completion by teachers: Preliminary findings. *J.Child Psychology and Psychiatry. 8*, 1-11

Sara, V R; King, T L; and Lazarus, L, (1976). The influence of early nutrition and environmental rearing on brain growth and behaviour *Experientia. 32*, 1538- 1540

Schalling, D., Asberg, M., Edman, G. and Oreland, L. (1987). Markers for vulnerability to psychopathology: temperament traits associated with platelet MAO activity. *Acta Psychiatrica Scandinavica 76*, 172–182.

Schneider, JS., Anderson, DW., Wade, TV., Smith, MG., Leibrandt, P., Zuck, L., Lidsky, TI. (2005). Inhibition of progenitor cell proliferation in the dentate gyrus of rats following post-weaning lead exposure.*Neurotoxicology. 26*, 141-145.

Sever, Y., Ashkenazi, A., Tyano, S., Weizman, A.(1997). Iron treatment in children with attention deficit hyperactivity disorder. A preliminary report. *Neuropsychobiology 35*,178–180.

Shih, JC., Chen, K. (1999) MAO-A and -B gene knock-out mice exhibit distinctly different behavior. *Neurobiology 2*, 235-246.

Shoham, S., Youdim, MB (2002). The effects of iron deficiency and iron and zinc supplementation on rat hippocampus ferritin.: *J Neural Transm.109*, 1241-1256.

Sluyter, F., Jamot, L., van Oortmerssen, GA., and Crusio, WE. (1994). Hippocampal mossy fiber distributions in mice selected for aggression. *Brain Res.16, (64)*:145-148.

Smart, J. L. (1986) Undernutrition, learning and memory: review of experimental studies. In: *Proceedings of the 13th Congress of Nutrition* (Taylor, T. G. and Jenkins, N. K., eds.), pp. 74-78. Libbey, London, UK.

Smit, EN., Muskiet, FA., and Boersma, ER.(2004). The possible role of essential fatty acids in the pathophysiology of malnutrition: a review. *Prostaglandins Leukot Essent Fatty Acids. 71*, 241-250.

Smith, J., Lensing, S. Horton, JA., Lovejoy, J., Zaghloul, S., Forrester, I., McGee, BB., and Bogle, ML (1999). Prevalence of self-reported nutrition-related health problems in the Lower Mississippi Delta. *Am J Public Health 89*, 1418-1421.

Soderstrom, H., Tullberg, M., Wikkelsoe, C., Ekholm, S., Forsman, A. (2000). Reduced regional cerebral blood flow in non-psychotic violent offenders. *Psychiatry Research: Neuroimaging 98,* 29–41.

Stalenheim, E. G., von Knorring, L. and Oreland, L. (1997) Platelet monoamine oxidase activity as a biological marker in a Swedish forensic psychiatric population. *Psychiatry Research 69,* 79–87.

Stevens, L.J. Zentall, S.S. M.L. Abate, T. Kuczek and J.R. Burgess (1996). Omega-3 fatty acids in boys with behavior, learning, and health problems. *Physiol. Behav. 59,* 915–920.

Tikal, K., Benesova, O., and Frankova, S. (1976). The effect of pyrithioxine and pyridoxine on individual behavior, social interactions, and learning in rats malnourished in early postnatal life. *Psychopharmacologia, 46,* 325-332.

Tu, J. B., Shafey, H., and VanDewetering, C. (1994). Iron deficiency in two adolescents with conduct, dysthymic and movement disorders. *Canadian Journal of Psychiatry, 39,* 371-375.

Venables, P. H. (1978). Psychophysiology and psychometrics. *Psychophysiology, 15,* 302-315.

Venables, P. Raine, A. Dalais, C. Liu, J. and Mednick, SA (2006) Malnutrition, cognitive ability, and Schizotypy. In A. Raine (ed). *Crime and schizophrenia: Causes and cures.* New York: Nova Science Publishers.

Virkkunen, M., Goldman, D., Nielsen, D. A., and Linnoila, M. (1995). Low brain serotonin turnover rate (low CSF 5-HIAA) and impulsive violence. *Journal of Psychiatry and Neuroscience, 20,* 271-275.

Volavka, J., Crowner, M., Brizer, D., Convit, A., Van Praag, H., and Suckow, RF.(1990). Tryptophan treatment of aggressive psychiatric inpatients. *Biol Psychiatry. 15,* 728-732.

Voigt, R.G., Llorente, A.M., Jensen, C. L., Fraley, J. K., Berretta, M. C., and Heird, WC. (2001). A randomized, double-blind, placebo-controlled trial of docosahexaenoic acid supplementation in children with attention-deficit/hyperactivity disorder, *J. Pediatr. 139,* 189–196.

Walsh, W. J., Isaacson, H. R., Rehman, F., and Hall, A. (1997). Elevated blood copper/zinc ratios in assaultive young males. *Physiology and Behavior, 6,* 327-329.

Watts, D.L., (1990). Trace elements and neuropsychological problems as reflected in tissue mineral analysis (TMA) patterns. *Journal of Orthomolecular Medicine 5,* 159–166.

Werbach, MR. (1992). Nutritional influences on aggressive behavior. *J Orthomolecular Med.7,* 45–51

Wechsler, D. (1967). *Wechsler Preschool and Primary Scale of Intelligence* San Antonio: The Psychological Corporation.

Weiser, M., Levkowitch, Y., Neuman, M., and Yehuda, S. (1994). Decrease of serum iron in acutely psychotic schizophrenic patients. *Int J Neurosci., 78,* 49-52.

Wienk, KJ., Marx, JJ., and Beynen, AC. (1999). The concept of iron bioavailability and its assessment. *Eur J Nutr. 38:*51-75.

Wurtman, RJ. (1990). Ways that foods can affect the brain (pp. 106-113) in Ornstein, Robert Evan (ED) and Swencionis, Charles (ED).*The healing brain: A scientific reader New York, NY, US:* Guilford Press.

World Health Organization (WHO) (2001), Iron deficiency anaemia: assessment, prevention and control. *A Guide for Program Managers*. World Health Organization, Geneva.

World Health Organization (WHO) (2000) World Health Organization Dept. of Nutrition for Health and Development: *Nutrition for Health and Development: a Global Agenda for Combating Malnutrition*. Geneva World Health Organization

Young, S. N. (1996). Behavioral effects of dietary *neurotransmitter* precursors: Basic and clinical aspects *Neuroscience and Biobehavioral Reviews. 20*, 313-323

Young, S. N, and Leyton, M. (2002). The role of serotonin in human mood and social interaction insight from altered tryptophan levels. *Pharmacol Biochem Behav. 71,* 857-865.

In: Nutrition Research Advances
Editor: Sarah V. Watkins, pp. 103-136

ISBN 1-60021-516-5
© 2007 Nova Science Publishers, Inc.

Chapter IV

THE EFFECT OF SHORT AND LONG TERM ANTIOXIDANT TREATMENTS ON REDOX HOMEOSTASIS ON EXPERIMENTAL AND CLINICAL STUDIES

Anna Blázovics[1],*, Ágota Kovács[2] and Andrea Lugasi[3]

[1]Semmelweis University, [2]Péterfy Hospital, [3]National Institute for Food Safety and Nutrition, Budapest, Hungary.

ABSTRACT

Research justified, that natural antioxidants and bioactive agents related to antioxidant effects could act on signal transduction pathways and/or phase II enzyme activities directly and/or indirectly. These molecules can also influence the apoptotic genes.

In the case of plant extracts, which contain several active compounds, one might consider it is impossible to discover the single mechanism of action. This problem becomes even more complicated, when we bring the obtained data of in vitro and in vivo experiments into consideration. Therefore the multifactorial actions must be analyzed in short and long term in vivo studies on redox homeostasis.

The questions are: - can the absorbed compounds of natural extracts from the gastrointestinal tract influence the changed cellular redox states in experimental bowel disease in all parts of gut, and how can these molecules act on the redox homeostasis of blood in IBD patients?

---

* Correspondence concerning this article should be addressed to:
  Dr. Ph.D. D.Sc. Anna Blázovics: Semmelweis University, Faculty of Medicine, 2nd Department of Medicine; H-1088 Budapest, Szentkirályi Str. 46., email: *blaz@bel2.sote.hu*.
  Dr. Ph.D. Ágota Kovács: Péterfy Hospital, Department of Gastroenterology, H-1074 Budapest, Alsóerdõsor Str. 7., email: *kovacs_agota@yahoo.com*.
  Dr. Ph.D. Andrea Lugasi: National Institute for Food Safety and Nutrition, 1097 Budapest, Gyáli rd. 3/a., email: *lugasi@oeti.antsz.hu*.

Our aim was to present the protective effect of natural polyphenols and flavonoids of the *Sempervivum tectorum* extract (2g/bwkg/day for 10 days) on alimentary induced bowel disease in rats, and the isothiocyanate-rich *Raphanus sativus* niger based granule (0.2 g/die Raphacol) in a twelvemonth clinical study in patients suffered from IBD.

The redox balance did not change significantly, when the health animals were treated with the *Sempervivum tectorum* extract. In fat rich diet induced bowel disease the treatment caused a beneficial change in reducing power of ileum and H-donating ability was significantly better in all large bowel parts. The data of scavenger capacity were better in part of short bowel and enormous changes were detected in parts of large bowel in sick animals. The *Sempervivum tectorum* treatment was beneficial. We concluded from these results that antioxidant compounds (after bacterial and non bacterial enzymatic transformation) take part in redox homeostasis.

Raphacol treatment did not influence the activity of IBD. Beside beneficial subjective judgement, bile acid level was elevated continuously and the values of redox parameters were decreased in the plasma during treatment. The granule diminished the erythrocyte chemiluminescence significantly and the HbA_{1c}-level moderately until the beginning of the ninth month. After this, the trend has changed until the end. Data showed, that antioxidant and isothiocyanate-rich granule could influence the redox homeostasis of IBD patients even at low dose.

Keywords: natural antioxidants, isothiocyanates, Sempervivum tectorum, Raphanus sativus, redox homeostasis, experimental bowel disease, inflammatory bowel diseases.

ABBREVIATIONS

ABTS = 2,2'-azinobis-(3-ethylbenzothiazoline-6-sulfonic acid; ALP = alkaline phosphatase; AP-1 = transcription factor; APC = activated protein C; ARE = antioxidant responsive element; BRJ = black radish root (*Raphanus sativus* L. *var. niger)* BUN = blood urea nitrogen; COX2 = cyclooxygenase 2; CD = Crohn disease; CHOL = cholesterol; CU = ulcerative colitis; CREA = creatinin; EPR = electron spin resonance; f = female; GOT = aspartate aminotransferase; GPT = alanine aminotranferase; GS = glucosinolate; GSH = glutathione; γGT = gamma-glutamil transpeptidase; HDL-cholesterol = high density lipoprotein–cholesterol; HDA = H-donor activity; IBD = inflammatory bowel diseases; K-ras = onco gene ; IL-1β, IL-6, = interleukines; iNOS = induced nitric oxide synthase; ITC = isothiocyanate; JNK/SAPK = c-Jun N-terminal kinases; LOX = lipoxygenase; m = male; MAPK-s = mitogen activated protein kinases (serine/threonine kinases); NAD(P)H = nicotine amide adenine dinucleotide reduced form; NF-κB = nuclear transcription factor κB; Nrf2 = nuclear factor E2-related factor 2; p38, p53 = nuclear transcription factors; PERK = pancreatic endoplasmic reticulum kinase; PI3K = phosphoinositol 3-kinase; PKC = proteine kinase C; RLU or RLU% = relative light unit or ~ %; PRP = plasma reducing pover; RBC = red blood cell; SOD = superoxide dismutase; TBIL = total bilirubin; TG = triglycerides; TNF α = tumor necrosis factor; TSC/CLI = total scavenger capacity/chemiluminescence intensity.

INTRODUCTION

Redox homeostasis is very important for the equilibrium between tissue regeneration and apoptosis, when the balance is injured, cancer and/or necrosis may develop. The moderate dietary habits with natural antioxidants can help to restore to the normal function of gastrointestinal tract, but the immoderate consumption of vitamins and polyphenol type antioxidant molecules is contraindicated. Unhealthy dietary habits (lipid rich diet, indigestible foods, alcohol etc.) could result in inflammatory processes and necrosis in the gastrointestinal tract in which free radical reactions involved (Blázovics et al., 1992, Fehér et al., 1992, 1998, Powis et al., 1997, Sípos et al., 2001, Mózsik et al., 2001).

Polyposis is associated with high frequency gastrointestinal cancer. The duodenum is the second commonest site of polyp development after the colon. Adenomas tend to be noted in the duodenum approx. 15 years after colonic polyps occurance. The prevalence of gastric cancer is very high not only in the Western but in the Japanese and the Korean family (in which people consume green tea and other polyphenols) as well. Genetic alterations (mutation of genes: p53, K-ras, APC) are in the background of tumorous processes. Mucosal exposure to bile favours cancer development both in the duodenum and colon (Lee et al., 2002, Kim et al., 1993, Lin et al., 1995, Wallace & Phillips, 1998). It is generally agreed that the composition of diet plays as fundamental role in the induction of these types of cancers. Persons on high fat diet excrete three times as much bile acids as vegetarians (Seymour et al., 1989). At the same time bile acids are very important to prevent of absorption of bacterial endotoxin on colonic mucosa (Bertók, 1998).

Inflammatory bowel diseases are multifactorial heterogenous diseases with extreme variability in their clinical course. These diseases are conditions that persist throughout the life of the patients. The extension of the involved area occurs in up to 70 % of the cases and therefore malnutrition is a characteristic symptom in IBD, which affects the free radical/antioxidant balance of the organism (Buffinton & Doe 1995, Tragnone et al., 1995, Nielsen et al., 1996, McKenzie et al., 1996, Blázovics et al., 1999).

Janus faced oxyradicals are secunder messengers of intracellular signal transduction pathways but also cytotoxic agents of cells. Oxygen free radicals have several functions in the expression of cytokines associated inflammatory bowel disease. The molecular mechanism between activation and inhibition participants of signal transduction are excellently controlled. The antioxidant - prooxidant balance of the cells can be traced back to the concentration of free-SH and its oxidised form, - S-S- (Jacobson et al., 1985, McKenzie et al., 1996, Buffinton et al., 1995, Dalekos et al., 1998)

Several nutritional polyphenols (the secondary metabolites of plants) are COX2 and/or LOX inhibitors and iNOS activators. Antioxidant vitamins (vitamin A, C, E) and polyphenols (e.g. flavonoids) are signaling molecules. Flavonoids may affect beneficially or as like toxic actions on cells via signaling cascades (Polya et al., 2002, Lunec et al., 2002, Zingg et al., 2004, Azzi et al., 2004, Gebhardt, 2004)

Prostaglandins have proinflammatory and anti-inflammatory effects on the immune system. NF-κB is responsible among others for the cytokine production, and cytokines stimulate the action of NF-κB in circulus vitiosus. NF-κB and AP-1 are proteins regulated by reactive oxygen radicals under numerous pathogenic conditions (Schulze-Osthoff et al.,

1997). For example, hydrogen peroxide induces the activation of NF-κB (Meyer et al., 1993). In contrast to NF-κB, the DNA binding of AP-1 is only weakly induced by hydrogen peroxide (Lander et al., 1995).

In in vitro studies epigallocatechin-3-gallate antioxidant treatments caused cell cycle deregulation and the apoptosis of several cancer cells may be mediated through NF-κB inhibition, although not in the case of normal cells. The inhibition of NF-κB constitutive expression and activation in normal human epidermal keratinocyte was observed only at high concentration (Ahmad et al., 2000).

Phenolic type antioxidants activate mitogen activated protein–kinase (MAPK), which may lead to the induction of genes producing protection and survival mechanisms leading to apoptosis (Kong et al., 1998). MAP kinases (JNK and p38 pathways) may participate in the regulation of NF-κB transcriptional activity (Schulze-Osthoff et al., 1997).

Cytotoxic activity of hydrolysable tannins was observed against human oral squamous cell carcinoma and salivary gland tumour cell lines, but not against normal cells. Several macrocyclic ellagtannin oligomers showed cytotoxic activity. These compounds induced apoptotic cell death characterized by DNA fragmentation, but macrocyclic compounds in higher concentrations produce their own radicals and become prooxidants (Sakagami et al., 2000). Flavonoids are inhibitors and enhancers of the cytotoxicity of TNF-alpha in L-929 cells. The magnitude of protection and potentiation by flavonoids is concentration dependent (Habtemariam, 1997).

A lot of polyphenols, especially tannins precipitate proteins, depending on their dosage, and therefore cannot penetrate the mucous membranes (Lugasi, 2000).

Higher plants have many free radical scavenger molecules and anti-inflammatory compounds in important variations (Manach et al., 1997, Tarr, 2002). *Sempervivum tectorum L. (Crassulaceae)* species are well known plant in folk medicine. In the Mediterranium, its leaves are consumed as salad for ages. The juice of fress leaves is used as antiphlogistic in ear inflammation (Penso, 1982, Bremnes, 1995, Stevens et al., 1996, Blaschek et al., 1998). Antimicrobial activity of *Sempervivum* was also justified (Abram & Donko, 1999).

In previous in vitro and in vivo studies we gave account of antioxidant, scavenger (by EPR technique) membrane protecting, immune stimulating, serum lipid level lowering and HDL-cholesterol enhancing properties of *Sempervivum tectorum* extractum in concordance with literature. Liver protecting effect was also justified in alimentary induced fatty liver in rats (Kéry et al., 1992, Blázovics et al., 1993a,b, 1994). This extract was able to modify the fatty acid ratio in the liver in cases of hyperlipidemy and this fact and the lipid lowering activity of *Sempervivum tectorum* contribute together to membrane restitution (Blázovics et al., 1992, 2000). It was established that activities of NAD(P)H reductases and the content of cytochrome P450 were normalised in hyperlipidemic rat liver microsomes, if the animals were treated with the *Sempervivum tectorum* extractum. Fatty acid composition was changed beneficially examined by HRGLC analysis. At the same time *Sempervivum tectorum* had no significant influence on PSMO system in normolipidemic animals and on cytochrome b5 concentration of microsome fractions of hyperlipidemic rats (Blázovics et al., 2000).

The detoxicating property of *Sempervivum tectorum* was shown by eliminating Al, Ba, Ni and Ti from the fatty liver of the rat. The element concentration of liver and bile was determined by inductively coupled plasma optical emission spectrometry (ICP-OES) (Szentmihályi et al., 2000).

Recently we have described the immunostimulatory activity of the hepatoprotectant *Sempervivum tectorum* in hyperlipidemic rats similarly to the most commonly used natural antioxidants, Vitamin E and silibinin (Blázovics et al., 1994, Fehér et al., 1996). Their interactions in cytokine production in hyperlipidemia concludes us to think, that their immunostimulatory effects may be most satisfactory in regulation of lipid metabolism. Generally, the favourable changes in the immune system observed are attributable to antioxidant property (Kéry et al., 1992, Blázovics et al., 1994).

Partial hepatectomy significantly influences immune reactivity. A marked increase in spontaneous TNF-alpha, IL-1 production and blast transformation of spleen cells could be detected after the 72nd hour of lobectomy. Neither TNF-alpha by LPS, nor blast transformation by Con A were not inducible at 72 hours after partial hepatectomy. Therefore we concluded, that the cellular immune function was depressed in an early period after the operation. The *Sempervivum tectorum* extract treatment influenced the Con-A stimulated blast transformation, LPS triggered TNF-alpha activity of spleen macrophages of operated rats beneficially. The decreased blast transformation of splenocytes induced by Con-A is increased by this extract treatment significantly. TNF-alpha activities (untreated and treated with LPS) were changed in contrary in early regeneration period in *Sempervivum tectorum* extract treated rats. LPS induced TNF-alpha activity was significantly increased in this treated group, while the extract does not influence the LPS induced higher IL-1 activity as a consequence of the operation in this system. The regeneration of liver tissue was faster in treated group too, which could be appreciated by the changes of serum parameters and liver weight/body weight ratio (Blázovics et al., 2002). Therefore it can be established, that the absorbed and/or metabolised flavonoid and phenoloid components of the *Sempervium tectorum* extract can modify the cellular immune responses by multifactorial steps not only in the necrotising (in fatty liver of hyperlidemic animals) (Blázovics et al., 1994, 2000), but in the regenerating liver after partial hepatectomy. It can also accelerate the regression and regeneration processes. Presumably, the protection and modification of membrane surfaces by the influence of the cytokine production can be dependent on antioxidant property compounds of *Sempervivum tectorum* extract. The above mentioned is proven. Micronutrients (K, Ca, Mg) content can contribute of maintenance the normal membrane potential compensate the inhibitory effect of flavonoids on the plasma membrane ATP-ases (Blázovics et al., 1989). Collectively these results indicate, that the immunostimulating effect of this extract is appeared in the modification of cellular immune responses of spleen macrophages after lobectomy in early time regerneration.

Besides, results showed that this extract administered actually 5 days before and 3 days after operation, did affect the regeneration processes in the liver. ALP, GOT, GPT, γGT activities of the sera were lowered as well as cholesterol, triglycerides, TBIL, but BUN, CREA, and sugar were not changed by the treatment (Blázovics et al., 2002). Significant differences were detected in the liver weight/body weight ratio. Control group: $100 \pm 5.88\%$, *Sempervivum tectorum* extract treated group without operation $93.8 \pm 7.206\%$, the ratio after parial hepatectomy was changed $78.22 \pm 9.53\%$ and the successfulness was significant in the operated and antioxidant treated group: $93.22 \pm 2.96\%$ (Blázovics et al., 2002).

In folk medicine black radish *(Raphanus sativus L.* var. *niger)* root has been also used since antiquity as food and spice and also as a natural drug against abdominal flatulence, insufficient digestion and for the inhibition of gallstone formation and for the stimulation of the bile function (Weiss, 1985, Jakobey, 1988). In the regions where radish is frequently used in nutrition a smaller prevalence of gallbladder diseases was observed (Pahlow, 1989). Radish juice increases bile excretion and it is an efficient agent against inflammation (Hänsel, 1985). It is supposed that black radish has not got a direct effect on bile juice drainage, but it is much more probable that the drug can beneficially modify the tonicity of the muscles in the gallbladder wall, intestine and stomach, as well, thus contribute to the more efficient peristaltic movement (Lutomski & Speichert, 1952, Ritter, 1984). Chronic dyskinesis and dyspepsia with serious obstipation may be successfully treated with the freshly prepared juice from 100-150 g black radish daily during a long-term administration (Weiss, 1985). Although Popovic et al., (1993) did not found significant protective effect of black radish juice in acute liver injury caused by paracetamol in rats, there was no doubt that some parameters like bile excretion and hematochrit indicated some beneficial effect of the drug pre-treatment against paracetamol toxicity. Vargas et al., reported a significant antiurolithiatic activity of black radish on rats (1999).

Black radish root contains different glucosinolate compounds, essential oils, flavonoids and other phenolic compounds (Jakobey et al., 1988). Concentration of the glucosinolates in the fresh root is very high (1.0-1.1 mg/100g f.w.) but these compounds can be hydrolysed by myrosinase during the storage (Ciska, et al., 1994, Lugasi et al., 1998).

The glucosionolate glucoraphanin was initially coined for an antibacterial principle isolated from radish *(Raphanus sativus* L.) (Ivanovics & Horvath, 1947). Sulphoraphane is the cognate isothiocyanate of glucoraphanin. Sulforaphane has received much recent interest lately, since it was found to be the most potent naturally-occuring inducer of phase II enzymes and inhibitors chemically induced mammary tumours (Zhang et al., 1994). Sulforaphane is not supposed to be a direct-acting antioxidant or prooxidant, since it is very unlikely that the isothiocyanate group can participate in oxidation or reduction reactions under physiological conditions. There is, however, substantial and growing evidence that sulforaphane administration acts indirectly to increase the antioxidant capacity of animal cells, and their abilities to cope with oxidative stress.

Isothiocyanates (ITCs) are a class of small molecules, available often abundantly from many cruciferous vegetables, and may play a significant role in affording the cancer-preventive activity of these vegetables. They are synthesized and stored as glucosinolates (GSs) in plants and are released from the latter when the plant tissue is damaged. The conversion is catalyzed by myrosinase, a thioglucoside glucohydrolase that coexists with but is physically separated from GSs under normal conditions (Fenwick et al., 1983, Fahey et al., 2001). However, GSs that escape the plant myrosinase may also be hydrolysed in the intestinal tract, as the microflora is known to possess a myrosinase activity (Getahun et al., 1999). Many ITCs are potent inhibitors of tumorigenesis in a variety of organs in rodents (Hecht, 2000, Conaway et al., 2002). More recently, several epidemiological studies have reported that dietary consumption of ITCs inversely correlates with the risk of developing lung, breast, and colon cancers (London et al., 2000, Zhao et al., 2001, Fowke et al., 2003), providing further evidence that these compounds may prevent cancer in humans. ITCs are capable of both inhibiting the formation of a cancer cell and eliminating an existing one, in line with their known mechanisms, which include inhibition of carcinogen-activating cytochrome P450 monooxygenases, induction of carcinogen detoxifying enzymes, induction of apoptosis, and the inhibition of cell cycle progression (Zhang 2004, Yu et al., 1998). However, it also has become increasingly apparent that ITCs are double-edged swords in the modulation of cellular oxidative stress. While there is clear evidence that ITCs stimulate many enzymes and nonenzyme proteins that have antioxidative/anticarcinogenic properties, studies also show that these compounds can cause oxidative stress and even damage to cells, although ITCs probably do not participate in any direct oxidation/reduction reactions in cells (Kassie, 2000). Ironically, ITC-induced stress appears, at least in part, to be the initiating event for achieving their chemoprotective activity.

It appears that significant portion of the chemopreventive effects of isothiocyanates may be associated with the inhibition of the metabolic activation of carcinogens by cytochrome P450s (Phase I), coupled with strong induction of Phase II detoxifying and cellular defensive enzymes (Barcelo et al., 1996, Keum et al., 2004). Inductions of Phase II cellular enzymes are largely mediated by the antioxidant responsive element (ARE), which is regulated by the transcriptional factor, Nrf2 (Zhang & Gordon, 2004, Nguyen et al., 2003). Zhang and Talalay (1994) reported that many isothiocyanates raise tissue reduced glutathione level by stimulating antioxidant response elements in the 5'-upstream region of the gene for the heavy subunit of γ-glutamylcysteine synthetase, the enzyme that catalyses the rate-limiting step in GSH synthesis. Sulforaphane induce glutathione transferases (Gerhauser et al., 1997) from which some have well-defined (selenium-independent) glutathione-peroxidase activities. Additional potent regulatory mechanisms of Nrf2 include the different signalling kinase pathways (MAPK, PI3K, PKC and PERK) as well as other non-kinase dependent mechanisms (Keum et al., 2003, Zhang et al., 2005). Moreover, apoptosis and cell cycle perturbations appear to be yet another potential chemopreventive mechanisms elicited by isothiocyanates, especially with respect to the effects on pre-initiated or initiated tumor cells. Finally, modulation of other critical signaling mediators, including the NF-κB and AP-1 by a wide array of chemopreventive agents including isothiocyanates may also contribute to the overall chemopreventive mechanisms (Yu et al., 1998, Young et al., 2003, Jeong et al., 2004).

Table 1.

elements	concentrartion, µg/g	elements	concentration, µg/g
Al	4.20 ± 0.03	K	2118 ± 20
B	1.01 ± 0.001	Mg	105 ± 0.4
Ca	167.7 ± 11.5	Mn	0.375 ± 0.003
Cr	0.02 ± 0.006	Na	166 ± 12.9
Cu	0.076 ± 0.003	P	241 ± 2.3
Fe	0.318 ± 0.012	S	416 ± 2.6
		Zn	0.76 ± 0.01

An industrially prepared cold press juice of black radish contained antioxidant compounds such as tocopherols, ascorbic acid and phenolics. Chemical screening of the juice showed the following substances in 100 ml: dry material (4.46 g), ascorbic acid (5 mg), β-carotene (0.02 mg), tocopherols (0.31 mg), total polyphenols (25.5 mg), sugars (fructose, glucose) (1.5 g), quercetin (0.066 mg), kaempferol (0.495 mg), but glucosinolates were not detectable (Lugasi, 1998, Lugasi, 2001). Relatively low element concentrations can be seen in the juice and no concentrations higher than the detection limit were measured in toxic (As, Cd, Hg, Pb) and in some other elements (Co, Mo, V). Relatively high potassium concentration (2118 ± 20 μg/g) was found in the extract compared to other element concentrations (Table 1.) (Szentmihályi et al., 2000, Lugasi, 2001).

The squeezed juice of black radish expressed significant antioxidant and free radical scavenging properties that were investigated by spectrophotometry and luminometry. Investigated juice exhibited strong hydrogen-donating ability, reducing power, copper (II)-chelating property and showed radical scavenging effect in the H_2O_2/•OH-luminol system (Lugasi et al., 1998, Lugasi, 2001, Lugasi et al., 2002). The effects of black radish juice in alimentary induced hyperlipidaemia were intensively studied in animal experiments. Black radish juice had a beneficial effect on cholesterol, LDL-cholesterol, triglyceride, and malondialdehyde levels in the sera, significantly inhibited the oxidation of cholesterol in steatotic liver and improved the antioxidant enzymatic defence system in erythrocytes and the liver of hyperlipidaemic rats (Lugasi et al., 1999, Kocsis et al., 2002, Lugasi et al., 2002, Lugasi et al., 2005). Black radish juice had a beneficial effect on free radical scavenging capacity of the bile fluid and on biochemical characteristics of intestinal mucosa in rats fed with a fat rich diet (Lugasi et al., 1996, Szentmihályi et al., 2000, Sipos et al., 2001, 2002).

Raphacol granule is a natural product with curative effects. The effective compounds of the product are coming from the squeezed juice of black radish root and aetherolum foeniculi. Both plant products contain biologically active compounds that improve quality of life related to digestive system. The effects of this product were studied in diabetic patients during a 6 months' intervention period while subjects consumed regularly 0.6 g/day *Raphacol granule*. After 6 months the lipid peroxidation characteristics such as thiobarbituric acid reactive substances, uric acid and total sulfhydryl-groups in sera, catalase and glutathione peroxidase activities in erythrocytes and the radical scavenging capacity in plasma changed beneficially (Lugasi et al., 2001). The most routine laboratory serum parameters such as glucose, hemoglobin A1c, glycohemoglobin, cholesterol, and triglyceride levels improved (Lugasi et al., 2000). The majority of the patients in both diabetic groups reported the elimination of the abdominal inconveniences such as insufficient digestion, inflation, nausea, obstipation or diarrhoea, repletion, wind colic, abdominal pressing. Results suggest that regular consumption of *Raphacol granule* helps to prevent atherosclerosis via the decrease of the serum cholesterol level, and results in a more comfortable life for them as well. Quality improvement of lipid peroxidation characteristics might help to prevent the gallstone formation and other clinical alterations that have high prevalence in diabetic patients and in which free radicals are involved such as other gastrointestinal disorders or atherosclerosis (Lugasi et al., 2000, 2001).

MATERIALS AND METHODS

Materials

Stable radical 1,1-diphenyl-2-picrylhydrasyl (DPPH) luminol, hydrogen peroxide and microperoxidase were obtained from SIGMA (St.Luis), serum bovine albumin from CALBIOCHEM AG (Lucerne). Haemisol kit was HUMAN product (Budapest) and Ca-, Na- and K-diadnostic kits were obtained Diagnosticum Rt, (Budapest). The total antioxidant status (TAS) was measured using a kit manufactured by Randox Laboratories Ltd. (Mississauga, Canada). All other reagents were purchased from Reanal Chemical Company (Budapest).

Sempervium tectorum

The lyophilised extract of *Sempervivum tectorum L.S. ruthenicum L (Crassulaceae)* is used as a standardised preparation by 207657/1993 Semmelweis University Patent. This extract contains approximately 20 different flavone and flavonol mono-and diglycosides (0.7%w/w), mainly quercetin and kaempherol glycosides, polyphenolic compounds (4.2%w/w), e.g. proanthocyanides, phenol carboxylic acids, ascobic acid, 11.2%w/w polysaccharides and micronutrients, mainly Ca (76.52mg/g), K (40.47mg/g), Mg (17.85mg/g). Characteristic monosaccharides are rhamnose, arabinose, xylose, mannose, galactose, uronic acids after strong hydrolysis (Kéry et al., 1992). Alcaloids could not be detected in any examined samples (Blázovics et al., 2000).

Data for toxicity after i.p. administration are: in male rats LD50 value is 2276 mg/bwkg and in female rats LD50 value is 2098 mg/bwkg, maximal tolerance i.p. 500 mg/bwkg and p.o. 5000 mg/bwkg. in both sexes. These data indicate that the administration of STF1 extract represents a very low risk (Blázovics et al., 2000).

Raphanus sativus / Raphacol Bile-Granule /

The standardized squeezed juice from black radish root (*Raphanus sativus L. var. niger*)(BRJ) was prepared by Parma Product Company (Budapest) under the control of the Institute of Pharmacognosy, Semmelweis University, Budapest (Hungary). Chemical screening of the juices were from five different squeezing showing the following substances in 1000 ml: dry material (44.6 g), ascorbic acid (50 mg), β-carotene (0.2 mg), tocopherols (3.1 mg), total polyphenols (255 mg), sugars (fructose, glucose) (15 g), quercetin (0.66 mg), kaempferol (4.95 mg), and glucosinolates were not detectable (Lugasi et al., 1998, Lugasi, 2001).

Raphacol bile-granule contains squeezed juice from 60 g of fresh black radish root and 0.25 g *aetherolum foeniculi* completed with granulum simplex to 100 g.

According to the leaflet attached to the product it is suggested to be used against abdominal discomfort, indigestion, inflation and for the increase of the bile secretion. Recognized gallstone disease is contraindicated because of the high risk of occlusion as a result of the high bile juice flux. The drug is produced by Parma Product Company, (Hungary) and registered by the National Institute of Pharmacology (OGYI-090/1988).

Animal Experiments

Forty Wistar rats (150-200g) (obtained from Charles River Hungary Kft.) were divided into four groups: control and fat rich diet fed and treated with extract in two adequate groups. 10 animals were in each group. Lipid rich diet (2% cholesterol 0.5% cholic acid, 20 % sunflower oil added to the rat chow) was applied for the experiments. Normal diet was obtained from BIOFARM PROMT Kft (BFP. Gödöllő, Hungary). The extract of *Sempervivum tectorum* was dissolved (2 g/bwkg) in the daily drinking water and added parallel with feeding for 10 days. The animals were operated and bile was collected from common bile duct after laparatomy in deep pentobarbital narcosis (55 mg/bwkg). The bile was collected for 2 hours into plastic tube. After exsanguination bowel parts were isolated and prepared.

Human Study

Valuable data came from 32 patients from 50 sick volunteers (13 males, 19 females) suffering from moderately active IBD, and the half of patients were treated with 0.2 g/die granule for 12 months. In measuring times the processed data of granule treated patients were from 6 male and 10 female patients suffering from moderate IBD. The patients in the control IBD group (withouth granule treatment) were randomly choosen and the data of them were analysed only in the case of 7 males and 9 females moderately sick patients. All these patients were observed during the whole term (Table 2-3).

Table 2. Grouping of IBD patients
I.

group	sex	age (year)	diagnosis
control IBD (n=25)	10 male; 15female	47,5 ± 15,7	11 CU; 14 CD
granule treated IBD (n=25)	10 male;15 female	42,5 ± 12,7	9 CU; 16 CD

Red Blood Cell Separation

Blood was put into vacutainer tubes containing citrate for the plasma and into native tubes for the sera (Greiner). The plasma and sera were centrifuged immediately at 4 °C at 3000 rpm for 10 min using a standard method. The red blood cells (RBC) were separated and washed 3 times with 0.9% NaCl solution. After washing and centrifugation (10 min; 3000 rpm) the haemoglobin content of RBC was determined by Haemisol kit. The haemoglobin content was adjusted to 1%, uniformly.

Table 3. Grouping of IBD patients
II.

group	sex	extension	activity, type	treatment
control IBD patients (N=25)				
CU patients	5 m.; 6 f.	left colon	Rachmilewitz 6-10	aminosalicilic acid
CD patients	6 m.; 8 f.	small and large bowel	CDAI 150-250 fistula 9 stricture 5	aminosalicilic acid Imuran
granule treated IBD patients (N=25)				
CU patients	4 m.; 5 f.	left colon	Rachmilewitz 6-10	aminosalicilic acid
CD patients	7 m.; 9 f.	small and large bowel	CDAI 150-250 fistula 11 stricture 5	aminosalicilic acid Imuran

Preparation of Mucosa Homogenates

After the identification of bowel parts (duodenum, jejunum, ileum, coecum, colon, rectum) the bowel was cut and the content of actual bowel was eliminated tenderly and washed three times with isotonic ice-cold NaCl solution. Mucosa was harvested by tender power with blunt knife using microscopic control.

Biochemical measurements: The redox-status of duodenum, jejunum, ileum, coecum, colon and rectum homogenates of sick animals and antioxidant treated rats was determined by H-donating ability, reducing power property and tissue chemiluminescent intensity measurements. The biochemical changes were controlled by histological examinations and compared with adequate control groups. (Permission number: 59/1996)

Four simple redox measurements, H-donating ability, reducing-power property, free SH-group and stimulated chemiluminescent intensity of plasma and erythrocytes were performed to evaluate the redox homeostasis in IBD compared to the control values. (Permission number: 24/1996)

H-donating Ability

The hydrogen-donating ability (HDA) of the sample was estimated in the presence of 1,1-diphenyl-2-picrylhydrazyl (DPPH) radical according to the method of Hatano et al., (1988). The characteristic was expressed as I_{50}, that is the amount of the sample that results in a 50% decrease of the colour intensity of DPPH at 517 nm.

Free SH-group

Free SH-groups were determined by the Sedlack method based on the Ellmann reaction (Sedlak, 1985).

Reducing Power

Oyaizu's method was adopted for the analysis of the reducing power of plasma (RP). The change in absorbance was measured, which accompanied Fe^{3+}-Fe^{2+} transformation at 700 nm, and the P(RP) was compared to that of ascorbic acid (Oyaizu 1986).

Copper (II) and Fe(II) Chelating Ability

The chelating ability of *Sempervivum tectorum* on metallic ions was measured as described by Shimada et al., (1992) with a minor modification. Chelating activity was determined as the absorbance ratio at 485 vs 530 nm in hexamine buffer in the presence of tetramethylmurexide and in the presence and absence (control) of the sample. The control showed the highest ratio. The lowest ratio is the strongest chelating ability.

Superoxide Radical Scavenging Capacity

The superoxide radical scavenging capacity of BRJ was determined according to McCord and Fridovich (1968). Superoxide radical was generated by a xanthine - xanthine oxidase system. Cytochrome c was reduced by superoxide radical during colour development at 550 nm. Colour intensity significantly decreased as a result of scavenging superoxide radicals by antioxidant molecules.

Inhibition of the Linoleic acid Autoxidation

The inhibition of the linoleic acid autoxidation at 40°C was studied with the use of the thiocyanate method described by Masude and co-workers (1992). The absorbance of the reaction mixture was read at 500 nm.

Total Antioxidant Status

In TAS kit, metmioglobin reacts with H_2O_2 to form the radical species ferrilmioglobin. A chromogen, 2,2'-azinobis-(3-ethylbenzothiazoline-6-sulfonic acid) (ABTS), is incubated with the ferrilmioglobin to produce the radical cation species ABTS$\cdot^+$. This has a relatively stable blue-green colour, which is measured at 600 nm. (Miller et al., 1993). Antioxidants in the added sample cause suppression of this colour production to a degree, which is proportional to their concentration. The assay is calibrated using 6-hydroxy-2,5,7,8-tetramethylchromane-2-carboxylic acid (Trolox), a synthetic form of vitamin E.

Plasma and Erythrocyte Luminometry

A recently developed chemiluminescence assay adapted to a Berthold Lumat 9501 instrument, which was applied for the determination of the total scavenger capacity of the plasma and erythrocytes to assess the antioxidant deficiency in patients with intestinal diseases. The scavenger capacity of the samples obtained from healthy individuals and patients were expressed in RLU or RLU% (relative light unit or ~ %) of the standard (basic chemical reaction) (Blázovics et al., 1999). The plasma and the erythrocytes of the patients were separated by centrifugation (see above).

The scavenger capacity of the samples obtained from healthy individuals and patients was expressed in RLU or RLU% (relative light unit or ~ %) of the standard (basic chemical reaction).

Chemiluminescence of Tissue Homogenates and Bile Juice

Light emission was measured by Blázovics et al., (1999) which was carried out using a Berthold Lumat LB 9501 luminometer (see before), The composition of the reaction mixture was as follows: 300 µl hydrogen peroxide (10000 x dilution), 300 µl microperoxidase ($3x10^{-7}$ M), 50 µl luminol ($7x10^{-7}$ M), tissue sample was 50 or 100 µl (protein content 10 mg/ml using bovine albumin as standard) and bidestilled water in different volume. The total volume was 850 µl. The intensity of the chemiluminescence light is given as the relative light unit (RLU) reduced by free radical scavenging substances or tissue homogenates. In bile examination the system did not have microperoxidase (Blázovics 2005).

Protein Content

Protein contents of sample homogenates were measured by Lowry et al., (1951).

Routine Laboratory Measurements

Together with other redox parameters as reducing power, H-donating ability, free SH groups and IL-6-, IL-1-, TNF-alpha, bile acids, cholesterol, triglycerides, red blood cell chemiluminescence and HbA_{1c} level were determined.

Other laboratory parameters in IBD were used to calculate the BEST index and the CU activity index: total protein, albumin, gamma-glutamyltransferase, alanine aminotransferase, aspartate aminotransferase, alkaline phosphatase, glucose, creatinin, total and direct bilirubin, C-reactive protein, red cell distribution, platelet, white blood cell, lymphocytes granulocytes, erythrocytes, haemoglobin, mean corpuscular volume (MCV), mean cell haemoglobin (MCH), mean corpuscular haemoglobin concentration (MCHC), hematocrite, Ca, Na and K. Laboratory studies were performed on a HITACHI 717 Analyser.

Mathematical Statistical Analysis

In these studies 5 parallel measurements were carried out, and in the animal experiments 2-2 parallel were in each measuring point in each animal., In human study, 2 parallels were determined in each measuring system.Significance was established p<0.05.

One-way ANOVA statistical analysis was applied to evaluate significance levels between the different groups. Pearson's correlation matrix was used to evaluate the correlation between measured parameters.

RESULTS AND DISCUSSION

In Vitro Antioxidant and free Radical Scavenging Properties of *Sempervivum tectorum* Extract

The concentration dependent antioxidant activity of *Sempervivum tectorum* extract was verified. H-donating ability, reducing power and chelating ability were detected in in vitro studies (Figure 1-4).

The extract of *Sempervivum tectorum* exerted proton-donating ability in the presence of DPPH stable radical as a function of concentration. The extract exhibited reducing power, which was measured on the basis of Fe(III) to Fe(II) redox reaction. The reducing power was expressed in ascorbic acid equivalent (ASE/ml). The chelating activity of the extract of *Sempervivum tectorum* was justified as well (Figure 3, 4). These experiments streghtened the earlier results (Blázovics et al., 1993, 1994).

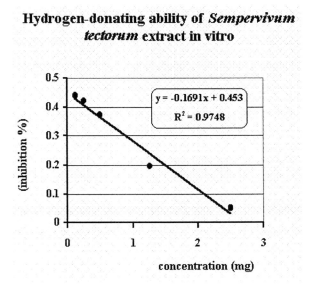

Figure 1.

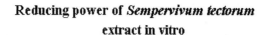

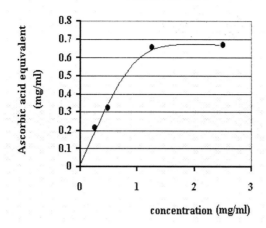

Figure 2.

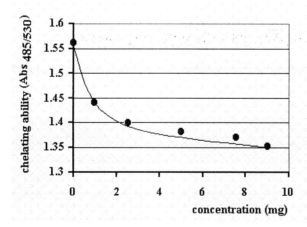

Figure 3.

In Vitro Antioxidant and free Radical Scavenging Properties of Black Radish Juice

As it can be seen on Figure 5 black radish juice significantly inhibited the reduction of cytochrome c caused by superoxide radical generated in xanthine-xanthine oxidase system. This effect showed a concentration-depending manner. The result suggests that BRJ may have a superoxide radical scavenging property. In a study carried out by Ramarathnam and co-workers, a very strong superoxide radical scavenging activity of *Cruciferae* species such as broccoli, Brussel sprouts and radishes were observed using a hypoxanthine-xanthine oxidase superoxide generating and an electron spin resonance measuring system (Ramarathnam et al., 1997). It was also reported that lipid peroxidation can be inhibited by flavonoids possibly acting as a strong superoxide radical scavenger (Yuting et al., 1990). There is no doubt that other biologically active compounds in BRJ such as carotene can also scavenge superoxide radicals (Coon et al., 1992).

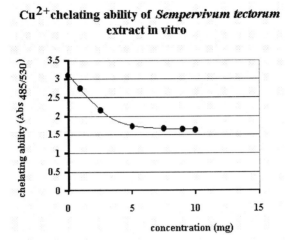

Figure 4.

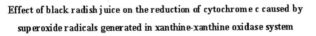

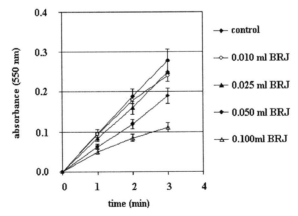

Figure 5.

In the autoxidation process of linoleic acid at 40°C, BRJ acted as an effective antioxidant. On Figure 6 it can be read that BRJ could retard the oxidation of the fatty acid caused by the elevated temperature. The induction time of the oxidation measured by the thiocyanate method was longer when the sample was present in the reaction mixture. The induction period was dependent from the concentration of the juice. It has been proposed that flavonoids react with lipid peroxil radicals leading to the termination of radical chain reactions. The autoxidation of linoleic acid and methyl linoleate was inhibited by flavonoids such as catechin, quercetin, rutin, luteolin, kaempferol and morin (Kandaswami & Middleton, 1997). Morin and kaempferol were the most effective inhibitors. From the inhibition of the formation of trans-trans hydroperoxide isomers of linoleic acid by flavonoids, inhibition of autoxidation of fatty acids by radical chain reaction termination was discerned.

The sample exhibited strong antioxidant property as a result of TAS measurement. The TAS value of the black radish juice expressed as Trolox equivalent was 70.5 ± 13.7 mmol/l. Other juices from different vegetables having high polyphenol content do not show such high TAS activity. For example 100% juices of beetroot, vegetable mixture, and carrot having 529, 316 and 264 mg polyphenols in 1000 ml, showed only 7.95, 1.0, and 0.45 mmol/l TAS activity, respectively (Lugasi, unpublished data). We supposed that biologically active compounds represent a special mixture in black radish juice to exhibit a strong antioxidant activity. Presence of other important antioxidants in the juice is also possible.

Effect of black radish juice on the autoxidation of linoleic acid

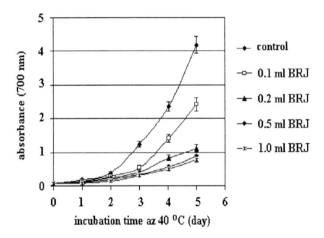

Figure 6.

Animal Experiments

The judgement of biological and pharmacological effects of quercetin and kaempherol is extreme in literature, similarly to the polyphenolic compounds their mutagenicity and carcinogenicity in biological relevant pH. In spite of, that these two antioxidant types of flavonoids are findable in almost every plant originated foods (György et al., 1992; Tarr, 2002). In previous studies we established that *Sempervivum tectorum* extract had no toxic effect on the whole body in spite of its high quercetin and kaempherol contents in this applied concentration (2g/bwkg/day for 10 days) (Blázovics et al., 2000).

Since cells and tissues have specific defence mechanism against pathological free radical processes, certain activities or concentrations of antioxidants themselves (enzymes, vitamins or function groups) do not represent the total antioxidant states of specimens. Therefore three non-specific biochemical measurements (PRP; HAD; TSC/CLI) were applied for the detection of antioxidant states of bowel parts to evaluate the redox states of mucosa homogenates (Blázovics et al., 2003).

The redox balance was not changed significantly, when the normolipidemic animals were treated with this extract. (it cannot be shown). H-donating ability, reducing power and total scavenger capacity of duodenum, jejunum, ileum were significantly higher than in coecum, colon, and rectum. There was no significant difference between measured parameters of the large bowel parts in H-donating ability and the reducing power, but significance was observed in total scavenger capacity between coecum, colon and rectum. Ileum homogenate could scavenge free radicals the best way, but the H-donating ability and the reducing power were not unambiguous. (High RLU % means low scavenger capacity of the tissue.) (Figure 7-12)

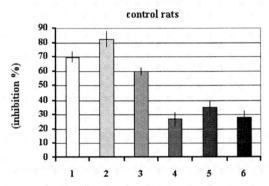

1: doudenum, 2: jejunum, 3: ileum, 4: coecum, 5: colon, 6: rectum

Figure 7.

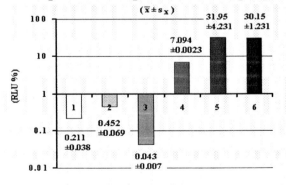

1: doudenum, 2: jejunum, 3: ileum, 4: coecum, 5: colon, 6: rectum

Figure 8.

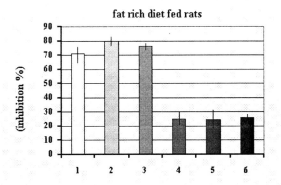

Figure 9.

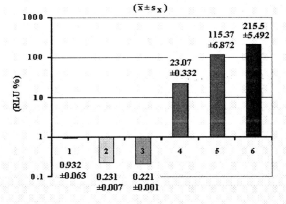

Figure 10.

Antioxidant treatment caused a beneficial change in reducing power of ileum homogenate and H-donating ability was significantly better in all large bowel parts (Blázovics et al., 2003). The data of total scavenger capacity was very beneficial in part of short bowel and enormuous changes were detected in parts of large bowel and rectum. We concluded from these results that antioxidant compounds (after bacterial enzymatic transformation) take part in redox homeostasis of bowel tissues. It is known from the literature, the fenolic acids, sourced from flavonoids can absorb in large bowel (Lugasi, 2000, Hollmann et al., 1997). Reducing power was very high in the duodenum of fat rich diet fed animals, but the data were not changed in jejunum, ileum, coecum, colon and rectum (Blázovics et al., 2003). H-donating ability was better in the colon of normolipidemic animals and ileum of hyperlipidemic ones consequence of lipid metabolism. Total scavenger capacity was very wrong in all parts of short and large bowel and rectum in hyperlipidemia, but the differences were enormuous between upper and lower parts compared to the control ones.

The total antioxidative status of doudenum, jejunum and ileum were injured less than coecum, colon and rectum. Antioxidant treatment caused faurable change in redox states of all measured bowel parts, especially in coecum, colon, and rectum. Active components or their derivates of *Sempervivum tectorum* (in its natural and/or transformed forms by bacterial metabolism) come into the circulation (Blázovics et al., 2000; 2002) and secrete into the bile fluid. The antioxidant activity of these compounds can be obtained in the cannulated bile juice of rats, in particular in hyperlipidemic animals, where the activity approximately with 36 % is better than that of normolipidemic rats. This is explained the absorption of active compounds in injured bowel membranes and bacterial activity (Figure 13).

H-donating ability in homogenates of small and large bowel mucosa

fat rich diet fed and antioxidant treated rats

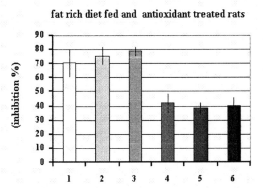

1: doudenum, 2: jejunum, 3: ileum, 4: coecum, 5: colon, 6: rectum

Figure 11.

Enhanced chemiluminescence intensity of small and large bowel homogenates in fat rich diet fed and antioxidant treated group

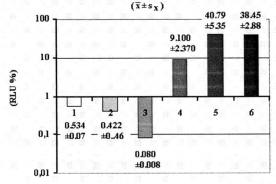

1: doudenum, 2: jejunum, 3: ileum, 4: coecum, 5: colon, 6: rectum

Figure 12.

On the basis of our experimental data we prove that the antioxidant power of this drug extract is manifested both in the bowel parts and in the secreted bile juice harvested from cannulated ductus choledochus. Therefore membrane protective and anti-inflammatory properties of this natural plant extract can be detectable primarily and secondarily.

Histological studies supported that enormous changes happened both in the liver and in jejunal mucosa of fat rich diet fed animals. The *Sempervivum tectorum* extract in that treatments could restore the tissue structures (Fehér et al., 1992; Blázovics et al., 1992).

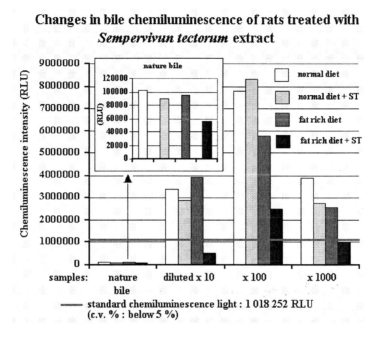

Figure 13.

Human Studies

A lot of research strenghtened, that biopsies obtained from inflammatory parts of mucosa both in Crohn's disease and in ulcerative colitis showed lower levels of urate, glutathione and ubiquinol-10 antioxidants (Bhaskar et al., 1995, D'Odorico et al., 2001, McKenzie et al., 1996). Ascorbic acid concentration was also decreased in samples obtained from the inflammatory bowel of IBD patients (Buffinton et al., 1995a). Furthermore, reduction of dehydroascorbic acid by GSH/NADPH dependent dehydroascorbic acid reductase significantly decreased in inflammed mucosa, whereas alpha tocopherol content remained unchanged compared to controls (Buffinton et al., 1995a,b). A scavenger isoenzyme glutathione-S-transferase mu, is dominantly inherited and is expressed in approximately half of the population. Lower incidence of GST expression was detected in patients with ulcerative colitis and Crohn's disease (Hertervig et al., 1994). This finding is associated with a more severe clinical course leading to colectomy. Superoxide dismutase and catalase enzyme activities were also decreased in the inflammatory bowel. In the rectal tissue myeloperoxidase activity was increased due to neutrophyl infiltration, but malondialdehyde concentration was unchanged. Metallothionein content in mucosa was also less in active state of IBD (Mulder et al., 1994).

The antioxidant defence mechanism depends on the concentration of metal elements, which determines enzyme activities. It seems that nutritional supplementation and adequate therapy restore ion homeostasis, although, Zn overdose may cause disturbance in iron metabolism and consequently influences erythrocyte functions (Blázovics et al., 2004a).

Healthy erythrocytes and plasma are rich in antioxidants, although their types of protection differ significantly. The long life erythrocytes have several antioxidant enzymes, vitamins and glutathione, which is the main redox molecule of the cells. The main trace metal elements of erythrocytes are Fe, Cu, Zn and Se. In bowel diseases, the concentrations of these paremeters are significantly low therefore the antioxidant defence system is injured. The circulating erythrocyte is strongly sensitive for oxidative stress and lipid peroxidation (Blázovics et al., 1999, 2000, 2003). In an earlier study, decreased total scavenger capacity (TSC) of plasma and erythrocyte was observed in ulcerative colitis and Crohn's disease, depending on the severity of the illness (Blázovics et al., 1999). H-donor activity and reducing-power were found to change parallel in the plasma and antiparallel with the chemiluminescence intensity. Free SH-group concentration of the plasma was not a significant index for IBD (Blázovics et al., 1999).

Age related normal range of erythrocyte total scavenger capacity was calculated by the remnant chemiluminescent intensity of the measuring system in RLU or RLU%. The range of healthy people was 35 – 60 RLU% (age: 20 – 50 year). 50 – 80 RLU% were the chemiluminescent intensity of the erythrocytes in different severe IBD. 100 ± 10 RLU% was the severe IBD (age independently). The given data are in correlation with the changes of activity of erythrocyte superoxide dismutase and glutathione peroxidase as well as concentrations of plasma reducing power and H-donating ability. The low level of uric acid (UA) in plasma does not favour the erythrocyte antioxidant capacity. High erythrocyte chemiluminescence intensity (EryCL) indicates low antioxidant capacity, therefore haemoglobin (HGB), haematocrit (HTC), C-reactive protein (CRP), HDA and the RP in the plasma change opposite to the free radical intensity. Consequently it may be concluded that total antioxidant capacity was influenced by the parameters mentioned above (Blázovics et al., 2004a). Plasma chemiluminescence studies rather show only momentary improvement in the course of the IBD therapy (Blázovics et al., 1999).

While in the conditions of Crohn-disease and ileum resection, gallbladder formation is frequent, therefore choleretic and cholekinetic Raphacol granule is useful in IBD. The granule is made of a black radish juice, which has antioxidant, scavenger, antiinflammatory and lipid peroxidation decreasing properties. For these, it can minimize the oxidative stress in IBD. The isothiocynates are formed from glucosinolates of black radish and are potent cancer-preventive agents.

It was supported, that polyphenols, flavonoids, isothiocyanates and vitamin (A,C,E) contents of the natural product influence the redox condition of bowel mucose, and through them influence the redox homeostasis of the organism. The bactericid and fungicid properties of the Raphacol granule are also effective in the defence of normal bacterial flora of the bowel. On the basis of these beneficial effects, we were interested in the complement therapeutic application of the granule in IBD. We were curious to know, when its beneficial or side effects would appear. For deciding these questions, we applied some global (spectrophotometric and luminometric) methods to measure the changes of the redox homeostasis in the plasma and erythrocytes. Table 4. shows the significant correlations of redox parameters in the plasma and in the erythrocyte of IBD patients.

Table 4. Significant correlations in IBD

positive correlation		negative correlation	
in blood			
UA–HGB	(r=0.7913; p=0.004)	EryCL–UA	(r=-0.7743; p=0.009)
UA–HCT	(r=0.8332; p=0.001)	EryCL – HGB	(r =-0.8214; p=0.004)
UA–PHDA	(r=0.6328; p=0.020)	EryCL – CRP	(r =-0.8987; p<10^{-4})
UA–PRP	(r=0.6229; p<10^{-4})	EryCL – PHDA	(r =-0.8281; p=0.003)
PFSHG–Na	(r=0.7472; p=0.013)	EryCL –PRP	(r =-0.8942; p<10^{-4})
PHDA– PRP	(r=0.8780; p<10^{-4})	EryCL –HTC	(r =-0.8131; p=0.004)
RBC–HCT	(r=0.6103; p=0.046)	PHDA – TP	(r =-0.5783; p=0.038)
PHDA-K	(r =0.7040; p=0.016)		
CRP = C-reactive protein; EryCL = erythrocyte chemiluminescence; HGB = haemoglobin; HTC = haematocrit; K = potassium; Na = sodium; PFSHG = plasma free SH group; PHDA = plazma H-donating ability; PRP = plasma reducing power; RBC = red blood cell; TP = total protein; UA = uric acid;			

(Blázovics et al., 2004b)

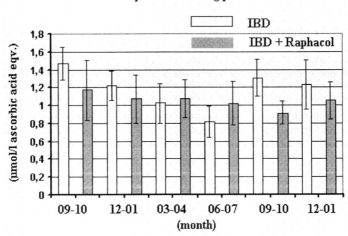

Figure 14.

The plasma reducing power decreased gradually till the 12th month, than after the leaving of Raphacol, the reducing power increased moderaterly (Figure 14.). Figure 15 shows, that the concentration of free SH group increased significantly after the 9th month of supplementary treatment in the plasma, and even after leaving the Raphacol treatment, this high concentration remained. It can be seen in Figure 16, that the H-donating ability from food was the smallest during winter months. H-donating active compounds of Raphacol granule did not cause significant changes.

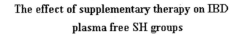

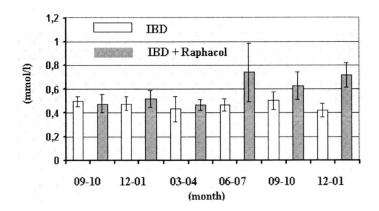

Figure 15.

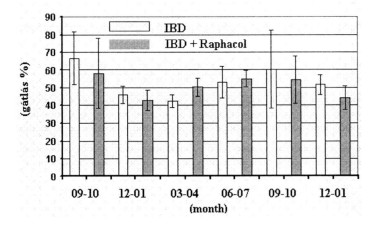

Figure 16.

The chemiluminescence of red blood cells also decreased gradually, although at 12th month the trend was changed so as can be seen in Figure 17. After leaving of Raphacol treatment the scavenger capacity also decreased to the start stay. The level of free radical was elevated during the treatment after the beginning, but the variance was large. After 3 months of the complementary treatment, the starting level was detected. This data of control IBD patients showed the same change, but the variance was moderate (Figure 18.). IL-6 concentration of the plasma was decreased after different changes during the supplementary treatment. After 3 months of ending of treatment the level of this cytokins was lower than that of control IBD patients (Figure 19.). Raphacol treatment caused an unfavourable elevation of the bile acid level in the plasma opposingly the beneficial subjective judge: flatulance, nausea, digestion) (Figure 20).

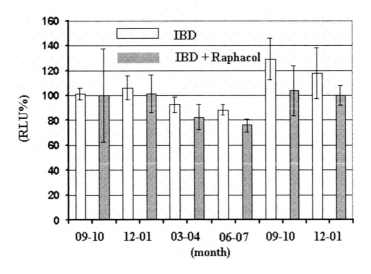

Figure 17.

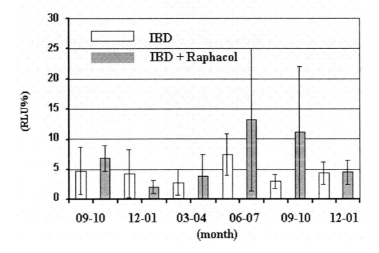

Figure 18.

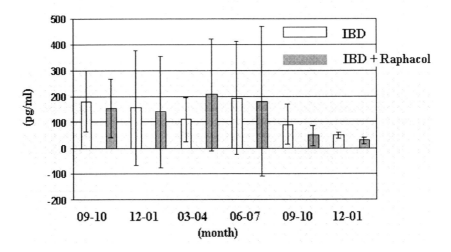

Figure 19.

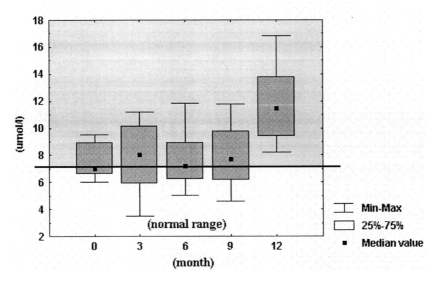

Figure 20.

HbA1c level was reduced from June to October in the red blood cells (Figure 21.). After the third mounth of the treatment, this positive change became unassured.

As a summary, the Raphacol treatment did not influence the activity of IBD. Beside beneficial subjective judgement, bile acid level was elevated continuously and the values of redox parameters were decreased in the plasma during research. The granule diminished the erythrocyte chemiluminescence significantly until the beginning of the ninth month. After this, the trend has changed and stood that way until the end. Data showed, that antioxidant and isothiocyanate-rich granule could influence the redox homeostasis of IBD patients even at a low dose.

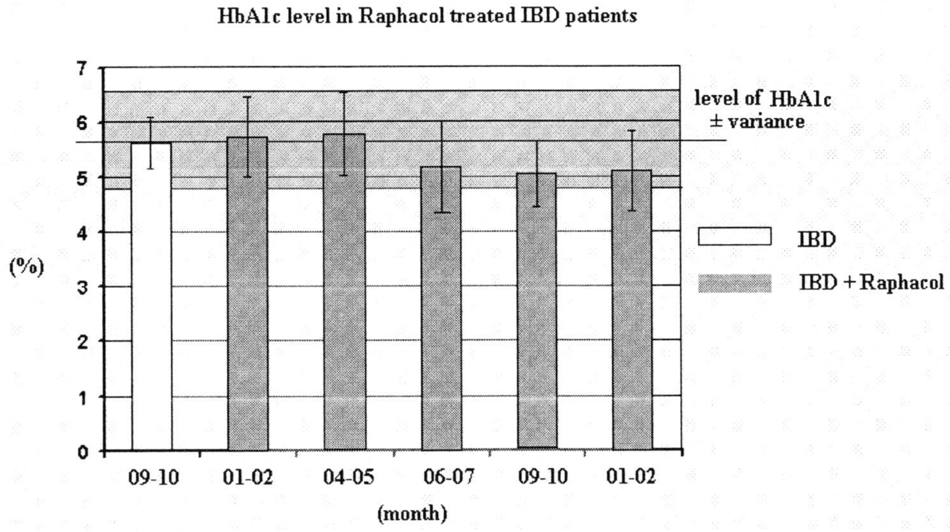

Figure 21.

CONCLUSION

In short term animal experiments e.g. as in alimentary induced bowel disease the high dose of natural antioxidants can act beneficialy. These active components inhibit the free radical induced necrotic processes because of their radical scavenging effect and H-donating property. Natural polyphenols, such as flavonoids modify the PG biosynthesis pathways and cytokine production, therefore influence the lipid metabolism (Blázovics et al., 2004a, Sher et al., 1995).

We supposed that tissues modify the red-ox balance, and compensate the antioxidant overflow in long term antioxidant and/or antioxidant related treatments. Based on the above, the treatments with natural polyphenols and isothiocyanate can modify the redox-homeostasis and should be called as compensatory effects of altered tissues.

According to the mentioned actions and literature, direct and indirect effects of natural antioxidants on the signal transduction process can be assumed (Lunec et al., 2002, Keum et al., 2003, 2004, Azzi et al., 2004, Johnson, 2002, Gebhardt, 2004).

ACKNOWLEDGEMENTS

Authors express their thanks to Prof. Dr. Ágnes Kéry, Zsolt Pallai and Timea Kurucz for consultations and supportings and to Mrs. Edina Pintér and Mrs. Sarolta Bárkovits for their excellent technical assistances. Researches were supported by NKFP 1/016, 1B/047, OTKA

T-043537 and ETT 002/2003, 012/2006 Projects. Raphacol granule was a gift from the Parma Product Company, Budapest.

REFERENCES

Abram, V. & Donko, M. (1999). Tentative identification of polyphenols in *Sempervivum tectorum* and assessment of the antimicrobial activity of *Sempervivum* L. *J Agric Food Chem, 47.* 485-489.

Ahmad, N., Gupta, S. & Mukhtar, H. (2000). Green tea polyphenol epigallocatechin-3-gallate differentially modulates nuclear factor-∎B in cancer cells versus normal cells. *Arch Biochem Biophys, 376.* 338-346.

Azzi, A., Gysin, R., Kempná, P., Munteanu, A., Villacorta, L., Visarius, T. & Zingg, J.M. (2004). Regulation of gene ecpression by alpha tocopherol. *Biol Chem, 385.* 585-591.

Barcelo, S., Gardiner, J. M., Gescher, A. & Chipman, J. K. (1996). CYP2E1-mediated mechanism of anti-genotoxicity of the broccoli constituent sulforaphane. *Carcinogenesis, 17.* 277-282.

Bertók, L. (1998). Bakteriális endotoxinok és hatásaik. /Bakterial endotoxins and their effects./ Orvosi Hetilap /*Hungarian Medicinal Journal/, 139.* 1947-1953.

Bhaska, L., Ramakrishna, B.S. & Balasubramanian, K.A. (1995). Colonic mucosal antioxidant enzymes and lipid peroxide levels in normal subjects and patients with ulcerative colitis. *J Gastroenterol Hepatol, 10.* 140-143.

Blaschek, W., Hansel, R., Keller, K., Reichlig, J., Rimpler, H. & Schneider, G. (1998). (Hrsg). *Hagers Handbuch,* Drogen L-Z, Springer, 535-539.

Blázovics, A., Fehér, E., Kéry, Á., Petry, G. & Fehér, J. (1993a). Liver protecting and lipid lowering effects of *Sempervivum tectorum* in the rats. *Phytotherapy Research, 7.* 98-100.

Blázovics, A., González–Cabello, R., Barta, I., Gergely, P. & Fehér, J. (1994). Effect of liver-protecting *Sempervivum tectorum* extract on the immune reactivity of spleen cells in hyperlipidemic rats. *Phytotherapy Research, 8.* 33-37.

Blázovics, A., Fehér, E. & Fehér, J. (1992). Role of free radical reactions in experimental hyperlipidemia in the pathomechanism of fatty liver, In. *Free Radicals and Liver,* Spinger-Verlag, Berlin, 98-126.

A., Kovács, Á., Lugasi, A., Hagymási, K., Bíró, L. & Fehér, J. (1999). Antioxidant defence in erythrocytes and plasma of patients with active and quiescent Crohn's disease and ulcerative colitis. A chemiluminescent study. *Clin Chem, 45.* 895-896.

Blázovics, A., Lugasi, A., Hagymási, K., Szentmihályi, K. & Kéry, A. (2002). Natural antioxidants and tissue regeneration; Curative effect and reaction mechanism, In. *Phytochemistry and Pharmacology. Vol. 8.* SCI TECH Publishing LLC, Texas, USA, 93-134.

Blázovics, A., Lugasi, A., Kemény, T., Hagymási, K. & Kéry, Á. (2000). Membrane stabilizing effects of natural polyphenols and flavonoids from S. tectorum on hepatic microsomal P450 system in hyperlipidemic rats. *J Ethnopharmacology, 73.* 479-485.

Blázovics, A., Lugasi, A., Szentmihályi, K. & Kéry, A. (2003). Reducing power of the natural polyphenols of Sempervivum tectorum in vitro and in vivo. *Acta Biologica Szegediensis, 47.* 99-102.

Blázovics, A., Prónai, L., Kéry, Á., Petri, G. & Fehér, J. (1993b). Natural antioxidant extract from Sempervivum tectorum. *Phytotherapy Research, 7.* 95-97.

Blázovics, A., Sipos, P., Örsi, F. & Abdel Rahman, M. (2005). Ambivalent property of bilirubin in human bile juice, *Egypt J Hosp Med, 18.* 66-72.

Blázovics, A., Szentmihályi, K., Prónai, L., Hagymási, K., Lugasi, A., Kovács, Á. & Fehér J. (2004a). Redox-homeosztázis gyulladásos bélbetegségekben. *Orvosi Hetilap, 28.* 1459-1466.

Blázovics, A., Szentmihályi, K., Vinkler, P. & Kovács, Á. (2004b). Zn overdose may cause disturbance in the iron metabolism. *Trace Elem Electrol, 21.* 240-247.

Bremnes, L. (1994). Herbs, Dorling Kindersley Ltd. London

Buffinton, G.D. &   Doe, W.F. (1995). Depleted mucosal antioxidant defenses in inflammatory bowel disease. *Free Radic Biol Med, 19.* 911-918.

Buffinton, G.D. & Doe, W.F. (1995). Altered ascorbic acid status in the mucosa from inflammatory bowel disease patients. *Free Radic Res, 22.* 131-43.

Ciska, E., Piskula, M., Waszczuk, K. & Kozlowska, H. (1994). Glucosinolates in Cruciferous vegetables grown in Poland. In. Kozlowska, H., Fornal, J. & Zdunczyk, Z. Bioactive substances in food of plant origin. Polish Academy of Science, Olsztyn, 36-39.

Conaway, C. C., Yang, Y. & Chung, F-L. (2002). Isothiocyanates as cancer chemopreventive agents. their biological activities and metabolism in rodents and humans. *Curr Drug Metab 3.* 233–255.

Coon, P.F., Lambert, C., Land, E. J., Schalch, W. & Truscott, T.G. (1992). Carotene-oxygene radical interactions. *Free Radical Res Comm, 16.* 401-408.

D'Odorico, A., Bortolan, S., Cardin, R., D'Inca, R., Martines, D., Ferronato A. & Sturniolo, G.C. (2001). Reduced plasma antioxidant concentrations and increased oxidative DNA damage in inflammatory bowel disease. *Scand J Gastroenterol, 36.* 1289-1294.

Fahey, J. W., Zalcmann, A. T. & Talalay, P. (2001). The chemical diversity and distribution of glucosinolates and isothiocyanates among plants. *Phytochemistry, 56.* 5 –51.

Fehér, J., Blázovics, A., Gonzalez-Cabello, R., Horváth, M.É. & Grergely, P. (1996). Effects of silibinin and vitamin-E on lipid peroxidation and cellular immunoreactivity in experimentally induced fatty liver of rats. *Med Sci Monit, 2.* 397-403.

Fehér, E., Blázovics, A., Horváth, É.M., Kéry, Á., Petry, G. & Fehér, J. (1992). Effect of *Sempervivum tectorum* extract in the experimental hyperlipidemia and alcoholism. A histological study in the liver and jejunum, In. *Role of Free Radicals in Biological Systems*. Akadémiai Kiadó, Budapest, 45-57.

Fehér, J., Lengyel, G. & Blázovics, A. (1998). Oxidative stress in the liver and biliary tract diseases. *Scand J Gastroenterol, 33. Suppl.*, 228-238.

Fenwick, G. R., Heaney, R. K. & Mullin, W. J. (1983). Glucosinolates and their breakdown products in food and food plants. *CRC Crit Rev Food Sci Nutr, 18.* 123– 201.

Fowke, J. H., Chung, F.L., Jin, F., Qi, D., Cai, Q., Conaway, C. C., Cheng, J-R, Shu, X.O., Gao, Z-T. & Zhang, W. (2003). Urinary isothiocyanate levels, brassica, and human breast cancer. *Cancer Res, 63.* 3980– 3986.

Gebhardt, R. Differential inhibition of protein kinases and matrix metalloproteinases by natural flavonoids, a general survey. COST 926 Meeting Budapest, 2004.

Gerhauser, C., You, M., Liu, J., Moriarty, R. M., Hawthorne, M., Mehta, R. G., Moon, R. C. & Pezzuto, J. M. (1997). Cancer chemopreventive potential of sulforamate, a novel analogue of sulforaphane that induces phase II drug-metabolizing enzymes. *Cancer Res, 57.* 272-278.

Getahun, S.M. & Chung, F.L. (1999). Conversion of glucosinolates to isothiocyanates in humans after ingestion of cooked watercress. *Cancer Epidemiol Biomark Prev, 8.* 447–451.

György, I., Antus, S., Blázovics, A. & Földiák, G. (1992). Substituent effects in the free radical reactions of silybin radiation-induced oxidation of the flavonoid at neutral pH. *Int J Radiat Biol, 61.* 603-609.

Habtemariam, S. (1997). Flavonoids as inhibitors or enhancers of the cytotoxicity of tunor necrosis factor alpha in L-929 tumor cells. *J Nat Prod, 60.* 775-778.

Hänsel, R. (1985). Pflanzliche Cholagoga. *Deutsche Apotheker Zeitung, 125.* 1373-1378.

Hatano, T., Kagawa, H., Yasuhara, T. & Okuda, T. (1988). Two new flavonoids and other constituents in licore root, their relative astringency and radical scavenging effects. *Chem Pharm Bull. 36,* 2090-2097.

Hecht, S. S. (2000). Inhibition of carcinogenesis by isothiocyanates. *Drug Metab Rev, 32.* 395–411.

Hertervig, E., Nilsson, A. & Seidegard, J. (1994). The expression of glutathione transferase mu in patients with inflammatory bowel disease. *Scand J Gastroenterol, 29.* 729-735.

Hollman, P.C.H. (1997). Bioavailability of flavonoids, *Eur J Clin Nutr, 51.* S66-S69.

Ivanovics, G. & Horvath S. (1947). Raphanin, an antibacterial principle of the radish (*Raphanus sativus*). *Nature, 160.* 297-298.

Jakobey, H., Habegger, R. & Fritz, D. (1988). Gemüse als Arzneipflanze. Sekundere Pflanzenstoffe im Gemüse mit Bedeutung für die menschliche Gesundheit. 2. Mitteilung. Gemüse aus der Familie der Brassicaceae und der Familie der Apiacae, *Ernährungs-Umschau, 35.* 275-279.

Jeong, W. S., Kim, I. W., Hu, R. & Kong, A. N. (2004). Modulation of AP-1 by natural chemopreventive compounds in human colon HT-29 cancer cell line. *Pharm Res. 21.* 649–660.

Johnson, I.T. (2002). Anticarcinogenic effects of diet-related apoptosis in the colorectal mucosa. *Food Chem Toxicol, 40.* 1170-1178.

Kandaswami, C. & Middleton, E. (1997). Flavonoids as antioxidants. In. Shahidi, F. Natural Antioxidants. *Chemistry, Health effects and Application.* AOCS Press, Champaign, IL, 182-203.

Kassie, F. & Knasmüller, S. (2000). Genotoxic effects of allyl isothiocyanate (AITC). and phenethyl isothiocyanate (PEITC). *Chem Biol Interact, 127.* 163–180.

Kéry, Á., Blázovics, A., Rozlosnik, N. & Fehér, J. (1992). Antioxidative properties of extracts from Sempervivum tectorum, *Planta Medica Suppl, 58.* 1. A661-A662,

Keum, Y-S., Jeong, W-S. & Kong, A. N. T. (2004). Chemoprevention by isothiocyanates and their underlying molecular signaling mechanisms. *Mutation Res, 555.* 191–202.

Keum, Y. S., Owuor, E. D., Kim, B. R., Hu R. & Kong A. N. (2003). Involvement of Nrf2 and JNK1 in the activation of antioxidant responsive element (ARE). by chemopreventive agent phenethyl isothiocyanate (PEITC). *Pharm Res, 20.* 1351–1356.

Kim, J.H., Choi, J.J., Noh, SH., Roh, J.K., Min, J.S., Youn, J.K., Yoo, N.C., Lim, H.Y., Carbone, D.P., Gazdar, A.F. & et al., (1993). Comparison of p53 gene mutations in paired primary and metastatic gastric tumor tissues. *J. Korean Med Sci, 8.* 187-191.

Kocsis, I., Lugasi, A., Hagymási, K., Kéry, Á., Fehér, J., Szőke, É. & Blázovics, A. (2002). Beneficial properties of black radish root (*Raphanus sativus* L. var. *niger*). squeezed juice in hyperlipidemic rats. Biochemical and chemiluminescence measurements. *Acta Alim Hung, 31.* 185-190.

Kong, A.N.T., Yu, R., Lei, W., Mandlekar, S., Tan, T.H. & Ucker, D.S. (1998). Differential activation of MAPK and ICE/Ced3 protease in chemical-induced apoptosis. The role of oxidative stress in the regulation of mitogen-activated protein kinases (MAPKs) leading to gene expression and survival or activation of caspases leading to apoptosis, *Restor Neurol Neurosci, 2-3.* 63-70.

Lander, H.M., Ogiste, J.S., Teng, K.K. & Novogrodsky, A. (1995). p21ras as a common signaling target of reactive free radicals and cellular redox stress. *J Biol Chem, 270.* 21195- 21198.

Lee, J.H., Abraham, S.C., Kim, H.S., Nam, J.H., Choi, C., Lee, M.C., Park, C.S., Juhng, S.W., Rashid, A., Hamilton S.R. & Wu, T.T. (2002). Inverse Relationship between *APC* Gene Mutation in Gastric Adenomas and Development of Adenocarcinoma. *Am J Pathol, 161.* 611-618.

Lin, S.Y., Chen, P.H., Yang, M.J., Chen T.C., Chang C.P. & Chang J.G. (1995). Ras oncogene and p53 gene hotspot mutations in colorectal cancers. *J Gastroenterol Hepatol, 10.* 119-124.

London, S. J., Yuan, J.M., Chung, F.L., Gao, Y.T., Coetzee, G. A., Ross, R. K. & Yu, M. C. (2000). Isothiocyanates, glutathione S-transferase M1 and T1 polymorphisms, and lung-cancer risk, a prospective study of men in Shanghai, China. *Lancet, 356.* 724– 729.

Lowry, A.H., Rosenbrough, N.J., Farr, A.L. & Randall, R.J. (1951). Protein measurement with the Folin-phenol reagents. *J Biol Chem, 193.* 265-275.

Lugasi, A. (2000a). Az élelmiszer eredetű flavonoidok potenciális egészségvédő hatása, Orvosi Hetilap/*Hungarian Medicinal Journal/, 141.* 1751-1761.

Lugasi, A. (2001). Thesis of Ph.D. Semmelweis University, Faculty of Medicine, Budapest, Hungary

Lugasi, A., Blázovics, A., Fehér, E., Szaleczky, E., Dworschák, E. & Fehér, J. (1996). Effect of lipid rich diet on free radical reactions of intestine in rats. *Z. Gastroenterol, 34.* 321.

Lugasi, A., Blázovics, A., Hagymási, K., Kocsis, I. & Kéry Á. (2005). Antioxidant effect of squized juice from black radish (*Raphanus sativus* L. var. niger). in alimentary hyperlipidaemia in rats. *Phytother Res, 19.* 587-591.

Lugasi, A., Blázovics, A., Kéry, Á., Kocsis, I., Kassai-Farkas, S. & Horváth, T. (2000). A fekete retek hatóanyagú *Raphacol* epegranulátum hatása cukorbetegek szérum paramétereire. (Effect of *Raphacol* bile-garnule containing black radish on serum parameters of diabetic patients). *Fitoterápia, 5.* 72-77.

Lugasi, A., Blázovics, A., Kéry, Á., Kocsis, I., Kassai-Farkas, S. & Horváth, T. (2001). A fekete retek hatóanyagú *Raphacol* epegranulátum hatása cukorbetegek lipidperoxidációs paramétereire. (Effect of *Raphacol* bile-garnule containing black radish on lipid peroxidation parameters of diabetic patients). *Fitoterápia, 6.* 12-18.

Lugasi, A., Blázovics, A., Lebovics, V. K., Kocsis, I. & Kéry, Á. (2002). Beneficial health effect of black radish and in vivo experimental conditions. In. *Phytochemistry and Pharmacology. Vol. 2.* SCI TECH Publishing LLC, Texas, USA, 365-375.

Lugasi, A., Dworschák, E., Blázovics, A. & Kéry, Á. (1998). Antioxidant and free radical scavenging properties of squeezed juice from black radish (*Raphanus sativus* L. var niger). root. *Phytother Res, 12.* 502-506.

Lugasi, A., Lebovics, V. K., Kocsis, I., Hagymási, K. & Blázovics A. (1999). Black radish juice modifies the cholesterol metabolism in animal experiment. Z. *Gastroenterol, 37.* 431.

Lunec, J., Holloway, K.A., Cooke, M.S., Faux, S., Griffits, H.R. & Evans, M.D. (2002). Urinary 8-oxo-2'-deoxyguanosine. Redox regulation of DNA repair in vivo. *Free Rad Biol Med, 33.* 875-85.

Lutomski, J. & Speichert, H. (1982). Black radish as a source of various phytopharmaceuticals. *Pharm Unserer Zeit, 11.* 151-155.

Manach, C., Morand, C., Demigné, C., Demigne, C. & Texier, O. (1997). Bioavailability of rutin and quercetin in rats. *FEBS Letter, 409.* 12-16.

Masude, T., Isobe, J., Jitoe, A. & Nakatani, N. (1992). Antioxidative curcuminoids from rhizomes of Curcuma xanthorrhiza. *Phytochemistry, 31.* 3645-3647.

McCord, J. M. & Fridovich, I. (1968). The reduction of cytochrome c by milk xanthine oxidase. *J Biol Chem, 243.* 5753-5760.

McKenzie, S.J., Baker, M.S., Buffinton, G.D., & Doe, W.P. (1996). Evidence of oxidant-induced injury to epithelial cells during inflammatory bowel disease. *J Clin Invest, 98.* 136-41.

Meyer, M., Schreck, R. & Baeuerle, P.A. (1993). H_2O_2 and antioxidants have opposite effects on activation of NF-□B and AP-1 in intact cells. AP-1 as secondary antioxidant responsive factor. *EMBO J, 12.* 2005-2015.

Miller N. J., Rice-Evans, C., Davies, M. J., Gopinathan, V. & Milner, A. (1993). A novel method for measuring antioxidant capacity and its application to monitoring the antioxidant status in premature neonates. *Clin Sci, 84.* 407-412.

Morel. Y. & Barouki, R. (1999). Repression of gene expression by oxidative stress. *Biochem J, 342.* 481-86.

Mózsik, G., Bodis, B., Figler, M., Király, A., Karádi, O., Par, A., Rumi, G., Sütõ, G., Tóth, G., & Vincze, A. (2001). Mechanisms of action of retinoids in gastrointestinal mucosal protection in animals, human healthy subjects and patients. *Life Sci, 69.* 3103-12.

Mulder, T.P., van der Sluys Veer A., Verspaget, H.W., Griffioen, G., Pena, A.S., Janssens, A.R. & Lamers, C.B. (1994). Effect of oral zinc supplementation on metallothionein and superoxide dismutase concentrations in patients with inflammatory bowel disease. *J Gastroenterol Hepatol, 9.* 472-77.

Nguyen, T., Sherratt, P. J. & Pickett, C. B. (2003). Regulatory mechanisms controlling gene expression mediated by the antioxidant response element. *Ann Rev Pharmacol Toxicol, 43.* 233–260.

Nielsen, O.H. & Rask-Madsen, J. (1996). Mediators of inflammation in chronic inflammatory bowel disease. *Scand J Gastroent Suppl, 216.* 149-59.

Oyaizu, M. (1986). Studies on products of browning reaction prepared from glucosamine. *Jpn J Nutr, 44.* 307-315.

Pahlow, M. (1989). *Heilpflanze heute.* Grafe und Unzer GmbH, München, 249.

Penso G. (1982). *Index Plantanum Medicinalium,* O.E.M.F. Milano, p. 872.

Polya G.M., Polya Z. & Kweifio-Okai G. (2002). Biochemical pharmacology of anti-inflammatory plant secondary metabolites, In. *Recent Progress in Medicinal Plants Vol. 8.* SCI TECH Publishing, LLC, Texas, USA, 1-22.

Popovic, M., Lukic, V., Jakovlevic, V. & Mikov, M. (1993). The effect of the radish (Raphanus sativus ssp. niger). juice on liver function. *Fitoterapia, 64.* 229-231.

Powis, G., Gasdanska, J.R. & Baker A. (1997). Redox signalling and the control of cell growth and death. *Adv Pharmacol, 38.* 329-58.

Ramarathnam, N., Ochi, H., & Takeuchi, M. (1997). Antioxidant defense system in vegetable extracts. In. Shahidi, F. Natural Antioxidants. *Chemistry, Health effects and Application.* AOCS Press, Champaign, IL, 76-87.

Ritter, U. (1984). Therapie mit Choleretika and Cholekinetika. *Med Monatsch Pharmacol, 7.* 99-104.

Sakagami, H., Jiang, Y., Kusama, K., Atsumi, T., Ueha, T., Toguchi, M., Iwakura, I., Satoh, K., Ito, H., Hatano, T. & Yoshida, T. (2000). Cytotoxic activity of hydrolysable tannins against human oral tumor cell lines. A possible mechanism. *Phytomed, 7.* 39- 47.

Sedlak, J. & Lindsay, R.H. (1985). Estimation of total protein bound and non protein sulfhydryl groups in tissues with Ellmann's reagent. *Anal Biochem Biophys, 25.* 192-205.

Seymour, I., Schwartz I., Shires, G.T., Spencer, F.C. & Husser, W.C. (1989). *Principles of surgery,* McGraw-Hill Inc, New York, 1270.

Schulze-Osthoff, K., Ferrari, D., Riehemann, K. & Wesselborg, S. (1997). Regulation of NF-κB activation by MAP kinase cascades. *Immunbiol, 198.* 35-49.

Sher, M.E., D'Angelo, A.J., Stein, T.A., Bailey, B., Burns, G. & Wise, L. (1995). Cytokines in Crohn's colitis. *Am J Surg, 169.* 133-36.

Shimada, K., Fujikawa, K., Yahara, K. & Nakamura T. (1992). Antioxidant properties of xanthan on the autoxidation of soybean oil in cyclodextrin emulsion, *J Agric Food Chem, 40,* 945-948.

Sipos, P., Hagymási, K., Lugasi, A., Fehér, E. & Blázovics, A. (2002). Effect of black radish root *(Raphanus sativus* L. var niger). on the colon mucosa in rats fed a fat rich diet. *Phytother Res, 16.* 677-679.

Sipos, P., Hagymási, K., Lugasi, A., Fehér, E., Örsi, F. & Blázovics A. (2001). Direct effect of bile colon mucosa in alimentary induced hyperlipidemy in rats, *Acta Alimentaria, 1,* 25-35.

Stevens, J., Hart, H., Elema, E.T. & Bolck A. (1996). Flavonoid variation in Eurasian *Sedum* and *Sempervivum. Phytochemistry, 41.* 503-512.

Szentmihályi, K., Blázovics, A., Lugasi, A., Kéry, Á., Lakatos, B. & Vinkler P. (2000). Effect of natural polyphenol-type antioxidants (*Sempervivum tectorum* and *Raphanus sativus* L. var. niger extracts). on metal ion concentrations in rat bile fluid. *Curr Topics Biophys, 24(2).* 203-207.

Tarr, F. (2002). *A flavonoidok.* /Flavonoids/, Nyíregyháza-Debrecen, ISSBN. N0 9636409765, 1-214.

Tragnone, A., Valpiani, D., Miglio, F., Elmi, G., Bazzocchi, G., Pipitone, E. & Lafranchi G. A. (1995). Dietary habits as risk factors for inflammatory bowel disease. *Eur J Gastroenterol Hepatol, 7.* 47-51.

Young, M. R., Yang, H. S. & Colburn, N. H. (2003). Promising molecular targets for cancer prevention. AP-1, NF-kappa B and Pdcd4. *Trends Mol Med, 9.* 36–41.

Yu, R., Mandlekar, S., Harvey, K. J., Ucker, D. S. & Kong, A. N. (1998). Chemopreventive isothiocyanates induce apoptosis and caspase-3-like protease activity. *Cancer Res, 58.* 402–408.

Yuting, C., Rongliang, Z., Zhonghan, J. & Yong, J. (1990). Flavonoids as superoxide scavengers and antioxidants. *Free Rad Biol Med, 9.* 19-21

Vargas, R., Perez, R. M., Perez, S., Zavala, M. A. & Perez, C. (1999). Antiurolithiatic activity of Raphanus sativus aqueous extract on rats. *J Ethnopharmacol, 68.* 335-38.

Wallace, M.H., & Phillips, R.K.S. Upper gastrointestinal disease in patients with familial adenomatous polyposis. *Br J Surg, 85.*742-750.

Weiss, R. F. (1985). *Lehrbuch der Phytotherapie. 4.* Auflage. Hippokrates-Verlag, Stuttgart, 125.

Zhang Y. (2004). Cancer-preventive isothiocyanates. measurement of human exposure and mechanism of action. *Mutat Res, 555.* 173–190.

Zhang, Y. & Gordon, G. B. (2004). A strategy for cancer prevention. stimulation of the Nrf2-ARE signaling pathway. *Mol Cancer Ther, 3.* 885–893.

Zhang, Y., Kensler, T. W., Cho, C. G., Posner, G. H. & Talalay, P. (1994). Anticarcinogenic activities of sulforaphane and structurally related synthetic norbornyl isothiocyanates. *Proc Natl Acad Sci USA, 91.* 3147-3150.

Zhang, Y., Li, J. & Tang, L. (2005). Cancer-preventive isothiocyanates. dichotomous modulators of oxidative stress. *Free Rad Biol Med, 38.* 70-77.

Zhang, Y. & Talalay, P. (1994). Anticarcinogenic activities of organic isothiocyanates. chemistry and mechanism. *Cancer Res, 54S.* 1976S-1981S.

Zhao, B., Seow, A., Lee, E. J. D., Poh, W.T., Teh, M., Eng, P., Wang, Y.T., Tan, W.C., Yu, M. C. & Lee, H-P. (2001). Dietary isothiocyanates, glutathione S-transferase-M1, -T1 polymorphisms and lung cancer risk among Chinese women in Singapore. *Cancer Epidemiol Biomark Prev 10.* 1063– 1067.

Zingg, J.M. & Azzi A. (2004). Non-antioxidant activities of vitamin E, *Current Medicinal Chemistry, 11.* 1113-1133.

In: Nutrition Research Advances
Editor: Sarah V. Watkins, pp. 137-160

ISBN 1-60021-516-5
© 2007 Nova Science Publishers, Inc.

Chapter V

METABOLIC/NUTRITION PROGRAMMING OF ENZYME SYSTEMS OF DIGESTIVE AND NON-DIGESTIVE ORGANS

N. M. Timofeeva, V. V. Egorova and A. A. Nikitina

Laboratory of Physiology of Nutrition, Pavlov Institute of Physiology, Russian Academy of Sciences, St. Petersburg, Russia.

ABSTRACT

We have found that the quality of nutrition during pregnancy, lactation or early ontogeny induces changes in a functioning of enzyme systems of the digestive and non-digestive organs in the adult rat posterities not only of the first generation, but also of the subsequent ones. These researches develop the ideas of academician A.M. Ugolev – a discoverer of the membrane digestion. It has been shown that protein deficiency in nutrition of pregnant or lactating rats results in significant reduction of activities of some digestive enzymes in the small intestine, and of the same enzymes in the large intestine, liver and kidney in the rat posterities of 2- and 4-months old. Activities of the enzymes in the rat posterities of 6-months old do not restore their levels in control animals, receiving a standard diet during the development. Various changes of enzymes activities in the digestive and non-digestive organs take also place in the adult posterities of the second (and the third) generations, born by rats, whose "mothers" (and "grandmothers") received a low protein diet during pregnancy or lactation. The protein excess in the diet of the lactating rats results in significant reduction of activities of the digestive enzymes in the small intestine and of the same enzymes in the large intestine, the liver and kidney in the posterities of 2- and 6-months old. On the contrary, an increase of the enzymes activities has been observed in the posterities of 4-months old. A restriction of protein in the diet of rat pups during their transition from the mixed to the definitive nutrition leads to increase of activities of some enzymes and to decrease some other ones in adult life of the rat pups and in adult life of their posterities. It has been concluded that such a stress factor, as deficiency or excess of the protein in nutrition of animals during pregnancy or lactation, and in early ontogeny as well, results in disorders of formation of enzyme systems in the digestive and non-digestive organs and in changes of their functioning in adult life of themselves and in adult life of their posterities. These processes seem to realize at genetic or epigenetic levels. The epigenetic phenomena may involve the altered packaging and activation of a variety of the genes. The unfavorable early nutrition programming of enzymatic systems of the digestive and non-digestive organs may be a key event in the disorders of various metabolic reactions, therefore promoting a development of chronic diseases.

INTRODUCTION

At present, much attention has been paid to the rapidly developing problem of the "early metabolic/nutrition programming". According to this problem, alimentary effects on maternal organism at critical periods of the prenatal (pregnancy) and early postnatal development (lactation) of offspring determine its health not only in early ontogenesis, but also during the adulthood and even determine health of subsequent generations. It is before birth and at early periods after it that structural and functional characteristics of organs and systems are being formed [1-6]. Studies on this subject are of great importance, particularly when taking into consideration the problem of balanced nutrition. Life at all levels of its organization is associated with expenditure of substances and energy. Therefore, the necessary condition of existence of biological systems of any level is the supply from outside of new alimentary substrates providing energy and plastics needs. Effect of disturbances of diet at early stages of human development was revealed several decades ago [7]. It was established that there was a brief period in the rat postnatal life when nutrition manipulations (achieved by altering litter size) produced effects of programming on growth and body size of offspring. Subsequent numerous studies on animals showed a pronounced diversity of long programming effects on metabolism, arterial pressure, diabetes, obesity, atherosclerosis, behavior and learning as well as on lifespan [8-16].

Many authors studied effects of quality of maternal nutrition during pregnancy or lactation on growth and size as well as on functions of various organs of offspring in early ontogenesis and adulthood. It follows from analysis of the literature data that changes of quality of nutrition during pregnancy, especially of the higher or lower ratio of proteins to carbohydrates seem to lead to disturbances of a number of metabolic reactions, which activates development in the offspring adult life of various diseases [10-14,16-21]. It is obvious that the poor mother's nutrition not only prevents normal development of fetus, but "programs" a child to the appearance of various chronic diseases in the adult life due to irreversible alterations in pancreas, liver, kidney, cardiovascular system, and other organs. D.J.P. Barker states that conditions of intrauterine development produce their effect not in the early life period, but beginning from the age of 50. It is the conditions of intrauterine life for 9 months, which determine decades later the greater or lower probability of heart attacks, diabetes, and chronic high arterial pressure [22]. A particular role is played by alimentary proteins. Protein deficit has been known to be widely spread among the globe population. It can be produced by protein starvation, chronic diseases producing it, pregnancy toxicoses, medicament treatment that can be accompanied by loss of appetite or disturbances of alimentary substrate assimilation [3-20, 23-27].

It has been shown that in rats on a low-protein diet during pregnancy, offspring is born with lower body sizes; during adulthood it has a high blood pressure [28-30]. In pregnant women consuming both a low-protein and a high-carbohydrate diet as well as a diet with the reverse ratio of these components, children were found to have in their future a high arterial blood pressure [15,31]. The offspring was observed to have a low body weight on birth, which is a risk factor for development of cardiovascular diseases, diabetes, and other pathologies.

The child's health is affected by life conditions not only of mother, but also of grandmother at the time when she was pregnant by the future mother. When studying twelve rat generations submitted to protein starvation, a significant mass reduction of the body and a number of visceral organs was established [8]. Recovery of the body and organ sizes as well as of behavior to the level of control animals occurred only after refeeding in three rat generations [9].

Disbalance of nutrition, especially of the protein one, during pre- and postnatal development produces essential morpho-functional alterations in various organs and tissues, including the intestinal one [3,32-34]. It is to be noted that the digestive system is the first to contact alimentary substrates whose splitting leads to formation of carbohydrate, protein, and lipid metabolites able to affect enzyme activities, possibly at the pre- or posttranslation levels. Such processes might have been responsible for a decrease of synthesis of enzyme proteins and for an increase of their degradation or an opposite change of these processes.

Studies of effects of protein deficit and protein rehabilitation on synthesis of lactase phlorizin hydrolase (LPH) have shown that protein malnutrition decreases the LPH synthesis rate by altering posttranslational events, whereas the jejunum responds to rehabilitation by increasing LPH mRNA relative abundance, which suggests pretranslational regulation [35].

Such prerequisites stimulated studies on metabolic programming of enzyme systems of digestive, while later also of some non-digestive organs, during a change of the quality of nutrition (protein deficit or excess) at critical periods of development of offspring (pregnancy, lactation, transition from lactotrophic to definite nutrition) not only in the first generation ("children"), but also in the subsequent ones ("grandchildren", "great-grandchildren"). In our experiments on pregnant and lactating females we used isocaloric diet, but with a 2.5-fold decreased or increased amount of its protein (casein) [33].

PROTEIN DEFICIT IN MATERNAL NUTRITION DURING PREGNANCY AND LACTATION AND INTESTINAL ENZYME ACTIVITIES OF OFFSPRING IN EARLY ONTOGENESIS

We have established that protein deficit in rat nutrition during pregnancy and lactation produces a decrease of activities of membrane and soluble sucrase forms in jejunum and especially in ileum of the 30-day old rat pups, which indicates a retardation of induction of this enzyme synthesis [36]. A delay in maltase induction in jejunum, although less pronounced as compared with sucrase, also was observed. However, the membrane form of this enzyme in jejunum rose markedly (more than 3 times) in the 20- and 30-day old rat pups as compared with the enzyme activity in the rat pups of the corresponding age born by the mothers that were kept on the full-scale ration. This is most likely to be due to substrate regulation of the enzyme activity, since females of the experimental group, on the background of protein deficit, were given an excess of carbohydrates (starch) [37].

Activity of the lactase membrane form fell markedly in the 21-day old rat pups of the experimental group in jejunum, while in the 20-30-day old pups, only in ileum. Changes of the enzyme soluble form were less pronounced. However, the lactase soluble form activity decreased markedly in jejunum and ileum. In the experimental group rat pups there was an earlier formation (as early as in the 20-day old animals) of the "adult" type of distribution of the alkaline phosphatase activity along jejunum, i.e. the activity increased in the proximal and decreased in the distal jejunum parts.

Astonishing was a rise of the membrane form activities of peptide hydrolases (aminopeptidase M and glycyl-L-leucinedipeptidase) in jejunum of the 20-day-old experimental group rat pups, which is paradoxical under conditions of protein deficit in nutrition. Based on the theory of substrate regulation, a reduction of these enzyme activities should have been expected due to a decrease of protein in the maternal ration. However, B.Lonnerdal [38] states that the protein and lactose content of maternal milk are constant regardless of quality of her nutrition reduction. Mammalian milk contains a large set of biologically active substances, trophic factors, hormones (including thyroxin, glucocorticoids, and insulin) [39,40]. These substances produce modulating effects on functional characteristics of jejunal mucosa. The revealed disturbances of the rate of induction of the sucrase and maltase membrane forms and repression of lactase can be explained by a change of levels of glucocorticoids and thyroxin at certain periods of offspring development due to protein deficit in maternal nutrition. An increase of peptidehydrolase activities presumably due to activation of synthesis of enzyme protein is likely to occur at the expense of the maternal organism under conditions of insufficient protein nutrition. It is commonly accepted that changes in the maternal organism are the main ones, determining the success of the fetal development and its further well-being [41]. The lack of a decrease of activities of some intestinal enzymes, which we observed by the 30th day after birth at a transition to the normal nutrition, indicates compensatory-adaptive possibilities of maternal organisms, which are aimed at maintaining homeostasis of the developing fetus [36]. The maternal organism tries to "sacrifice its resources", so that the offspring could survive and become adapted to conditions of the existence in environment, which is of biological significance.

At the same time there is the point of view that in a certain situation it is the fetus that takes over function of the poorly functioning maternal organs. Under these conditions the fetal organs start working prematurely, the mother as if "exploits the fetus" to force its systems to function for preservation of pregnancy. The premature development can also lead to a premature wear of organs at the period of postnatal development, which will certainly produce a negative effect on functioning of organs in the adult life [41,42]. This point of view agrees with the earlier repression of lactase and formation of the adult type of the distribution gradient of the alkaline phosphatase activity, which we observed in the offspring of mothers on the low-protein diet during pregnancy and lactation, as compared with control.

The effect of adverse factors, including protein deficit in maternal nutrition, is known to lead to negative consequences during the offspring development [25,33,34,41,43]. A change of the maternal diet during pregnancy or nursing has been shown to affect negatively ontogenesis of intestine [44]. Pronounced changes in offspring can appear only in the cases when the maternal adaptive reactions turn out to be insufficient. For instance, the low-calory food during the offspring prenatal development inhibits formation of its physiological systems and physical development [23].

CONSEQUENCES OF PROTEIN DEFICIT IN NUTRITION DURING PREGNANCY OR LACTATION FOR FUNCTIONING OF ENZYMES OF DIGESTIVE AND NON-DOGESTIVE ORGANS IN ADULT OFFSPRING

We carried out studies of structural parameters (body mass, the mass of mucosa of various parts of small and large intestines, and the length of small intestine) and of activities of digestive enzymes (maltase, alkaline phosphatase, aminopeptidase M, and glycyl-L-leucinedipeptidase) as well as of the corresponding hydrolases of liver and kidney in the adult offspring (2, 4, and 6 months) whose mothers were for 21 days of pregnancy (the 1st group) or of lactation (the 2nd group) on the 2.5-fold reduced protein ration [33].

In both groups of experimental animals we have revealed changes of structural parameters. In the 2-month old offspring of the 1st group the body mass increased (by 26%), while the length of the small intestine decreased (by 15%). In the 4-month old offspring the mass of duodenal mucosa and of kidney decreased (by 43% and 22%, respectively). In the 6-month old offspring the mass of the body decreased by 28%, of jejunal mucosa by 26%, of colonic mucosa by 43%, of kidney by 25%, and of liver by 37%.

The body mass also changed in the 2nd group offspring: it increased in the 2- and 4-month old rat pups by 61% and 65%, respectively, but decreased by 20% in the 6-month old offspring. In the 2-month old rat pups the kidney mass rose by 35%, while in the 4-month old animals the mass of jejunal mucosa, by 60%. In the 6-month old offspring no changes of the mass of the organs have been revealed.

We also found statistically significant changes of activities of intestinal enzymes, as well as of the same enzymes in liver and kidney (table 1). In the 2-month old rat pups of all experimental groups, activity of maltase decreased markedly in all small intestine parts. In large intestine, the activity was lower in animals of the 1st experimental group than in control animals, whereas it remained unchanged in animals of the 2nd experimental group. In kidney the enzyme activity did not change in rats of the 1st experimental group, but was higher than in control in animals of the 2nd experimental group. In the 4-month old animals of both experimental groups the maltase activity decreased essentially in duodenum, jejunum, ileum, and large intestine as well as in kidney. In the 6-month old rats of the 1st experimental group the maltase activity decreased markedly in each small intestine part and slightly, in the large intestine. In the 6-month old animals of the 2nd experimental group the enzyme activity, on the contrary, decreased essentially in duodenum and kidney and slightly, in jejunum (table 2).

In duodenum of the 2-month old rat pups of both experimental groups the maltase activity decreased to approximately the same degree, while remained unchanged in jejunum and ileum. In large intestine and kidney the enzyme activity decreased only in animals of the 2nd experimental group as compared with the corresponding control. In the 4-month old rats of both experimental groups, activity of alkaline phosphatase decreased statistically significantly in each of the studied organs, the most markedly in all small intestine parts and in large intestine in animals of the 1st experimental group, while in kidney, in rats of the 2nd experimental group. In the 6-month old rats of the 1st experimental group the alkaline phosphatase activity decreased to a significant degree only in large intestine, while in rats of the 2nd experimental group, in duodenum and kidney.

Table 1. Activity (μmol/min per g of protein) of enzymes in the different parts of the small intestine, in colon, kidneys and liver of the 2- and 4-month old rats, whose mothers received a control (C) and a low-protein diets during pregnancy (1) or lactation (2)

Enzymes	Age, month	Group of the rats	Parts of the small intestine			Colon	Kidneys	Liver
			duodenum	jejunum	ileum			
Maltase	2	C	241±28	437±40	388±48	52±7	169±11	2.1±0.9
		1	149±19*	309±29*	227±24*	33±2*	133±19	23±5*
		2	161±4*	366±4	305±3	50±5	239±18*	7.4±0.7*
	4	C	301±35	547±65	681±83	71±8	235±37	10±2
		1	129±9*	239±14*	248±12*	50±2*	53±6*	14±3
		2	136±16*	271±39*	275±17*	50±3*	113±24*	11±3
Alkaline phosphatase	2	C	178±10	98±15	15±2	12±2	18±1	2±0.2
		1	103±12*	76±16	19±4	8±1	9±2*	1±0.2*
		2	102±14*	77±7	12±3	10±2	24±1*	2±0.1
	4	C	165±14	80±21	36±6	14±2	29±3	2±0.5
		1	74±12*	50±2	10±0.6*	5±0.4*	17±2*	0.8±0.07*
		2	86±23*	67±13	23±8	8±1*	11±2*	0.6±0.1*
Aminopep-tidase M	2	C	47±8	114±22	73±13	25±5	140±18	14±2
		1	15±5*	60±7*	47±11	11±0.8*	67±16*	7±2*
		2	18±6*	48±8*	38±5*	10±1*	130±4	16±2
	4	C	50±7	112±11	123±15	35±7	129±12	21±2
		1	15±3*	49±5*	52±13*	7±2*	63±11*	3±0.6*
		2	17±4*	49±4*	54±3*	7±1*	85±10*	7±2*
Glycyl-L-leucine-dipeptidase	2	C	370±70	860±150	740±70	290±20	610±130	240±20
		1	390±110	1480±200*	1140±95*	420±50*	900±200	570±120*
		2	270±40	900±100	1180±110*	470±75*	1470±260*	530±100*
	4	C	580±80	1610±190	1760±210	690±70	1520±150	560±60
		1	130±40*	370±10*	500±120*	260±60*	420±170*	130±60*
		2	410±110	610±20*	470±140*	410±75*	590±150*	250±40*

*- p<0.05 in comparison with control

In each of the studied organs in rats of both experimental groups, activity of aminopeptidase M decreased statistically significantly, except for liver and kidney in which this activity did not change in rats of the 2nd experimental group as compared with control animals. This decrease was also similar in duodenum and jejunum in the 2- and 4-month old rats of both experimental groups. In ileum, colon, kidney, and liver this decrease of the enzyme activity was more pronounced in the 4-month than in the 2-month old rats of both experimental groups. In the 6-month old rats of the 1st experimental group the aminopeptidase M activity decreased markedly in duodenum, kidney, and liver, but slightly increased in jejunum. In rats of the 2nd experimental group the enzyme activity decreased significantly in duodenum and jejunum and to a lesser degree in kidney.

Table 2. Activity (μmol/min per g of protein) of enzymes in the different parts of the small intestine, in colon, kidneys and liver of the 6-month old rats, whose mothers received a control (C) an a low-protein diets during pregnancy (1) or lactation (2)

Enzymes	Group of the rats	Duodenum	Jejunum	Ileum	Colon	Kidneys	Liver
Maltase	C	390±51	684±15	428±46	51±1	198±16	24±4
	1	699±71*	1383±71*	814±74*	65±6*	184±14	22±3
	2	138±1*	355±6*	343±41	49±1	96±7*	6±1*
Alkaline phosphatase	C	184±26	99±20	24±6	6±0.4	30±1	1.4±0.2
	1	135±16	110±12	15±2	4±0.6*	26±2	1±0.2
	2	55±5*	60±9	18±3	12±1*	9±0.3*	1±0.3
Aminopeptidase M	C	48±4	76±7	80±9	14±4	164±15	15±3
	1	29±4*	95±4*	90±7	8±2	118±7*	7±1*
	2	20±7*	48±3*	45±6*	15±2	83±6*	6±0.2*
Glycyl-L-leucine-dipeptidase	C	158±20	381±70	488±82	155±18	10912±62	168±13
	1	178±31	454±34	865±80*	137±10	676±94*	201±28
	2	62±11*	157±16*	393±35	164±13	470±30*	122±11*

* - $p < 0.05$ in comparison with control

Changes of glycyl-L-leucinedipeptidase activity in the 2- and 4-month old rats of experimental groups were different. In duodenum of the 2-month old rats of all experimental groups the activity was the same as in control animals; in jejunum the activity rose in rats of the 1st experimental group, in ileum and colon in rats of both experimental groups, in kidney in rats of the 2nd and in liver in rats of the 1st and 2nd experimental groups. In the 4-month old animals of all experimental groups, activity of glycyl-L-leucinedipeptidase decreased statistically significantly in all studied organs. The most pronounced was a decrease of this enzyme in organs of rats of the 1st experimental group. In the 6-month old rats of the 1st experimental group this enzyme activity increased markedly in ileum and decreased considerably in kidney. In rats of the 2nd experimental group, the glycyl-L-leucinedipeptidase activity decreased markedly in duodenum, jejunum, kidney, and liver.

Thus, in the experimental animals there occurred changes of structural parameters and as a rule an essential decrease of digestive enzyme activities in various part of small and large intestines as well as of the corresponding hydrolases in liver and kidney in the 2- and 4-month old rats. In the 6-month old rats no complete restoration of the activities to control levels was observed in the studied organs of rats of both experimental groups. The most obvious changes of the enzyme activities were preserved in duodenum and kidney of rats of the both experimental groups.

Probably the protein deficit in maternal nutrition during pregnancy or lactation leaves a trace in biochemical memory in spite of that since the first hours after delivery or at once after lactation (at the 22nd day) the females with rat pups got the balance nutrition that was maintained till the beginning of experiment. We did not observe essential differences between effects of the protein deficit in maternal nutrition during pregnancy or lactation.

Our study of effects of protein deficit in nutrition of female rats during pregnancy and lactation (together) on enzyme activities of digestive and non-digestive organs of adult offspring (2, 4, and 6 months) has shown the changes of these activities to be practically the same as in the animals whose mothers were on a low-deficit diet either during pregnancy or during lactation [26].

REMOTE CONSEQUENCES OF PROTEIN DEFICIT IN NUTRITION OF PREGNANT OR LACTATING "GRANDMOTHERS" FOR FUNCTIONING OF ENZYMES OF DIGESTIVE AND NON-DIGESTIVE ORGANS IN "GRANDCHILDREN"

What were changes of the body and organ masses and of functioning of enzyme systems of digestive and non-digestive organs in the 2nd generation offspring ("grandchildren") born by female rats whose mothers were on a low-protein diet during pregnancy or lactation?

In the 2-month old "grandchildren" whose "grandmothers" experienced protein deficit in nutrition during pregnancy the mass of jejunal mucosa increased by 40%. Activity of maltase increased markedly in jejunum, but decreased in liver; activity of alkaline phosphatase decreased in duodenum, but increased in large intestine (table 3). Activities of amino- and dipeptidases changed considerably. The aminopeptidase M activity increased in duodenum and jejunum, but decreased in ileum and kidney; the glycyl-L-leucinedipeptidase activity decreased in duodenum, ileum, and colon, but increased in jejunum and kidney.

Thus, in the 2-month old rats whose "grandmothers" were on a low-protein diet during pregnancy, activities of most studied enzymes changed in duodenum (alkaline phosphatase, aminopeptidase M, and glycyl-L-leucinedipeptidase), in jejunum (maltase, aminopeptidase M, and glycyl-L-leucinedipeptidase), and in kidney (alkaline phosphatase, aminopeptidase M, and glycyl-L-leucinedipeptidase). In the 4-month old rats of this group there occurred a decrease of the mass of body (by 34%), of jejunum (by 25%), of large intestine mucosa (36%), of kidney (by 40%), and of liver (27%). Activities of maltase rose in jejunum and ileum, of alkaline phosphatase in kidney, of aminipeptidase M slightly (by 15%) only in duodenum. The glycyl-L-leucinedipeptidase activity decreased in all studied organs except for ileum in which it was at the level of control animals.

Table 3. Activity (μmol/min per g of protein) of enzymes in the different parts of the small intestine, in colon, kidneys and liver of the 2- and 4-month old 2nd generation offspring of rats, whose mothers received a control (C) or a low-protein diets during pregnancy (1)

Enzymes	Age, month	Group of the rats	Parts of the small intestine			Colon	Kidneys	Liver
			duodenum	jejunum	ileum			
Maltase	2	C	499±74	356±28	367±92	34±4	174±28	12±0.5
		1	510±63	669±87*	365±81	46±12	201±16	5.4±1.4*
	4	C	401±69	601±54	309±53	45±7	100±13	5.7±1.3
		1	500±60	957±129*	662±82*	45±5	77±8	4.3±1.8
Alkaline phosphatase	2	C	166±15	47±5	16±4	2.8±0.2	20±2	1.1±0.3
		1	98±9*	62±11	9±3	5.7±1*	10±1*	1.1±1.0
	4	C	127±9	83±7	16±2	4±0.03	12±1.3	0.7±0.1
		1	103±18	79±13	14±3	3.7±1.2	17±0.2*	0.5±0.2
Aminopep-tidase M	2	C	27±5	67±4	88±7	12±0.4	133±19	8±0.4
		1	41±2*	82±5*	56±0.5*	11.6±1.4	37±16*	9±1
	4	C	34±2	62±13	61±12	8.2±1.6	72±5	5.8±0.8
		1	39±0.8*	74±4	79±11	11±2	75±2	7.5±0.6
Glycyl-L-leucine-dipeptidase	2	C	580±58	395±42	624±63	245±27	526±52	218±26
		1	294±14*	592±23*	447±43*	135±16*	769±83*	181±36
	4	C	440±52	889±171	834±135	265±50	1191±211	204±13
		1	218±9*	471±13*	679±96	138±18*	515±38*	101±15*

* - p<0.05 as compared with control

Table 4. Activity (μmol/min per g of protein) of enzymes in the different parts of the small intestine, in colon, kidneys and liver of the 2- and 4-month old 2nd generation offspring of rats, whose mothers received a control (C) or a low-protein diets during lactation (2)

Enzymes	Age, month	Group of the rats	Parts of the small intestine			Colon	Kidneys	Liver
			duodenum	jejunum	ileum			
Maltase	2	C	163±28	261±26	198±38	55±2	74±6	9±1.5
		2	180±37	275±30	207±36	63±7	69±5	5.0±0.7*
	4	C	259±38	450±71	339±52	22±3	139±6	7±0.3
		2	319±30	483±39	300±25	29±6	105±8*	9±1
Alkaline phosphatase	2	C	50±20	30±7	13±6	10±0.4	8±1	0.8±0.2
		2	86±22	56±8*	17±3	13±2	10±0.6	0.9±0.1
	4	C	243±29	58±9	10±3	3±0.5	9±0.7	0.5±0.1
		2	139±29*	77±20	20±7	3±1	9±0.7	1±0.3
Aminopep-tidase M	2	C	15±3	42±15	24±0.4	15±3	54±4	8±1
		2	20±5	51±7	33±7	13±2	43±1*	6±0.4
	4	C	46±7	58±5	52±8	3±0.5	81±3	7±0.9
		2	34±3	64±6	57±3	4±0.9	72±2*	8±0.3
Glycyl-L-leucine-dipeptidase	2	C	37±9	371±13	323±123	210±24	600±103	145±9
		2	41±16	294±27*	213±34	120±24*	348±32*	102±3*
	4	C	49±12	111±9	250±39	63±16	540±80	262±10
		2	62±13	211±39*	190±12*	38±6	642±61	152±24*

* - p<0.05 as compared with control

In the 6-month old rats of this group the liver mass increased slightly (by 20%). The hepatic maltase activity rose 1.2 times. In the 10-month old rats whose "grandmothers" were on a low-protein diet during pregnancy, the jejunum length increased by 15% and mass of jejunal mucosa by 27%, while the colon mucosa mass rose by 60%. The enzyme activities in organs did not change as compared with control animals.

In the 2-month old rats whose "grandmothers" were on a low-protein diet during lactation (for the first 21 days) only the duodenal mucosa mass decreased (by 24%). Activities of maltase in liver, of aminopeptidase M in kidney, and of glycyl-L-leucinedipeptidase in jejunum, large intestine, kidney, and liver were shown to decrease, whereas of alkaline phosphatase in jejunum to increase (table 4). In the 4-month old rats of this group there was a decrease of the jejunum mass (by 8%), but an increase of mass of ileal mucosa (by 13%) and of kidney (by 15%). A significant decrease of activity of maltase was revealed in kidney, of alkaline phosphatase in duodenum, and of aminipeptidase M in kidney. The glycyl-L-leucinedipeptidase activity decreased in ileum and liver, while rose in jejunum.

In the 6-month old rats of this group the small intestine length decreased (by 11%), but mass of the colonic mucosa increased (by 60%). A decrease of alkaline phosphatase and aminopeptidase M activities was found in jejunum, while of maltase and glycyl-L-leucinedipeptidase, in ileum (table 5). In the 10-month old rats there was a decrease of the jejunal mucosa mass (by 12%). Activity of maltase increased in jejunum and colon, while of glycyl-L-leucinedipeptidase, in colon.

Table 5. Activity (μmol/min per g of protein) of enzymes in the different parts of the small intestine, in colon, kidneys and liver of the 6-month old 2nd generation offspring of rats, whose mothers received a control (C) and a low-protein diets during pregnancy (1) or lactation (2)

Enzymes	Group of the rats	Duodenum	Jejunum	Ileum	Colon	Kidneys	Liver
Maltase	C	490±73	560±35	470±50	112±12	116±5	9±0.9
	1	450±59	690±40*	410±37	92±9	125±9	8±0.6
	2	340±53	520±56	290±54*	97±7	136±11	8±2
Alkaline phospha-tase	C	150±17	80±5	32±5	16±2	21±2	2±0.2
	1	130±27	90±12	30±7	13±2	16±1	1±0.1*
	2	110±6	60±7*	30±5	11±2	17±2	1±0.3*
Aminopep-tidase M	C	90±10	120±14	110±13	32±5	135±11	9±0.9
	1	70±8	120±17	90±10	22±3	140±4	12±0.9*
	2	60±16	80±5*	90±9	20±3	140±11	8±1**
Glycyl-L-leucine-dipeptidase	C	290±45	400±41	470±88	232±39	720±12	220±20
	1	290±38	600±99	760±21*	240±6	880±160	320±58
	2	380±100	400±89	420±65**	383±147	700±120	186±25

* - p<0.05 as compared with control;

** - p<0.05 1 as compared with 2

Thus, at the later age (6 and 10 months), changes of enzyme activities in digestive and non-digestive organs were less pronounced than those in the 2- and 4-month old animals (tabl 3-5). It is to be noted that in the 10-month old offspring whose "grandmothers" experienced the low-protein starvation during lactation, changes of activities of some enzymes (maltase and glycyl-L-leucinedipeptidase) were revealed in ileum and large intestine, whereas in the offspring whose "grandmothers" were on the low-protein diet during pregnancy the enzyme activities remained unchanged, but structural parameters did change essentially.

Apparently, the negative effect of the protein deficit in nutrition of "grandmothers" during pregnancy and lactation on functioning of enzymes in digestive and non-digestive organs takes also place in "grandchildren".

ENZYME ACTIVITIES IN DIGESTIVE AND NON-DIGESTIVE ORGANS IN THE ADULTHOOD OF THE THIRD GENERATION OFFSPRING ("GREAT-GRANDCHILDREN") WHOSE "GREAT-GRANDMOTHERS" WERE ON A LOW-PROTEIN DIET DURING LACTATION

Experiments were carried out on the 4-month old male rats.

In the rats whose "great-grandmothers" experienced protein starvation during pregnancy the mass of body and of liver decreased by 6% and 13%, respectively. Activity of maltase decreased in jejunum and ileum, of alkaline phosphatase only in ileum, and of aminopeptidase M in liver (table 6).

In the rats whose "great-grandmothers" were on a low-protein diet during lactation there was a significant decrease of the body mass (by 38%), of the length of small intestine (by 12%), of the mucosa mass of duodenum (by 40%), of jejunum (by 18%), of ileum (by 31%), of large intestine (by 25%), and of the kidney and liver mass (by 39% and 35%, respectively) as compared with the rats whose "great-grandmothers did not experienced protein starvation during lactation. In rats of this group, activities of maltase and alkaline phosphatase in ileum increased, while the maltase activity in kidney decreased (table 6). Activity of aminopeptidase M decreased in ileum, while of glycyl-L-leucinedipeptidase in jejunum and kidney.

Thus, the negative effect of protein deficit in nutrition of the "great-grandmothers" on the body and organ mass as well as on formation and functioning of enzyme systems in digestive and non-digestive organs is also revealed in the third generation offspring, the changes of mass being especially pronounced in the animals whose "great-grandmothers" were on a low-protein diet during lactation.

Table 6. Activity (μmol/min per g of protein) of enzymes in the different parts of the small intestine, in colon, kidneys and liver of the 4-month old 3rd generation offspring of rats, whose mothers received a control (C) and a low-protein diets during pregnancy (1) or lactation (2). V. There are 7 tests in each series.

Enzymes	Group of the rats	Duodenum	Jejunum	Ileum	Colon	Kidneys	Liver
Maltase	K	251±11	373±21	266±16	51±2	153±11	13±0.4
	1	264±23	461±28*	313±2*	55±4	137±6	14±1
	2	215±12*	306±31	451±12*	52±2	102±13*	12±1
Alkaline phospha-tase	K	145±12	38±4	13±2	7±1	20±2	1±0.1
	1	137±12	95±8	7±1*	8±1	20±2	1±0.2
	2	126±9	92±6*	22±2*	9±1	20±3	1±0.1
Aminopep-tidase M	K	66±3	77±6	49±6	8±1	108±13	7±1
	1	42±6*	89±11	63±6	12±2	110±8	11±1*
	2	24±2	46±4*	34±4	9±1	98±7	6±1
Glycyl-L-leucine-dipeptidase	K	317±33	475±21	545±41	264±13	610±50	201±19
	1	287±25	393±17	456±36	240±21	636±92	216±29
	2	259±18	359±25*	451±25	237±11	439±48*	165±26

* - p<0.05 as compared with control

ENZYME ACTIVITIES IN DIGESTIVE AND NON-DIGESTIVE ORGANS IN THE ADULT OFFSPRING WHOSE MOTHERS WERE ON A HIGH-PROTEIN DIET DURING LACTATION

An increasing interest has been paid to a high-protein, low-carbohydrate diet that is used for weight loss. Problems of safety of use of such diet, especially for hepatic and renal functions, maintenance of calcium balance, and insulin sensitivity have being actively debated. A study was carried out on effect of consumption of a high-protein diet (50% protein) on many parameters of metabolism, such as body composition, plasma hormones and nutrients, liver and kidney histopathology, hepatic markers of oxidative stress, and calcium balance [45]. A significant decrease of the white adipose tissue and a low basal concentration of triglycerides, glucose, leptin, and insulin were reported. The authors concluded that a long consumption of a high-protein diet by male rats produced no negative effect and could prevent metabolic syndrome. There has also been shown that an elevation of the protein content in a carbohydrate-free diet leads to a pronounced increase of the fat loss [46].

Is it possible to change functioning of enzyme systems of digestive and non-digestive organs in the offspring due to the maternal nutrition with a ration with a protein excess and a carbohydrate deficit?

To solve this problem, we carried out experiments on the 30-day old rat pups and adult (the 2-, 4-, and 6-month old) Wistar male rats whose mothers during lactation (for 21 days) were on an isocaloric ration, but with a 2.5-fold elevated protein content. Then from the 22nd postnatal day to the onset of the experiment the experimental animals were on the normal ration. Control animals were rats of the same age that got normal nutrition during the pre- and postnatal development. Studied in experimental and control rats of the corresponding age were structural parameters and activities of membrane-bound enzymes (sucrase, maltase, alkaline phosphatase, and aminopeptidase M) and of predominantly intracellular glycyl-L-leucinedipeptidase in various parts of small intestine and in large intestine as well as activity of these enzymes in liver and kidney.

In the 30-day old rat pups the body mass did not change, the small intestine length increased (by 7%), the jejunal mucosa mass decreased (by 32%), but the mass of large intestine, of kidney, and of liver increased (by 13%, 27%, and 24%, respectively) as compared with the corresponding parameters in control rats.

In the experimental rat pups, activities of maltase in large intestine and of alkaline phosphatase in ileum and large intestine decreased. Activity of aminopeptidase M increased in duodenum, but decreased in the large intestine and kidney. Activity of glycine-L-leucyldipeptidase increased in duodenum, but decreased in kidney.

In the 2-month old experimental rat pups the body and liver masses increased by 35%. Activities of maltase decreased in jejunum and large intestine, of alkaline phosphatase in large intestine, of aminopeptidase M in large intestine and liver, and of glycyl-L-leucinedipeptidase in jejunum, ileum, large intestine, and kidney (table 7).

Table 7. Activity (μmol/min per g of protein) of enzymes in the different parts of the small intestine, in colon, kidneys and liver of the 2-month old rats, whose mothers received a control (C) and a high-protein diets during lactation (2)

Enzymes	Group of the rats	Parts of the small intestine			Colon	Kidneys	Liver
		duodenum	jejunum	ileum			
Maltase	C	412±37	856±38	383±51	138±21	139±19	64±2
	2	302±53	605±95*	318±39	65±10*	141±16	12±2*
Alkaline phosphatase	C	121±30	99±13	26±3	16±2	15±1	0.5±0.1
	2	103±19	63±14	19±5	12±1*	13±2	0.7±0.1
Aminopeptidase M	C	29±3	98±7	75±7	21±3	78±18	5.2±0.5
	2	21±6	70±15	63±11	13±1*	66±10	3.6±0.4*
Glycyl-L-leucine-dipeptidase	C	106±10	301±29	266±16	129±17	288±11	33±1
	2	86±7	197±13*	222±8*	68±5*	244±3*	34±3

* - $p<0.05$ as compared with control

In the 4-month old experimental rats the mass of mucosa of duodenum and of ileum increased (by 82% and 50%, respectively). The changes of enzyme activities in digestive and non-digestive differed from those in the 2-month old rats (table 8). Activities of all enzymes increased practically in all studied organs. An increase of the enzyme activities was marked in duodenum and less significant in jejunum and ileum. In large intestine, there was an elevation of activities of alkaline phosphatase and glycyl-L-leucinedipeptidase, while in kidney, of maltase, alkaline phosphatase and glycyl-L-leucinedipeptidase. In liver, only maltase activity rose.

Table 8. Activity (μmol/min per g of protein) of enzymes in the different parts of the small intestine, in colon, kidneys and liver of the 4-month old rats, whose mothers received a control (C) and a high-protein diets during lactation (2)

Enzymes	Group of the rats	Parts of the small intestine			Colon	Kidneys	Liver
		duodenum	jejunum	ileum			
Maltase	C	374±53	634±31	433±28	85±9	137±11	14±1
	2	809±100*	1011±120*	605±26*	99±13	247±27*	19±1*
Alkaline phosphatase	C	67±5	62±4	25±3	8±1	15±1	1±0.1
	2	229±23*	89±19	42±9*	17±2*	23±1*	1±0.1
Aminopeptidase M	C	25±2	57±3	45±4	13±1	75±6	10±1
	2	56±6*	84±8*	86±5*	18±3	101±16	11±1
Glycyl-L-leucine-dipeptidase	C	207±27	463±51	465±28	186±18	520±53	183±10
	2	607±49*	857±43*	1067±87*	283±18*	758±83*	164±10

* - p<0.05 as compared with control

No changes of structural parameters, as compared with control rats, were revealed in the 6-month old experimental rats. These, like the 2-monh old animals, were observed to have a decrease of several enzyme activities (of maltase in all studied organs, of aminopeptidase M in jejunum, ileum, large intestine, and in kidney, and of glycyl-L-leucinedipeptidase in large intestine and kidney (table 9). In some cases (for instance, in kidney) the decrease of the activities was quite pronounced.

Table 9. Activity (μmol/min per g of protein) of enzymes in the different parts of the small intestine, in colon, kidneys and liver of the 6-month old rats, whose mothers received a control (C) and a high-protein diets during lactation (2)

Enzymes	Group of the rats	Parts of the small intestine			Colon	Kidneys	Liver
		duodenum	jejunum	ileum			
Maltase	C	520±50	770±60	530±62	100±15	160±30	14±1
	2	350±30*	600±50*	360±30*	60±4*	90±7*	8±0.5*
Alkaline phosphatase	C	210±40	110±13	39±10	14±3	24±2	2±0.2
	2	170±30	120±10	40±9	10±8	16±2*	1±0.1*
Aminopeptidase M	C	80±20	120±10	110±10	30±5	130±20	11±1
	2	50±5	90±6*	70±3*	14±1*	70±10*	8±0.2*
Glycyl-L-leucine-dipeptidase	C	630±110	780±260	920±170	80±4	3800±130	160±30
	2	450±30	770±60	910±90	230±20*	780±110*	130±12

* - p<0.05 as compared with control

It is to be noted that the most marked changes involved activities of maltase (a decrease in all studied organs) and of aminopeptidase M (a decrease in all organs except for duodenum). Changes of activities of all enzymes were revealed in kidney, followed by large intestine (activity of alkaline phosphatase did not change as compared with control).

Thus, in experiments on rats it has been revealed that not only restriction of protein in nutrition of lactating females, but also its excess produce essential changes of enzyme activities in digestive and non-digestive organs that perform digestive and trophic-barrier functions.

CONCLUSION

Analysis of our data on effects of protein deficit during pregnancy and/or lactation or protein excess during lactation allows suggesting that any change of quality of nutrition at critical periods of embryonic (fetal) or early postnatal offspring development can possibly be considered as the general regularity leading to a disturbance of programming by triggering of a cascade of metabolic reactions, enzyme systems of digestive and non-digestive organs. Various disturbances of the nutrition quality due to malnutrition, pregnancy toxicoses, medicinal treatment, early or late weaning of newborns, obesity, and other situations can take place in real life.

We have also demonstrated that the protein deficit in nutrition of rat pups in early ontogenesis during transition from lactotrophic to definitive nutrition also leads to essential disturbances of functioning of the small and large intestine digestive enzymes as well as of the same hydrolases of liver and kidney in the adult life (2 and 4 months) of these animals [47].

However, the changes of enzyme activities differed from those in the animals whose mothers got protein-deficit nutrition during pregnancy or lactation. What can be the cause of differences in programming of the enzyme systems in digestive and non-digestive organs in the rats whose mothers were on a low-protein diet during pregnancy and/or lactation or in these animals themselves on this diet in early ontogenesis? These differences might possibly be accounted for by the difference in duration of alimentary protein restriction. The pregnant and lactating females got the low-protein ration for 21 days, whereas the rat pups, only for 10 days. Besides, in the programming of the enzyme systems of the studied organs, in the first variant the "mother-offspring" system participated, while in the second variant, only the offspring did.

How can such diverse changes of enzyme systems be explained in animals of different age when these animals themselves in early ontogenesis or their mothers, grandmothers or great-grandmothers during pregnancy or lactation got an isocaloric nutrition that however was non-balanced by protein (deficit or excess of protein)?

Is it possible to answer the question of how the early metabolic/nutritional programming of enzyme systems of digestive and non-digestive organs occurs in offspring during disturbances of nutrition quality at periods of prenatal and early postnatal development?

The entire sequence of the corresponding processes is hard to be traced. However, it is possible to suggest the following. Programming of enzymatic functions of various organs seems to be realized at the genetic level, which is also indicated by other authors [48]. By the example of enzymes responsible for maintenance of glucose homeostasis in insulin-sensitive organs (liver) it was shown that alongside changes of enzyme activities the liver mRNA level changed in the 3-month old offspring whose mothers experienced protein deficit in nutrition during pregnancy and lactation (for 21 days). However, it is not clear whether these changes can be attributed to changes in the mRNA transcription or to changes of mRNA stability. Moreover, the authors think their results to allow suggesting that the effect of metabolic programming involves not only protein biochemistry, but also regulation of gene expression. The fetal nutrition is suggested to possibly affect expression of enzymes before their genes obtain transcriptional activity. Mechanisms underlying changes in enzyme expression in offspring as a result of effect of protein deficit in maternal nutrition have remained unclear. Such changes of enzyme expression can be attributed to that in each cell the greater or lesser amount of enzyme can be expressed or that the number of cells can decrease [48]. The ontogenetic changes of intestinal enzymes are known to be produced by the replacement by a new enterocyte population rather than by the direct change of synthesis of enzymes. This leads to that changes of expression of the corresponding gene, which occur at the period of transition from lactotrophic to definitive nutrition, affect irreversibly undifferentiated cells of small intestine crypt villi.

Expression of the gene PepT1 of peptide transporter has been shown to increase under conditions of malnutrition in spite of atrophic alterations of intestinal mucosa [49]. It cannot be ruled out that such changes of activity of the peptide transporter gene PepT1 might affect absorption of peptide substrates formed as a result of hydrolysis of food proteins. The hydrolysis-dependent peptide transport can be accompanied by changes of peptide hydrolase activities, which remain in the offspring biochemical memory throughout adulthood.

We have also shown that protein deficit in maternal nutrition during pregnancy or lactation produces a significant decrease of glucose and glycine transport in small intestine in the adult life of the offspring first generation [50].

It is possible that in metabolic programming of enzyme systems of various organs a certain role is played by regulatory factors. An important role in formation of enzyme systems in various organs including the gastrointestinal tract is played by hormones of adrenal cortex and thyroid gland [1,2,5,51-54]. Function of these hormonal systems in coordination of enzymatic readjustment in intestine consists in that glucocorticoids induce synthesis of a number of intestinal glucosidases and simultaneously repress synthesis of lactase under effect of thyroxin. Exogenous administration of these hormones at the period of lactotrophic nutrition leads to a premature induction and repression of the corresponding enzymes. Dexamethazone (DM) and thyroxin (T4) have earlier been shown to change ratio of membranous and soluble forms of saccharase and maltase in the 10-day old rat pups in such a way that it becomes identical to their ratio in older rat pups, i.e. the proportion of the membrane form in these membrane-bound enzymes increases, while that of the soluble form decreases. On the contrary, in the rat pups whose mothers were for 21 days on a low-protein diet during lactation, the portion of activity of the soluble form under effect of hormones was higher than that in control rat pups whose mothers got the normal nutrition [55]. These results indicate a possibility of a delay in maturation of intestinal digestive enzymes. This difference was the most pronounced for sucrase, maltase, and peptidases [47].

However, it was shown that the K_M values of membrane and soluble forms of maltase, alkaline phosphatase, aminopeptidase M, and glycyl-L-leucinedipeptidase isolated from jejunum and ileum of the 10-day old rat pups in most cases little differed from those in control rat pups and in animals whose mothers were on the 2.5-fold decreased protein ration during lactation. Nor were the K_M values changed under effects of exogenous thyroxin and dexamethasone. It seems that under conditions of protein deficit in nutrition of lactating females as well as under action of exogenous hormones, no essential alterations occur in structure of synthesized enzymes in offspring [56].

At present, the low-protein nutrition of rats during pregnancy has been shown to induce development of hypertension in adult offspring [57]. Maternal glucocorticoids can program an increased risk of development of diseases in adult life [58]. The role of glucocorticoids in programming of hypertension was determined after administration of metyrapone (an inhibitor of 11b-hydroxylase protecting fetus from effect of maternal glucocorticoids) to pregnant rats that were on a diet of 18% or 9% casein. Activity of this enzyme was much lower in offspring whose mothers were on a low-protein diet. Metyrapone eliminated the hypertensive state in the 8-week old offspring of rats that were for 14 days on a low-protein diet (9% casein). These data agree with a hypothesis that alimentary modulations of fetal corticosteroids play a certain role in programming of hypertension in the adult life. However, Desai et al. [48] state that the role of glucagons and insulin hardly is probable in changes of expression of hepatic enzymes responsible for glucose homeostasis in rats whose mothers were on a low-protein diet during pregnancy and lactation.

It is to be noted that nutrition of pregnant rats with an isocaloric low-protein diet was reported to decrease insulin secretion by Langerhans' islets, these changes occurring at the exocytosis step in the insulin secretion cascade, but not in insulin pool of beta cells [59]. Administration of insulin to newborn mice [60] and rats [61] has been established to produce premature maturation and activation of expression of the brush border membranous (disaccharidases), lysosomal (N-acetyl-b-glucosaminidase), microsomal (sulfatase C), and cytosolic (lactate dehydrogenase) enzymes. The enzymatic response of immature enterocytes is mediated through binding of hormone to its receptors and is transduced to cells without synthesis *de novo* of polyamines [62]. Addition of insulin to diet of newborn animals can produce a trophic effect on the intestine mass and an increase of lactase activity [63]. However, it is not clear whether the intestinal changes result from the insulin specific action or from that mediated by release of corticosterone [64,65].

Insulin and insulin-related growth factors (IGF) are known to be hormonal mediators of fetal growth. Their effect is regulated by the alimentary supply of fetus. A decrease of glucose supply due to restriction of nutrition leads to a decrease of circulating insulin, of IGF concentration, and of fetal growth [13]. J.E.Harding (2001) claims that nutrition is important for regulation of the fetal growth, therefore it is an important candidate in development of programming stimuli by playing the key role in connection between the size at birth and subsequent risk of development of diseases. Insulin-related growth factors increase nutrient absorption in immature intestine characterized by a low level of glucose oxidation. Additions of insulin-related factors (IGF-1 and IGF-11) have been shown to increase the blood serum glucose content in immature rat pups nourished with an artificial formula and to change expression of jejunal glucose transporters [66].

It cannot be ruled out that various parts of gastrointestinal tract differ by sensitivity to regulatory factors whose effect during prenatal and early postnatal development can be different at protein restriction in nutrition at these periods. This can remain in the adult life of rats, which might account for different significance of changes of enzyme activities in different small intestine parts. It was earlier shown that lactase floridzine hydrolase encoded by the single gene in jejunum and colon was regulated differently. The lactase activity in colon is controlled at the pretranslational, while in jejunum at the posttranslational level. This can be due to different sensitivity of the intestine parts to regulatory factors and/or to differences in their receptors and effectors [67]. The rapid substrate-specific induction of intestinal angiotensin-converting enzyme (ACE) has been shown to have different regulation in the proximal and distal small intestine parts [68]. This was established on rats after a low-protein (4%) nutrition with subsequent transition to an isocaloric high-protein gelatin (50%) diet. The authors have come to conclusion that the dietary induction of the intestinal ACE is controlled at the level of mRNA translation. Such control of intestinal ACE along the longitudinal axis can be important for maintenance of its expression gradient. There are data that the translational control is an important parameter in regulation of numerous eukaryote genes [69]. At present, protein factors important for initiation of translation have been under investigation. Besides, phosphorylation plays a role in regulation of activity of some of these factors that in turn are associated with signal transduction pathways [70]. It is desirable to study such processes at alimentary disturbances (protein deficit or excess) at critical periods of development of offspring, which leads to alterations of functioning of enzymes of digestive and non-digestive organs in offspring not only of the first generation, but also in subsequent generations.

It can be suggested that information about protein deficit or excess in maternal nutrition during pregnancy or lactation and in early ontogenesis is laid into genetic code at critical periods of prenatal development and is transformed in genetic memory of adult offspring to produce diverse effects on expression of enzymes in the offspring adult life.

However, the different behavior of enzymes in different age groups of three offspring generation as if contradicts to this point of view. In the first generation of offspring whose mothers experienced protein starvation during pregnancy or lactation, we observed predominantly a marked decrease of enzyme activities of digestive and non-digestive organs in the 2- and 4-month old rats (with small exceptions), whereas in the offspring second generation the changes of enzyme activities in the studied organs were less pronounced and the activities either decreased or increased. In some organs there were revealed no changes of enzyme activities as compared with control. In the 10-month old, second generation offspring whose "grandmothers" were on a low-protein diet during pregnancy, only changes of structural parameters were found. In the 10-month old offspring whose "grandmothers" got the low-protein ration during lactation, mass of jejunal mucosa decreased, while activity of maltase increased in jejunum and large intestine and so did the glycine-L-leucyldipeptidase activity in large intestine. But, on the other hand, in the third generation offspring whose "great-grandmothers" were on a low-protein diet during pregnancy or lactation, essential changes both of structural parameters and of functional enzyme activities were revealed in all studied organs except for liver.

Studies of molecular grounds of heredity by non-genetic (epigenetic) mechanisms have recently begun to be carried out [13,71-73]. A similar epigenetic character of metabolic programming can include a change of packing and activation of various genes including those regulating synthesis of enzymes. One of examples is imprinting when activation of genes is under influence of parents. Genetically identical mice can have a different fur color depending on the fur color of their mothers [74]. Mechanism seems to consist in different methylation and hence activation of corresponding controlling genes regulating expression of fur color. From this, an important conclusion about perspectives of alimentary programming can be made: the degree of methylation and hence gene expression and the fur color can change when mothers are on a diet "with a considerable amount of methyl donors" during pregnancy (or lactation). Methylation of DNA has been shown to control all genetic processes in cells including replication, transcription, and reparation; therefore, it is very important for understanding and deciphering of processes of ontogenesis, species formation, evolution, and aging. Distortion of methylation produces cancer transformation of cells. It cannot be ruled out that disturbance of DNA methylation can occur at an early metabolic/nutritional programming in the case of a change of nutrition at critical periods of offspring development. DNA methylation is considered as an epigenetic control of genetic organism functions, as a principally new mechanism of regulation of gene expression and cell differentiation [72].

Understanding of the early metabolic/ nutrition programming needs unraveling of mechanisms of transport of nutrients, intracellular trafficking apoptosis, intracellular signalization, and role of such nutrients as calcium. Of a special significance is understanding of interaction of nutrients with gene expression and epigenetic regulation of gene expression by nutrient-dependent reactions (methylation, biotinylation, acetylation, and phosphorylation) [71].

Further studies are necessary on identification of factors determining fetal growth and affecting delivery of nutrients and oxygen to fetus. It is also necessary to find out how the fetus and newborn are adapted to restriction or excess of some alimentary component, how this affects programming of the body structure and physiology, and which molecular mechanisms are involved in changing gene expression by nutrients and hormones [11].

One of the prominent experts in the field of metabolic programming, Prof. J.E. Harding [13] states: "Ultimately all programming phenomena must have their basis in altered expression of genes. Further understanding of how fetal nutrition may alter gene expression by this and presumably other mechanisms will be helpful in clarifying the nutritional basis of the link between size at birth and adult disease risk".

In conclusion, it can be suggested that functioning of enzyme systems of digestive and non-digestive organs in a different regime (at a lower or higher level as compared with control animals) in adult offspring as a result of protein deficit or excess at periods of prenatal and early postnatal development due to an unfavorable early nutritional programming can play the key role in disturbances of various metabolic reactions. This in turn can activate development of chronic diseases (for instance, obesity or diabetes mellitus) and particularly of cardiovascular diseases (hypertension, ischemic diseases, and infarcts).

REFERENCES

[1] Koldovsky, O. *Development of the function of the small intestine in mammals and man.* Basel; New York: Karger; 1969.

[2] Henning, SJ. (1987). Functional development of the gastrointestinal tract. In: Ed. Johnson LR. *Physiology of the gastrointestinal tract.* NewYork: Raven Press; 1987; 17 p.

[3] Ugolev, AM. *Theory of adequate nutrition and trophology.* St. Petersburg: Science; 1991.

[4] Henning, SJ, Rubin, DC, Shulman, RJ. Ontogeny of the intestinal mucosa. In: Ed. Johnson LR. *Physiology of the gastrointestinal tract.* NewYork: Raven Press; 1994; 39 p.

[5] Timofeeva, N.M. (1995). Maturation of intestinal digestive enzymes in ontogeny. *Sechenov physiological journal, 78,* 21-28.

[6] Menard, D. (2004). Functional development of the human gastrointestinal tract: hormone- and growth factor-mediated regulatory mechanisms. *Can. J. Gastroenterol., 18,* 39-44.

[7] McCance, R.A. (1962). Food growth and time. *Lancet, 2,* 271-272.

[8] Stevart, R. J. C., Preece, R. F. & Sheppard, H. G. (1975). Twelve generations of marginal protein deficiency. *Br. J. Nutr., 33,* 233-253.

[9] Stevart, R. J. C., Sheppard, H.G., Preece, R. F. & Waterlow J.C. (1980). The effect of rehabilitation at different stages of development of rats marginally malnourished for ten to twelfe generations. *Br. J. Nutr., 43,* 403-412.

[10] Lucas, A. (1994). Role of nutritional programming in determining adult morbidity. *Arch. Dis. Child., 71,* 288-290.

[11] Godfrey, K. M.& Barker, D. J. P. (2000). Fetal nutrition and adult disease. *Am. J. Clin. Nutr., 71(suppl),* 1344-1352S.

[12] King, J.C. (2000). Physiology of pregnancy and nutrition metabolism. *Am. J. Clin. Nutr., 71(suppl),* 1218-1225S.

[13] Harding, J. E. (2001). The nutritional basis of the fetal origins of adult disease. *Int. J. Epidemiol., 30,* 15-23.

[14] Lucas, A., Morley, R. & Isaacs, E. (2001). Nutrition and mental development. *Nutrition Reviews, 59,* S24-S33.

[15] Rush, M. D. (2001). Maternal nutrition and perinatal survival. *Nutr. Rev., 59,* 315-326.

[16] Jones, J. H. (2005). Fetal programming: adaptive life-history tacties or making the best of bad start? *Am. J. Hum. Biol., 17,* 22-33.

[17] Baker, D, J. P. (1990). Fetal and infant origins of adult disease. *Br. Med. J., 301,* 1111.

[18] Barker, D. J. P. (1993). Fetal nutrition and cardiovascular disease in adult life. *Lancet, 341.* 938-941.

[19] Koldovsky, O., Hahn, P., Hromadova, V., Krecek, J. & Macho, L. (1995). Late effects of early nutritional manipulations. *Physiol. Res., 44,* 357-360.

[20] Lecours, A. R., Mandujano, M. & Romero, G. (2001). Ontogeny of brain and cognition: relevance to nutrition. *Nutrition Rewievs, 59,* S7-S12.

[21] Quesnel, H., Mejia-Guadarrama, C. A., Dourmad, J. Y., Farmer, C. & Prunier, A. (2005). Dietary protein restriction during lactation in primiparous sows with different life weights at farrowing: 1. Consequences on sow metabolic status and litter growth. *Reprod. Nutr. Dev., 45*, 39-56.

[22] Barker, D. J. P. (1998). *Mothers, babies and health in later life.* 2nd Edition. London: Churchill Livingstone; 1998.

[23] Kremer, J. N. *Biochemistry of protein nutrition.* Riga: Zinatne; 1965.

[24] Krasinski, S. D., Estrada, G., Yeh, K-Y., Yeh, M., Traber, P. G., Rings, E. H. H. M., Buller, H. A., Verhave, M., Montgomery, R. K. & Grand, R. (1994). Transcriptional regulation of intestinal hydrolase biosynthesis during postnatal development in rats. *Am. J. Physiol., 267*, G584-G594.

[25] Weaver, L.T., Desai, M., Austin, S., Arthur, H.M. & Hale, C.N. (1998). Effects of protein restriction in early life on growth and function of the gastrointestinal tract of the rat. J. Pediatr. *Gastroenterol., 27*, 553-559.

[26] Timofeeva, N. M. (2000). Metabolic/nutrition programming of the small intestine enzymes in posterity. *Rus. J. Physiol., 86*, 1531-1538.

[27] Wildman, R.E.C. & Medeiros, D.M. *Advanced human nutrition.* Boca Roton London, New York, Washington: CRS Press, 2000.

[28] Langley, R. S. & Jackson, A. A. (1994). Increased systolic blood pressure in adult rats induced by fetal exposure to maternal low protein diets. *Clin. Sci., 86*, 217-222.

[29] Langley-Evans, S. C. (1997). Hypertension induced by fetal exposure to a maternal low-protein diet, in the rat, is prevented by pharmacological blockade of maternal glucocorticoid synthesis. *J. Hypertens., 15*, 537-544.

[30] Sloan, N. L., Lederman, S. A., Leigton, J. & al. (2001). The effect of prenatal dietary protein intake on birth weight. *Nutr. Res.,* 129-139.

[31] Cambell, D. M., Hall, M. H., Barker, D. J. P., Cross, J., Shiell, A. W. & Godfrey, K. M. (1996). Diet in pregnancy and the offspring,s blood pressure 40 years later. *Br. J. Obstet. Gynaecol., 103*, 273-280.

[32] Timofeeva, N. M., Iezuitova, N. N., Egorova, V. V., Nikitina, A. A., Gromova, L. F. & Gordova, L. A. (1994). Protein deprivation and trophic-barrier function of enzyme and transport systems in digestive and non-digestive organs of adult and growing rats. *Sechenov Physiol. J., 80*, 91-103.

[33] Desai, M., Crowter, N. J., Lucas, A. & Hales, C. N. (1996). Organ-selective growth in the offspring of protein-restricted mothers. *Brit. J. Nutr., 76*, 591-603.

[34] Lucas, A., Baker, B.A., Desai, M. & Hales, C.N. (1996). Nutrition in pregnant or lactating rats programs lipid metabolism in the offspring. *Brit. J. Nutr., 76*, 605-612.

[35] Dudley, M. A., Schoknecht, P. A., Dudley, A. W., Jiang, L., Ferraris, R.P., Rosenberger, J. N., Henry, J. F. & Reeds, P. J. (2001). Lactase synthesis is pretranslationally regulated in protein-deficient pigs fed a protein-sufficient diet. *Am. J. Physiol., 280.* G621-G628.

[36] Timofeeva, N. M., Egorova, V. V., Nikitina, A. A., Iezuitova, N. N., Gordova, L. A. & Grusdkov, A. A. (1999). Effect of protein deficiency in female rats diet during pregnancy and lactation on tfe activity of membranes and soluble forms of digestive enzymes in small intestine of the rat pups. *Rus. J. Physiol., 85*, 1567-1573.

[37] *Adaptive-compensatory processes.* Leningrad: Science; 1991.

[38] Lonnerdal, B. (1986). Effects of maternal dietary intake on human milk composition. *J. Nutr., 116,* 499-513.

[39] Koldovsky, O. & Tohrnburg, W. (1987). Hormohes in milk. *J. Pediatr. Gastroenterol. Nutr., 6,* 172-196.

[40] Wunderlich, Sh. V., Baliga, B. S. & Munro, H. N. (1979). Rat placental protein synthesis and peptide hormone secretion in relation to malnutrition from protein deficiency or alcohol administration. *J. Nutr., 109,* 1534-1541.

[41] Serova, L. V. (1999). Influence of unfavourable factors of environment on the system of mother-fetus. *Usp. fiziol. Nauk., 30,* 62-72.

[42] Gromov, L. I. & Savina, E.A. (1964). Premature function of fetus as medical-biological problem. *Vestnik AMN SSSR, 6,* 10-17.

[43] Perin, N. M., Clandinin, M. T. & Thompson, A. B. R. (1997). Importance of milk and diet on the ontogeny and adaptation of the intestine. J. *Pediatr. Gastroenterol. Nutr., 24,* 419-425.

[44] Jarocka-Cyrta, E., Perin, E., Keelan, M., Wierzbiki, E., Clandinin, M. N. & Thompson, B. R. (1998). Early dietary experience influences ontogeny of intestine in response to dietary lipid changes in later life. *Am. J. Physiol., 275,* G250-G258.

[45] Lacroix, M., Gaudichon, C., Martin, A., Morens, C., Tome, D. & Huneau, J. F. (2004). A long-term high-protein diet markedly reduces adipose tissue without major side effects in Wistar male rats. *Am. J. Physiol., 287,* R934-R942.

[46] Marsset-Baglieri, A., Fromentin, G., Tome, D., Bensaid, A., Makkarios, L. & Even, P. S. (2004). Increasing the protein content in carbohydrate-free diet enhances fat loss during 35% but not 75% energy restriction in rats. *J. Nutr.,134,* 2646-2652.

[47] Timofeeva, N. M., Gordova, L. A., Egorova, V. V., Iezuitova, N. N. & Nikitina, A. A. (2003). Hormonal regulation of the activity of digestive enzymes of the small intestine in the rat litter following a low-protein ration for female rats during lactation. *J. evol. Physiol. and Biochem., 39,* 229-233.

[48] Desai, M., Byrne, C. D., Zhang, J., Petry, C., Lucas, A. & Hales, N. (1997). Programming of hepatic insulin-sensitive enzymes in offspring of rat dams fed a protein-restricted diet. *Am. J. Physiol., 272,* G1083-G1090.

[49] Ihara, T., Tsujikawa, T., Fujiyama, Y. & Bamba, T. (2000). Regulation of PepT1 peptide transporter expression in the rat small intestine under malnourished conditions. *Digestion, 61,* 59-67.

[50] Timofeeva, N.M., Gordova, L.A., Gromova, L.V., Egorova, V.V. & Nikitina, A.A. (2002). Effect restricted-protein diet during pregnancy on enzyme-transport function of the offspring. Trudi Vseros. conf. "Ot sovr. Fund. Biology k novim technologijam". Puschino, 134.

[51] Ugolev, AB., De Laey, P., Iezuitova, NN., Rakhimov, KR., Timofeeva, NM. & Stepanova, AT. Membrane digestion and nutrient assimilation in early development. In: Ed. Elliott K, Whelan J. *Development of mammalian absorptive processes.* Ciba Found. Symp. 70. Amsterdam etc.: Excerta Medica; 1979; 23 p.

[52] Hodin, R. A., Chamberlain, S. M. & Upton, M. P. (1992). Thyroid hormone differentially regulates rat intestinal brush border enzyme gene expression. *Gastroenterology, 103*, 1529-1536.

[53] Reisenauer, A. M., Lee, E. A. Castillio, R. O. (1992). Ontogeny of membrane and soluble aminooligopeptidases in rat intestine. *Fv. J. Physiol., 262*, 178-184.

[54] Quaroni, A., Tian, J. Q., Goke, M. & Podovsky, D. K. (1999)/ Glucocorticoids have pleiotropic effects on small intestinal crypt cells. *Am. J. Physiol., 277*, G1027-G1040.

[55] Gordova, L. A. & Timofeeva, N. M. (1999). Effects of dexamethasone and thyroxine on correlation of membranes and soluble forms of intestinal disacharidases in ontogeny of the rats. *Dokl. Ak. Nauk, 365*, 135-137.

[56] Egorova, V. V., Gordova, L. A., Iezuitova, N. N., Nikitina, A. A. & Timofeeva, N. M. (2002). Effects of thyroxine and dexamethasone upon kinetic characteristics of the small intestine enzymes in the rat litter following a low-protein ration for female rats during lactation. *Rus. J. Physiol., 88*. 1219-1224.

[57] Brawley, L., Torrens, C., Anthony, F. W., Wheeler, T., Jackson, A. A., Clough, G. F., Poston, L. & Hanson, M. A. (2004). Glycine rectifies vascular dysfunction by dietary protein imbalance during pregnancy. *J. Physiol., 554.2*, 497-504.

[58] Langley-Evans, S. C., Phillips, G. J., Gardner, D. S. & Jackson, A. A. (1996). Role of glucocorticoids in programming of maternal diet-induced hypertension in the rat. *Nutritional Biochemistry, 7*, 173-178.

[59] Cherif, H., Reusens, B., Dahri, S. & Remacle, C. (2001). A protein-restricted diet during pregnancy alters in vitro insulin secretion from islets of fetal Wistar rats. *J. Nutr., 131*, 1555-1559.

[60] Menard, D., Malo, C. & Calvert, R. (1981). Insulin accelerates the development of intestinal brush border hydrolytic activities of suckling mice. *Dev. Biol., 85*, 150-155.

[61] Buts, J. P., De Keyser, N. & Dive, C. (1988). Intestinal development in the suckling rat: effect of insulin on the maturation of villus and crypt cell functions. *Eur. J. Clin. Invest., 18*, 391-398.

[62] Buts, J. P., De Keyser, N., Kolanovski, J. & Vann Hoof. (1990). Hormonal regulation of the rat small intestine: responsiveness of villus and crypt cells to insulin during the suckling period and unresponsiveness after weaning. *Pediatr. Res., 27*, 161-164.

[63] Shulman, R. J. (1990). Oral insulin increases small intestinal mass and disaccharidase activity in the newborn miniature pig. *Pediatr. Res., 28*, 171-175.

[64] Henning, S. J. (1981). Ontogeny of enzymes in small intestine. *Ann. Rev. Physiol., 47*, 231-245.

[65] Martin,G. R. & Henning, S. J. (1984). Enzymic development of the small intestine. Are glucocorticoids necessary? *Am. J. Physiol., 246*, G695-G699.

[66] Lane, R. H., Dvorak, B., MacLennan, N. K., Dvorakova, K, Halpern, M. D., Pham, T. D. & Phillips, A. F. (2002). IGF alters jejunal transporter expression and serum glucose levels in immature rats. *Am. J. Physiol., 283*, R1450-R1460

[67] Freund, J. N., Duluc, I., Foltzer-Jourdainne, Ch., Gosse, F. & Raul, F. (1990). Specific expression of lactase in the jejunum and colon during postnatal development and hormone treatments in the rat. *Biochem. J., 268*, 99-103.

[68] Erickson, R. H., Yoon, B. C., Koh, D. Y., Kim, D. H. & Kim, Y. S. (2001). Dietary induction of angiotensin-converting enzyme in proximal and distal rat small intestine. *Am. J. Physiol., 281*, G1221-1227.

[69] Pain, V. M. & Hentze, M. V. (1996). Initiation of protein synthesis in eukaryotic cells. *Eur. J. Biochem., 236*, 747-771.

[70] Kleijn, M., Scheper, G. C., Voorma, H. O. & Thomas A. A. M. (1998). Regulation of translation initiation factors by signal transduction. *Eur. J. Biochem., 253*, 531-544.

[71] *Molecular nutrition.* Eds. Zemplini, J. & Daniel, H. Wallingford: CABI Publishing, United Kingdom; 2003.

[72] Vanyushin, B. F. (2005). Enzymatic DNA methylation is an epigenetic control for genetic functions of the cell. *Biochemistry, 70*, 598-608.

[73] Holliday, R. (2005). DNA methylation and epigenotypes. *Biochemistry, 70*, 612-617.

[74] Morgan, H. D., Sutherland, H. G. E., Martin, D.I. K. & Whitelaw, E. (1999). Epigenetic inheritance at the agouti of development in the mouse. *Nature Genetics, 23*, 314-318.

In: Nutrition Research Advances
Editor: Sarah V. Watkins, pp. 161-206

ISBN 1-60021-516-5
© 2007 Nova Science Publishers, Inc.

Chapter VI

Therapeutic Potential of Some Natural Plant and Dietary Constituents: A Review of the Available Scientific Evidence

Aamir Jalal Al-Mosawi[*]
University Hospital in Al-Kadhimiyia, PO Box 70025, Baghdad, Iraq.

Overview

There is now some scientific evidence largely obtained from experimental animal studies that certain natural dietary and plant constituents such as Nigella sativa seed, Ginsengs, and Caffeine could have a weak therapeutic or prophylactic potential .The main advantage of these agents is their low toxicity, as they had been used as food additives for decades and centuries without the occurrence of any serious toxicity or adverse effects.

Nigella Sativa(NS) seed has been reported in researches from many countries including USA, Canada, Germany, Spain, Japan, Sweden, Eygpt,Turkey, Iran and Saudia Arabia, to have many possibly beneficial therapeutic and prophylactic effects such as anti-inflammatory effect, analgesic effect, antioxidant effect, and anti-tumor effects.NS seed has also been reported to have a protective effect against nephrotoxixity,hepatotoxicity and diabetes. In particular, there is now a rather a convincing preliminary scientific evidence that NS seed component(s) could has a beneficial adjunctive role in the management of diabetes, and also in the management of some tumors especially colonic cancer, and clinical trials are particularly recommended in these fields. The anti-leukotrienes effect can also be clinically useful as there are very few drugs have this pharmacological effect; however this effect may need more experimental studies.

---

[*] Correspondence concerning this article should be addressed to University Hospital in Al-Kadhimiyia, PO Box 70025, Baghdad, Iraq Tel.: +96 414 431 760; almosawiAJ@yahoo.com.

The low toxicity of Nigella sativa fixed oil is evidenced by high LD50 values on experimental acute toxicity. There is no change in hepatic enzyme stability and organ integrity after 12 weeks of administration of large doses in which rats suggests a wide margin of safety for therapeutic doses of Nigella sativa fixed oil, but the changes in hemoglobin metabolism and the fall in leukocyte and platelet count must be taken into consideration when using large doses for a long time is required.

SECTION (1): NIGELLA SATIVA LINN (RANUNCULACEAE)

Composition

Nigella sativa (NS) belongs to the botanical family of Ranunculaceae and commonly grows in Europe, Middle East, and Western Asia. NS has been used as a flavoring additive to bread and prickles. The seeds of NS Linn (Ranunculaceae), commonly known as black seed or black cumin, contain both fixed and essential oils (32-40 %), proteins (16-19.9 %) arginine, glutamic acid, leucine, lysine, methionine, tyrosine, proline and threonine, etc., alkaloids (Nigellicine, nigellidine, nigellimine-N-oxide) and saponins (Alpha-hedrin triterpenes and steroidal saponins such as Steryl glucosides, acetyl-steryl-glucoside),coumarines (6-methoxy-coumarin,7-hydroxy-coumarin 7-oxy-coumarinMinerals(1.79-3.74 %) including calcium, phosphorous, potassium, sodium and iron Carbohydrates(33.9%)Fiber (5.5 %)water (6 %).

Oil analysis of NS yields 20 compounds. However, para-cymene (37.3%) and thymoquinone (13.7%) are the two major components of the essential oil. Much of the biological activity of the seeds has been shown to be due to thymoquinone (13.7%).

The extracted fixed oil (total fatty acid composition) and volatile oil of NS seeds are composed of eight fatty acids (99.5%).Thirty-two compounds (86.7%) have been identified in the fixed and volatile oils, respectively. The main unsaturated fatty acids of the fixed oil are linoleic acid (55.6%), oleic acid (23.4%) in addition to arachidonic, eicosadienoic, , linolenic, and almitoleic acid .The main saturated fatty acid is palmitic acid (12.5%) in addition to stearic and myristic acid.

The major compounds of the volatile oil were trans-anethole (38.3%), p-cymene (14.8%), limonene (4.3%), and carvone (4.0%). The major phospholipids (PL) classes are phosphatidylcholine followed by phosphatidylethanolamine (PE), phosphatidylserine (PS) and phosphatidylinositol (PI), respectively. Phosphatidylglycerol (PG), lysophosphatidylethanolamine (LPE) and lysophosphatidylcholine (LPC) were isolated in smaller quantities. The level of saturated fatty acids, namely palmitic $C16:0$ and stearic $C18:0$ acids, was considerably higher in PL classes than in the corresponding triacylglycerols [1,2,3,4,5,6,7,8,9,10,11,12,13,14,15].

Possible Therapeutic Potential

The crude extracts of the seeds and some of its active constituents, e.g. volatile oil and thymoquinone have been reported in experimental animal studies to have protective action against nephrotoxicity and hepatotoxicity induced by either disease or chemicals, and a protective effect against streptozocin induced diabetes. Anti-inflammatory, analgesic, antipyretic, antimicrobial and antineoplastic activity has also been reported. The oil decreases blood pressure and increases respiration. Treatment of rats with the seed extract for up to 12 weeks has been reported to induce changes in the haemogram that include an increase in both the packed cell volume (PCV) and hemoglobin (Hb), and a decrease in plasma concentrations of cholesterol, triglycerides and glucose. The seeds are characterized by a very low degree of toxicity. Two cases of contact dermatitis in two individuals have been reported following topical use. Administration of either the seed extract or its oil has not been shown to induce significant adverse effects on liver or kidney functions. Rats treated daily with an oral dose of 2 ml/kg body weight for 12 weeks didn't develop any change in hepatic enzymes levels, including aspartate-aminotransferase, alanine-aminotransferase, and gamma-glutamyl-transferase and no signs of histopathological toxicity (heart, liver, kidneys and pancreas) were observed.. The serum cholesterol, triglyceride and glucose levels and the count of leukocytes and platelets decreased significantly, compared to control values, while hematocrit and hemoglobin levels increased significantly. Transient coagulation abnormalities have also been reported when a large dose of NS is administered to rats. NS 180mg NS/kg rat/day administered to rats induced significant hyperfibrinogenemia (14%) after 4 weeks while the double dose induced significant transient prothrombin time PT prolongation (7.8%) and), thrombin time TT reduction (13%) after 2 weeks and the triple dose induced significant transient activated partial thromboplastin time (APTT),APTT reduction (16%), and TT reduction (13%) after 1 week. There was an increase in the albumin level and ALT activity paralleling that of fibrinogen. No changes were noticed in Anti-thrombin (AT) III level, and AST activity. Transient changes in the coagulation activity were associated with NS administration to rats.

A slowing of body weight gain was also observed in NS treated rats, as compared to control animals. The low toxicity of NS fixed oil was evidenced by high LD50 values. The key hepatic enzyme stability and organ integrity after 12 weeks of administration, suggests a wide margin of safety for therapeutic doses of NS fixed oil, but the changes in hemoglobin metabolism and the fall in leukocyte and platelet count must be taken into consideration. It would appear that the beneficial effects of the use of the seeds and thymoquinone might be related to their cytoprotective and antioxidant actions, and also to their effect on some mediators of inflammation [1,3,16,17,18,19].

Antioxidative Effect

Four components of NS thymoquinone, carvacrol, t-anethole and 4-terpineol demonstrated respectable radical scavenging (anti-oxidant). TQ, the main biologically active component of NS is acting mainly as a potent superoxide anion scavenger. The aqueous extract of NS seeds exhibits an inhibitory effect on nitric oxide.

Four components   thymoquinone (TQ), carvacrol, t-anethole and 4-terpineol demonstrated respectable radical scavenging (anti-oxidant) property when tested in the diphenylpicrylhydracyl assay for non-specific hydrogen atom or electron donating activity. They were also effective OH radical scavenging agents in the assay for non-enzymatic lipid peroxidation in liposomes and the deoxyribose degradation assay. GC-MS analysis of the essential oil obtained from six different samples of NS seeds and from a commercial fixed oil showed that the qualitative composition of the volatile compounds was almost identical. Differences were mainly restricted to the quantitative composition [20].

Thymoquinone: a Potent Superoxide Anion Scavenger

Thymoquinone (TQ), a natural main constituent of the volatile oil of NS seeds, and a synthetic structurally-related tert-butylhydroquinone (TBHQ), both efficiently inhibited iron-dependent microsomal lipid peroxidation in a concentration-dependent manner with median inhibitory concentration (IC50) values of 16.8 and 14.9 microM, respectively. TBHQ was stronger than TQ as a scavenger of 2, 2'-diphenyl-p-picrylhydrazyl radical (DPPH) (IC50 = 5 microM, 200 times more active than TQ) and as a scavenger of hydroxyl radical (OH*) with an IC50 of 4.6 microM (approximately 10 times more active than TQ). TQ was more active than TBHQ as a superoxide anion scavenger with IC50 of 3.35 microM compared to 18.1 microM for TBHQ. Only TBHQ significantly promoted DNA damage in the bleomycin-Fe(III) system. Both TQ and TBHQ have strong antioxidant potentials through scavenging ability of different free radicals. TQ is acting mainly as a potent superoxide anion scavenger [21].

Inhibitory Effect on Nitric Oxide Production

The aqueous extract of NS seeds exhibits an inhibitory effect on nitric oxide (NO) production by murine macrophages and the active component(s) is/are non-protein in nature. The Aqueous extract of NS seeds caused a dose-dependent decrease in NO production by murine macrophages was studied. Murine peritoneal macrophages pre-incubated with the extract and then activated with Escherichia coli lipopolysaccharide. NO production was measured after 24 hours by spectrophotometry. Dialyzed preparation of the extract did not affect NO production. However, the boiled fraction of the extract resulted in a dose-dependent inhibition of NO apparently comparable to that of the whole extract [22].

Free Radicals Scavenger

Aflatoxins, a group of closely related, extremely toxic mycotoxins produced by Aspergillus flavus and A, can occur as natural contaminants of foods and feeds. Aflatoxins have been shown to be hepatotoxic, carcinogenic, mutagenic and teratogenic to different animal species. The volatile oils of NS were able to scavenge free radicals generated during aflatoxicosis. Sixty male rats were divided into six treatment groups, including a control group, and the groups were treated for 30 days with NS and Syzygium aromaticum oils with or without aflatoxin. Exposure to aflatoxin resulted in hematological and biochemical changes typical for aflatoxicosis. Treatment with NS and Syzygium aromaticum oil of rats fed an aflatoxin-contaminated diet resulted in significant protection against aflatoxicosis. NS oil was found to be more effective than Syzygium aromaticum oil in restoring the parameters that were altered by aflatoxin in rats [23].

More Potent and Safer Antioxidant than Vitamin E

Reactive oxygen species cause cytotoxic effects. The body requires the uptake of exogenous compounds with antioxidant potential. The safety of the fractionated antioxidant compounds of NS and their potency was compared with pure thymoquinone and vitamin E on A549 cells in culture for 24, 48 and 72 hours.NS extracts and pure thymoquinone showed markedly reduced levels of malondialdehyde (MDA) for the duration of the study. The vitamin E dosage used led to greater toxicity and cellular damage rather than cell protection [24].

Anti-Inflammatory Activity

Both systemic and local administration of NS seed essential oil showed anti-inflammatory activity. Thymoquinone, as one of the major components of NS seed essential oil, probably has an important role in these pharmacological effects [2].NS seed essential oil was found to produce a significant analgesic effect in acetic acid-induced writhing, formalin and light tail flick tests. Naloxone, an opioid antagonist, could not reverse the analgesic effect observed in the formalin test. Anti-inflammatory activity; Oral administration of NS seed essential oil at doses of 100, 200 and 400 micro L/kg did not exert a significant anti-inflammatory effect in the carrageenan test-induced paw edemas in rats and croton oil-induced ear edemas in mice, i.p. injection of the same doses significantly ($p < 0.001$) inhibited carrageenan-induced paw edemas. NS seed essential oil at doses of 10 and 20 micro L/ear could also reduce croton oil-induced edemas. It seems that mechanism(s) other than opioid receptors is (are) involved in the analgesic effect of NS since Naloxone could not reverse this effect [3].

Favorable Effects in Experimental Diabetes

NS has protective and hypoglycemic effects on STZ induced diabetes. The pro-tective effect is attributed to a reduction in the oxidative stress, while the hypo glycemic effect is attributed to partial regeneration/proliferation of the beta-cells in the islets of Langerhans causing an increase in insulin secretion, a decrease in hepatic gluconeogenesis and stimulation of macrophage phagocytic activity, Insulinotropic, and insulin-sensitizing effects.

1-Pancreatic B cell protective effect has been shown in streptozocin (STZ) induced diabetes in association with a decrease in the oxidative stress [25]:

STZ injected intraperitoneally at a single dose of 50 mg/kg to induce diabetes induced a significant increase in serum nitric oxide (NO) and erythrocyte and pancreatic tissue malondialdehyde (MDA) levels, a marker of lipid peroxidation, and decreased antioxidant enzymes glutathione peroxidase (GSHPx), superoxide dismutase (SOD), and catalase (CAT)) in pancreatic homogenates. NS (0.2 ml/kg/day, i.p.) when injected for 3 days prior to STZ administration, and continued throughout the 4-week study provided a protective effect by decreasing lipid peroxidation and serum NO, and increasing antioxidant enzyme activity. Islet cell degeneration and weak insulin immunohistochemical staining was observed in rats with STZ-induced diabetes. Increased intensity of staining for insulin, and preservation of beta-cell numbers were apparent in the NS-treated diabetic rats. NS treatment exerts a therapeutic protective effect in diabetes by decreasing oxidative stress and preserving pancreatic beta-cell integrity.

2- Partial regeneration/proliferation of the beta-cells in the islets of Langerhans by Nigella sativa L. in streptozotocin [26].

Fifty male Wistar rats (200-250 g) were divided into two experimental groups (diabetics with no treatment and diabetics with NS. treatment), each containing twenty-five rats. Diabetes was induced in both groups by a single intraperitoneal injection of Streptozotocin (STZ) (50 mg/kg). The experimental animals in both groups became diabetic within 24 hours after the administration of STZ. The rats in NS treated group were given the daily intraperitoneal injection of 0.20 ml/kg of NS volatile oil for 30 days starting the day after STZ injection. Control rats received only the same amount of normal saline solution. The rats in both groups received the last injection 24 hours before the sacrification and 5 randomly selected rats in each group were sacrificed before, and the 1, 10, 20 and 30 days after the STZ injection to collect blood and pancreatic tissue samples. The NS treatment caused a decrease in the elevated serum glucose, an increase in the lowered serum insulin concentrations and partial regeneration/ proliferation of pancreatic beta-cells in STZ-induced diabetic rats with the elapse of the experiment. The hypoglycemic action of NS could be partly due to amelioration in the beta-cells of pancreatic islets causing an increase in insulin secretion.

3-Hypoglycemic effect has been shown in STZ in association with a decrease in hepatic gluconeogenesis and stimulation of macrophage phagocytic activity [27].

Diabetes was induced by intraperitoneal injection of 65 mg/kg body weight of STZ. Treatment with NS oil commenced 6 weeks after induction of diabetes at a dose of 400 mg/kg body weight by gastric gavage. NS oil reduced blood glucose from 391+/-3.0 mg/dl before treatment to 325+/-4.7, 246+/-5.9, 208+/-2.5 and 179+/-3.1 mg/dl after the first, second, third and fourth weeks of treatment, respectively. Hepatic glucose production from gluconeogenic precursors (alanine, glycerol and lactate) was significantly lower in isolated hepatocytes collected using collagenase in treated hamsters. Treatment with N. sativa oil significantly increased the phagocytic activity and phagocytic index of peritoneal macrophages (evaluated by injection of fluorescent latex (2 microM diameter) intraperitoneally, followed 24 h later by collection of peritoneal macrophages) and lymphocyte count in peripheral blood compared with untreated diabetic hamsters.

4- Insulinotropic effect of NS seeds [28]:

The insulin secretory effects of these extracts were evaluated individually at different concentrations (0.01, 0.1, 1 and 5 mg/mL), in vitro in isolated rat pancreatic islets in the presence of 8.3 mmol/L glucose. The results show that addition of the defatted whole extract or of the basic subfraction of the seed in the incubation medium significantly increased glucose-induced insulin release from the islets. In the case of the acidic and neutral subfraction, the stimulatory effect was observed only for the higher concentration (5 mg/mL). A clear concentration-dependent increase in insulin release from isolated pancreatic islets was observed for the basic subfraction.

Hypoglycemic effect of NS oil was also demonstrated in Streptozotocin plus Nicotinamide diabetic hamsters resulted. It was attributed at least partly to a stimulatory effect on beta cell function with consequent increase in serum insulin level [29].

Nicotinamide was injected intraperitoneally 15min before injection of Streptozotocin intravenously. Oral treatment with NS oil began 4 weeks after induction of diabetes. . Islets insulin was stained using anti-insulin monoclonal antibody. Significant decrease in blood glucose level together with significant increase in serum insulin level (measured by enzyme immunoassay) were observed after treatment with NS oil for 4 weeks. Big areas with positive immuno-reactivity for the presence of insulin were observed in the pancreases from NS oil-treated group compared to non-treated one using immunohistochemical staining function with consequent increase in serum insulin level.

5- insulin-sensitizing and hypolipedimic actions [30]:

A 4-week intragastric gavage with a petroleum ether extract of NS seeds was associated with lower fasting plasma levels of insulin and triglycerides, and higher HDL-cholesterol in the treated rats as compared controls. Fasting plasma glucose remained stable throughout NS treatment.

Response to insulin was evaluated in hepatocytes isolated from animals of all groups by Western blot analysis of phosphorylated MAPK p44/42erk and PKB. In vivo NS treatment resulted in greater dose-dependent activation of MAPK and PKB in response to insulin. In vivo treatment with the petroleum ether extract exerts an insulin-sensitizing action by enhancing the activity of the two major intracellular signal transduction pathways of the hormone's receptor.

In experimentally induced diabetic rabbits NS was associated with a decrease in lipid peroxidation, increase in the anti-oxidant defense system and also a protective effect against lipid-peroxidation-induced liver damage.

Fifteen New Zealand male rabbits were divided into three experimental groups: control, diabetic and diabetic and NS-treated. Diabetes mellitus was induced in the rabbits using 150 mg/kg of 10% alloxan. The diabetic + NS-treated group was given extract of NS seeds orally every day for 2 months after induction of DM. At the end of the 2-month NS decreased the elevated glucose and malondialdehyde concentrations, increased the lowered glutathione and ceruloplasmin concentrations, and prevented lipid-peroxidation-induced liver damage in diabetic rabbits [31].

Protective Effects Against Chemically-induced Hepatotoxicity and Nephrotoxicity

Renoprotective Effect

The pathogenesis of gentamicin (GM) nephrotoxicity has been shown to involve the generation of oxygen free radicals, and several free radical scavengers have been shown to ameliorate the nephrotoxicity. Oral treatment of rats with NS oil (0.5, 1.0 or 2.0 ml/kg/day for 10 days) was associated with amelioration of nephrotoxicity of GM (80 mg/kg/day given intramuscularly when used concomitantly with the NS oil during the last 6 days of treatment.GM treatment caused moderate proximal tubular damage, significantly increased the concentrations of creatinine and urea, and decreased total antioxidant status in plasma and reduced glutathione. Treatment with NS oil produced a dose-dependent amelioration of the biochemical and histological indices of GM nephrotoxicity that was statistically significant at the two higher doses used. Compared to controls, treatments of rats with NS did not cause any overt toxicity, and it increased GSH and TAS concentrations in renal cortex and enhanced growth [32].

Hepatoprotective Effects

It has been reported that NS oil possesses hepatoprotective effects in some models of liver toxicity. Aqueous suspension of NS was associated with a protective effect on carbon tetrachloride (CCL4)-induced liver damage. NS oil per se has also been associated with protective effect against hepatotoxicity induced by D-galactosamine or carbon tetrachloride and the hepatoprotective effect of TQ against tert-butyl hydroperoxide (TBHP) toxicity has also been shown in isolated rat hepatocytes.It has been shown that thymoquinone protects against carbon tetrachloride hepatotoxicity in mice via an antioxidant mechanism. The protective effect of NS on carbon tetrachloride (CCL4)-induced hepatotoxicity was superior to the effect of other antioxidants.

Aqueous suspension of the seeds was given orally at two dose levels (250 mg/kg and 500 mg/kg) for five days. CCL4 (250 microl/kg intraperitoneally / day in olive oil) was given to the experimental group on days 4 and 5, while the control group was only treated with the vehicles. Animals treated with CCL4 showed remarkable centrilobular fatty changes and moderate inflammatory infiltrate in the form of neutrophil and mononuclear cells when compared to the controls. This effect was significantly decreased in animals pretreated with N. sativa. Histopathological or biochemical changes were not evident following administration of N sativa alone. Serum levels of aspartic transaminase (AST), and L-alanine aminotransferase (ALT) were slightly decreased while lactate dehydrogenase (LDH) was significantly increased in animals treated with CCL4 when compared to the control group. LDH was restored to normal but ALT and AST levels were increased in animals pretreated with NS [33].

In an other study fifty Sprague-Dawley rats were allocated into five groups (I, IIA and B, IIIA and B) and CCl4 was injected biweekly to all groups. Group I (control, CCl4 only), group IIA and B (NS fixed oil and volatile oil), group IIIA and B (UD fixed oil and UD decoction extract) rats were killed at the end of week 12 and Histopathological and immunohistochemical examinations of liver tissues were performed. In the control group, coagulation necrosis and hydropic degeneration were marked in the periacinar regions (zone 3) associated with fibrosis in the periacinar regions and in the portal tracts. In groups IIA-B and IIIA-B (NS and UD), none of the serious Histopathological findings were detected except for sparse coagulation necrosis in the periacinar regions. ASMA-positive perisinusoidal cells with myo-fibroblastic transformation and lysosomal enzyme activity suggesting fibrogenesis were also significantly more common in the control group than in the NS and UD groups [34].

NS oil per se has also been associated with protective effect against hepatotoxicity induced by D-galactosamine or carbon tetrachloride. The daily administration of NS oil per se (800 mg/kg orally for 4 weeks) did not adversely affect the serum transaminases (ALT and AST), alkaline phosphatase, and serum bilirubin or prothrombin activity in normal albino rats. When the oil was given for 4 weeks prior to induction of hepatotoxicity by D-galactosamine or carbon tetrachloride, it was able to give complete protection against d-galactosamine and partial protection against carbon tetrachloride hepatotoxicity. NS oil showed a favorable effect on the serum lipid pattern where the administration of the oil (800 mg/kg orally for 4 weeks) caused a significant decrease in serum total cholesterol, low density lipoprotein, triglycerides and a significant elevation of serum high density lipoprotein level [35].

The Hepatoprotective effect of TQ against tert-butyl hydroperoxide (TBHP) toxicity has also been shown in isolated rat hepatocytes. TBHP (2 mM) was used to produce oxidative injury in isolated rat hepatocytes and caused progressive depletion of intracellular glutathione (GSH), loss of cell viability as evidenced by trypan blue uptake and leakage of cytosolic enzymes, alanine transaminase (ALT) and aspartic transaminase (AST). Pre-incubation of hepatocytes with 1 mM of either thymoquinone resulted in the protection of isolated hepatocytes against TBHP induced toxicity evidenced by decreased leakage of ALT and AST, and by decreased trypan blue uptake in comparison to TBHP treated hepatocytes. Both thymoquinone and silybin prevented TBHP induced depletion of GSH to the same extent [36]. It has been shown that TQ protects against carbon tetrachloride hepatotoxicity in mice via an antioxidant mechanism [37]. Comparing the effect of vitamins C and E, selenium and Nigella sativa (NS) on the prevention of carbon tetrachloride (CCl4)-induced liver fibrosis in rabbits. It was found that superoxide dismutase (SOD) values in all of the treated groups were significantly lower than those of the control at 12th week of experiment ($p < 0.05$), while at 6th week and 12th week of experiment glutathione peroxidase (GSH-Px) values in the vitamin C treated group were significantly different from the control ($p < 0.05$). Histopathologically, hepatocellular necrosis, degeneration and advanced fibrosis were found in the control group. Lesions were minor and only confined to midzonal regions without centrilobular necrosis and fibrosis in the NS treated animals. The lesions observed in the vitamin C treated animals were similar to that of the control group. Parenchymal changes with fibrosis were less in selenium and vitamin E treated animals than in those of the control, but more obvious than in NS group. Histopathological findings demonstrate that NS was superior in the prevention of liver fibrosis in rabbits than vitamin E and selenium [38].

Potential Anti-tumor Activity of NS

NS oil decreases the fibrinolytic potential of the human fibrosarcoma cell line(HT1080)in vitro.The volatile oil of NS inhibits colon carcinogenesis of rats in the post-initiation stage,whileThymoquinone extracted from NS seed inhibits the growth of colon cancer cells by triggering apoptotic cell death in human colorectal cancer cells via a p53-dependent mechanism.

TQ has anti-proliferative effect, induces apoptosis, disrupts mitochondrial membrane potential and triggers the activation of caspases 8, 9 and 3 in myeloblastic leukemia HL-60 cells.NS seeds fatty acids demonstrated in vitro 50% cytotoxic activities against Ehrlch ascites carcinoma Dalton's lymphoma ascites and sarcoma-180 cells and, in vivo completely inhibits Ehrlich ascites carcinoma tumor development in mice.

1- NS oil decreases the fibrinolytic potential of the human fibrosarcoma cell line (HT1080) in vitro [39]:

It is generally accepted that the fibrinolytic potential of tumor cells is related to their malignant phenotype. NS oil decreases the fibrinolytic potential of the human fibrosarcoma cell line (HT1080) in vitro, implying that inhibition of local tumor invasion and metastasis may be one such mechanism.

NS oil produced a concentration-dependent inhibition of tissue-type plasminogen activator (t-PA), urokinase-type plasminogen activator (u-PA) and plasminogen activator inhibitor type 1 (PAI-1). When subconfluent HT1080 cells were conditioned with oil, a concentration (0.0-200 microg oil/ml)-dependent decrease in t-PA, u-PA and PAI-1 antigen was observed. There was also a concentration-dependent decrease (from 0.0 to 112.5 microg oil/ml) in the confluent cultures.

2- The volatile oil of NS has the ability to inhibit colon carcinogenesis of rats in the post-initiation stage, with no evident adverse side effects, and that the inhibition may be associated, in part, with suppression of cell proliferation in the colonic mucosa [40]. Chemo-preventive effects of orally administered NS oil on the induction and development of 1,2-dimethylhydrazine-induced aberrant crypt foci (ACF), putative pre-neoplastic lesions for colon cancer was demonstrated in rats. In 344 Fischer rats, starting at 6 wk of age, 45 male rats (groups 1-3) were subcutaneously injected with DMH once a week for 3 wk. Group 1 (15 rats) served as a carcinogen control group without NS administration. Group 2 or 3 (15 rats each) were given the oil in the post-initiation stage or in the initiation stage, respectively. Animals of group 4 (11 rats) were injected with 0.9% saline and received N. sativa oil from the beginning until the termination. At sacrifice, 14 wk after the start, the total numbers of ACF as well as those with at least four crypts were significantly reduced in group 2 (P < 0.01). However, treatment with NS oil in the initiation stage (group 3) did not exhibit significant inhibitory effects except on foci with only one aberrant crypt. Immunohistochemical analysis of 5-bromo-2'.-deoxyuridine labeling in colonic crypts revealed the NS oil to have significant anti-proliferative activity in both initiation and post-initiation stages and especially in the latter. Histological examination revealed no pathological changes in the liver, kidneys, spleen, or other organs of rats treated with NS. In addition, biochemical parameters of blood and urine as well as body weight gain were not affected.

3- Thymoquinone extracted from NS seed triggers apoptotic cell death in human colorectal cancer cells via a p53-dependent mechanism [41].

Thymoquinone (TQ) inhibits the growth of colon cancer cells inhibition was correlated with G1 phase arrest of the cell cycle. TUNEL staining and flow cytometry analysis indicate that TQ triggers apoptosis in a dose- and time-dependent manner. Apoptosis induction by TQ was associated with a 2.5-4.5-fold increase in mRNA expression of p53 and the downstream p53 target gene, p21WAF1. Simultaneously a marked increase in p53 and p21WAF1 protein levels but a significant inhibition of anti-apoptotic Bcl-2 protein. Co-incubation with pifithrin-alpha (PFT-alpha), a specific inhibitor of p53, restored Bcl-2, p53 and p21WAF1 levels to the untreated control and suppressed TQ-induced cell cycle arrest and apoptosis. P53-null HCT-116 cells were less sensitive to TQ-induced growth arrest and apoptosis. TQ is antineoplastic and pro-apoptotic against colon cancer cell line HCT116. The apoptotic effects of TQ are modulated by Bcl-2 protein and are linked to and dependent on p53. TQ has the potential for the treatment of colon cancer.

4- Thymoquinone (TQ) exhibits anti-proliferative effect, induces apoptosis, disrupts mitochondrial membrane potential and triggers the activation of caspases 8, 9 and 3 in myeloblastic leukemia HL-60 cells. The apoptosis induced by TQ was inhibited by a general caspase inhibitor, z-VAD-FMK; a caspase-3-specific inhibitor, z-DEVD-FMK; as well as a caspase-8-specific inhibitor, z-IETD-FMK. Moreover, the caspase-8 inhibitor blocked the TQ-induced activation of caspase-3, PARP cleavage and the release of cytochrome c from mitochondria into the cytoplasm. In addition, TQ treatment of HL-60 cells caused a marked increase in Bax/Bcl2 ratios due to up regulation of Bax and down regulation of Bcl2 proteins. TQ-induced apoptosis is associated with the activation of caspases 8, 9 and 3, with caspase-8 acting as an upstream activator. Activated caspase-8 initiates the release of cytochrome c during TQ-induced apoptosis [42].

5- NS seed (fatty acids) at the dose of 2 mg/mouse per day for 10 days was associated with complete inhibition Ehrlich ascites carcinoma (EAC) tumor development in vivo. In vitro cytotoxic studies showed 50% cytotoxicity to Ehrlich ascites carcinoma, Dalton's lymphoma ascites and Sarcoma-180 cells at a concentration of 1.5 micrograms, 3 micrograms and 1.5 micrograms respectively with little activity against lymphocytes. The cell growth of KB cells in culture was inhibited by the active principle while K-562 cells resumed near control values on day 2 and day 3. Tritiated thymidine incorporation studies indicated the possible action of an active principle at DNA level. In vivo EAC tumor development was completely inhibited by the active principle at the dose of 2 mg/mouse per day x 10 [43].

6- In vitro cytotoxic activity of column fraction 5 (CC-5) of an ethanolic extract of NS seeds has been previously reported.

In vivo anti-tumor activity of CC-5 against intraperitoneally implanted murine P388 leukemia and subcutaneously implanted LL/2 (Lewis lung carcinoma) cells has been shown in BDF1 mice (C57BL/6 x DBA/2 mice). CC-5 at doses of 200 and 400 mg/kg body weight prolonged the life span of these mice by 153% compared to DMSO-treated control mice. The antitumor activity of a 21-day treatment of CC-5 against subcutaneously implanted LL/2 has been shown in mice. CC-5 at a dose of 400 mg/kg body weight produced significant tumor inhibition rate (TIR) values of 60% ($P < 0.001$) and 70% ($P < 0.001$) respectively. Alpha-hederin, a triterpene saponin isolated from CC-5, when given intraperitoneally for 7 days at doses of 5 and 10 mg/kg to mice with formed tumors, produced significant dose-dependent TIR values of 48% ($P < 0.05$) and 65% ($p < 0.01$) respectively on day 8 and 50% ($P < 0.01$) and 71% ($P < 0.001$), respectively, on day 15, compared to 81% ($P < 0.01$) on day 8 and 42% ($P < 0.01$) on day 15 in the cyclophosphamide (CP)-treated group [44].

A crude gum, a fixed oil and two purified components of NS seed, thymoquinone (TQ) and dithymoquinone (DIM), were associated in vitro with a cytotoxicity for several parental and multi-drug resistant (MDR) human tumor cell lines. Although as much as 1% w/v of the gum or oil was devoid of cytotoxicity, both TQ and DIM were cytotoxic for all of the tested cell lines (IC50's 78 to 393 microM). Both the parental cell lines and their corresponding MDR variants, over 10-fold more resistant to the standard antineoplastic agents doxorubicin (DOX) and etoposide (ETP), as compared to their respective parental controls, were equally sensitive to TQ and DIM. The inclusion of the competitive MDR modulator quinine in the assay reversed MDR Dx-5 cell resistance to DOX and ETP by 6- to 16-fold, but had no effect on the cytotoxicity of TQ or DIM. Quinine also increased MDR Dx-5 cell accumulation of the P-glycoprotein substrate 3H-taxol in a dose-dependent manner. However, neither TQ nor DIM significantly altered cellular accumulation of 3H-taxol. The inclusion of 0.5% v/v of the radical scavenger DMSO in the assay reduced the cytotoxicity of DOX by as much as 39%, but did not affect that of TQ or DIM. These studies suggest that TQ and DIM, which are cytotoxic for several types of human tumor cells, may not be MDR substrates, and that radical generation may not be critical to their cytotoxic activity [45].

A Potential Immunosuppressive Cytotoxic Agent

In long-Evans rats challenged with a specific antigen (typhoid TH).Antibody titre for the experimental animal was found to be 1280 as compared to the 2560 in the control rats. Treatment with NS volatile oil caused a significant ($p < 0.05$) decrease in splenocytes and neutrophils counts, but a rise in peripheral lymphocytes and monocytes in the experimental animals.

The cytotoxicity of NS volatile was compared to that of vinblastin and mitomycin C in a panel of five human cancer cell lines and a fibroblast line. The MTT assay was employed to estimate the cell mortality. Vinblastine sulphate and mitomycin C were used as the positive control. LC(50) values for NS volatile oil were 155.02 +/- 10.4, 185.77 +/- 2.9, 120.40 +/- 20.5, 384.53 +/- 12.1 and 286.83 +/- 23.3 micro g/ml respectively against the SCL, SCL-6, SCL-37'6, NUGC-4 cancer lines and 3T6 fibroblast line [46].

Anticonvulsant Effects of Nigella Sativa

The Anticonvulsant Effects of Thymoquinone

In pentylenetetrazole (PTZ)-induced seizure model. The Intracerebroventricular (i.c.v.) injection of thymoquinone at doses of 200 and 400 microM prolonged the time until onset and reduced the duration of tonic-clonic seizures. The protective effect of thymoquinone against lethality was 45% and 50% in the respective doses. In this study, flumazenil (1 nM, i.c.v.) reversed the anticonvulsant activity of thymoquinone. Also, pretreatment with naloxone (10 microM, i.c.v.) antagonized the prolongation of tonic-clonic seizure latency as well as the reduction in seizure duration induced by thymoquinone (200 microM, i.c.v.) [47]. In pentylenetetrazole (PTZ)-and maximal electroshock (MES)-induced seizure models, the intraperitoneally injection of thymoquinone with doses of 40 and 80 mg/kg, prolonged the onset of seizures and reduced the duration of myoclonic seizures. The protective effect of thymoquinone against mortality was 71.4% and 100% in the mentioned doses, respectively. In MES model, thymoquinone failed to reduce the duration of seizure, whereas exhibited a complete protection against mortality. In PTZ model, flumazenil (10 mg/kg, i.p.), an antagonist of benzodiazepine (BZD) site in the GABAA-BZD receptor complex, inhibited the prolongation of seizure latency, but did not show any effect on the duration of myoclonic seizures. Also, pretreatment with naloxone (0.1 and 03 mg/kg, i.p.) inhibited the prolongation of myoclonic seizure latency and antagonized the reduction of myoclonic seizure duration induced by thymoquinone (40 and 80 mg/kg) in the PTZ model. Moreover, thymoquinone (40 and 80 mg/kg) did not have any hypnosis effect in the pentobarbital-induced hypnosis, but impaired the motor coordination and reduced the locomotor activity Thymoquinone may have anticonvulsant activity in tonic clonic seizures and petit mal epilepsy probably through an opioid receptor-mediated increase in GABAergic tone [48].

Anti-Leukotriene Effect: 5-Lipoxygenase and Leukotriene C4 Synthase Inhibitor

Leukotriene B4 (LTB4) and the cysteinyl leukotrienes C4, D4 and E4 are the products of 5-lipoxygenase pathway of arachidonic acid metabolism. 5-lipoxygenase is found in cells of myeloid origin such as mast cells, eosinophils, basophils and neutrophils.

LTB4 is a potent chemo- attractant to neutrophils and eosinophils, wherease the cysteinyl LTs constrict bronchiolar smooth muscle, increase endothelial permeability, and promote mucus secretion. Few anti-leukotriene drugs (zileuton, zafirlukast and montelukast) have already been approved for the prophylaxis of asthma [49].

Leukotrienes (LTs) are important mediators in asthma and inflammatory processes TQ provoked a significant concentration-dependent inhibition of both LTC4 and LTB4 formation from endogenous substrate in human granulocyte suspensions with IC50 values of 1.8 and 2.3 microM, respectively, at 15 min. Major inhibitory effect was on the 5-lipoxygenase activity (IC50 3 microM) as evidenced by suppressed conversion of exogenous arachidonic acid into 5-hydroxy eicosatetraenoic acid (5HETE) in sonicated polymorphonuclear cell suspensions. In addition, TQ induced a significant inhibition of LTC4 synthase activity, with an IC50 of 10 microM, as judged by suppressed transformation of exogenous LTA4 into LTC4. In contrast, the drug was without any inhibitory effect on LTA4 hydrolase activity.

When exogenous LTA4 was added to intact or sonicated platelet suspensions pre-incubated with TQ, a similar inhibition of LTC4 synthase activity was observed as in human granulocyte suspensions. The unselective protein kinase inhibitor, staurosporine failed to prevent inhibition of LTC4 synthase activity induced by TQ. TQ potently inhibits the formation of leukotrienes in human blood cells. The inhibitory effect was dose- and time-dependent and was exerted on both 5-lipoxygenase and LTC4 synthase activity [50,51].

TQ caused a concentration-dependent decrease in the tension of the guinea-pig isolated tracheal smooth muscle pre-contracted by carbachol.The effects of TQ were significantly potentiated by pretreatment of the tracheal preparations with quinacrine, a phospholipase A2 inhibitor, nordihydroguiaretic acid, a lipoxygenase inhibitor and by pretreatment with methylene blue, an inhibitor of soluble guanylyl cyclase. On the other hand, the effects of TQ were not influenced by pretreatment of the tracheal preparations with indomethacin, a cyclooxygenase inhibitor, propranolol, a non-selective beta-adrenoceptor blocker or by the pretreatment with theophylline, an adenosine receptors antagonist. TQ totally abolished the pressor effects of histamine and serotonin on the guinea-pig isolated tracheal and ileum smooth muscles. TQ induced relaxation of pre-contracted tracheal preparation is probably mediated, at least in part, by inhibition of lipoxygenase products of arachidonic acid metabolism and possibly by non-selective blocking of the histamine and serotonin receptors. This relaxant effect of TQ, needs further experimental and clinical studies to confirm the possible therapeutic potential in the treatment of bronchial asthma [52].

Thymoquinone: Bone Healing Effect

In experimental femur defect model in rats treated with surgical implantation with TCPL capsule loaded with 0.02 grams of TMQ and 200 mg vancomycin. After 30 days of treatment, the healing pattern of animals in treatment group was better compared to control .Sustained levels of TMQ can enhance bone healing with little or no side effects on major vital and reproductive organs [53].

Anti-Inflammatory and Analgesic Effect

The crude fixed oil of NS and TQ inhibited cyclooxygenase and 5-lipooxygenase pathways of arachidonate metabolism in rat peritoneal leukocytes. The effect was demonstrated via the dose-dependent inhibition of the formation of thromboxane B_2 and leukotriene B_4. This effect was also confirmed using aqueous suspension of NS crushed seeds. In both studies formation of edema in rat hind paw was inhibited and these effects were comparable to those of indomethacin and aspirin, respectively [54]. The analgesic effect of aqueous susprion of NS seeds, comparable to aspirin, as measured by hot plate test conducted in rats. However the suspension did not relieve yeast-induced pyrexia in rats [55]. The mechanism of anti-inflammatory and analgesic effects has been attributed to inhibition of eicosanoid synthesis [3]. The analgesic action could be the result of the activation of supraspinal *mu* (1)- and *kappa*-opioid receptors subtypes, as elicited by the antagonistic effect of naloxone, naloxonazine and nor-binaltorphimine to antinociceptive effects of NS oil and thymoquinone [56].

Anti-Infective Properties

Bacterial Growth Inhibition

Filter paper discs impregnated with the diethyl ether extract of NS seeds (25-400 micrograms extract/disc) caused concentration-dependent inhibition of Gram-positive bacteria represented by Staphylococcus aureus. Gram-negative bacteria represented by Pseudomonas aeruginosa and Escherichia coli (but not Salmonella typhimurium) and a pathogenic yeast Candida albicans. The extract showed antibacterial synergism with streptomycin and gentamicin and showed additive antibacterial action with spectinomycin, erythromycin, tobramycin, doxycycline, chloramphenicol, nalidixic acid, ampicillin, lincomycin and sulphamethoxyzole-trimethoprim combination. The extract successfully eradicated a non-fatal subcutaneous staphylococcal infection in mice when injected at the site of infection [57].

Different crude extracts of NS demonstrated antimicrobial effectiveness against different bacterial isolates. These isolates comprised 16 gram negative and 6 gram positive representatives. They showed multiple resistance against antibiotics, specially the gram negative ones. Crude extracts of Nigella saliva showed a promising effect against some of the test organisms. The most effective extracts were the crude alkaloid and water extracts. Gram negative isolates were affected more than the grampositive ones [58].

Anti-Viral Effect

Antiviral effect of NS has been shown using murine cytomegalovirus (MCMV) as a model.

The viral load and innate immunity mediated by NK cells and Mφ during early stage of the infection were analyzed. Intraperitoneal (i.p.) administration of NSO to BALB/c mice, a susceptible strain of MCMV infection, strikingly inhibited the virus titers in spleen and liver on day 3 of infection with $1 \times 10(5)$ PFU MCMV. This effect coincided with an increase in serum level of IFN-gamma. Although NSO treatment decreased both number and cytolytic function of NK cells on day 3 of infection, it increased numbers of Mφ and CD4(+) T cells. On day 10 of infection, the virus titer was undetectable in spleen and liver of NSO-treated mice, while it was detectable in control mice. Although spleen of both control and NSO-treated mice showed similar CTL activities on day 10 after infection, serum level of IFN-gamma in NSO-treated mice was higher. Furthermore, NSO treatment upregulated suppressor function of Mφ in spleen. These results show that BSO exhibited a striking antiviral effect against MCMV infection which may be mediated by increasing of Mφ number and function, and IFN-gamma production [59].

Effect on the immune System

NS enhanced the production of interleukin-3 by human lymphocytes when cultured with pooled allogenic cells or without any added stimulator with an increase in interleukin-1 beta (IL-1β) suggesting that an effect on macrophages as well [60].

On mixed lymphocyte culture, NS seeds and its purified proteins demonstrated stimulatory as well as suppressive effects depending upon the donor and the concentration used. Stimulant effect was observed with fractionated NS proteins (P1 and P2) with a maximum effect at 10 ug/ml. Suppressive effect was observed with NS seeds and high concentrations of all of its four proteins when lymphocytes were activated with poked-weed mitogen. In culture medium with non-activated peripheral blood mononuclear cells and with allogenic cells whole, NS produced large quantities of IL-1 beta, but no effect was seen on IL-4 secretion. The effect on IL-8 production was variable. However, a stimulatory effect of whole NS and its fractionated proteins was noticed on the production of TNF-α in both non-activated and mitogen activated cells [61].

The ethyl-acetate chromatographic fraction of ethanolic extract of N Shas also been reported to potenciate cellular immune responses [62].

REFERENCES

[1]   Ali BH, Blunden G. Pharmacological and toxicological properties of Nigella sativa. *Phytother Res*. 2003 Apr;17(4):299-305.

[2]   Nickavar B, Mojab F, Javidnia K, Amoli MA. Chemical composition of the fixed and volatile oils of Nigella sativa L. from *Iran.Z Naturforsch [C]*. 2003 Sep-Oct;58(9-10):629-31.

[3]   Hajhashemi V, Ghannadi A, Jafarabadi H. Black cumin seed essential oil, as a potent analgesic and antiinflammatory drug. *Phytother Res*. 2004 Mar;18(3):195-9.

[4]   Ramadan MF, Morsel JT.Characterization of phospholipid composition of black cumin (Nigella sativa L.) seed oil. *Nahrung*. 2002 Aug;46(4):240-4.

[5]   Gad AM, El-Dakhakhany M, Hassan MM. Studies on the chemical constitution of Egyptian Nigella sativa L oil. *Planta Med* 1963; 11 (2): 134-8.

[6]   Babayan VK, Koottungal D, Halaby GA. Proximate analysis, fatty acid and amino acid composition of Nigella sativa L seeds. *J Food Sci* 1978; 43 (4): 1314-5.

[7]   Salama RB. Sterols in the seed oil of *Nigella sativa. Planta Med* 1973; 24 (4):375-7.

[8]   Menounos P, Staphylakis K, Gegiou D. The sterols of Nigella sativa seed oil. *Phytochemistry* 1986; 25: 761-3.

[9]   El-Zawahry BH. Isolation of new hypotensive fraction from Nigella sativa seed. *Kongr Pharm Wiss* 1964; 23: 193-203.

[10]   Ata-ur-Rehman, Malik S, Ahmed S, Chaudhry I, Habib-ur-Rehman. Nigellimine-N-Oxide, a new isoquinoline alkaloid from seeds of Nigella sativa. *Heterocycles* 1985; 23: 953-5.

[11]   Ata-ur-Rehman, Malik S, Cun-Hung H, Clardy J. Isolation and structure determination of nigellicine, a novel alkaloid from seeds of Nigella sativa. *Tetrahedron Lett* 1985; 26: 2759-62.

[12]   Atta-ur-Rehman, Malik S. Nigellidine, a new indazole alkaloid from seeds of Nigella sativa. *J Res Iinst* 1995; 36: 1993-6.

[13]   Drozed AG, Komissarenko FN, Litvinenko EA. Coumarins of some species of Ranunaulaceae family. *Farm ZH* 1970; 25 (4): 57-60.

[14] Kumara SS, Huat BT. Extraction, isolation and characterization of anti-tumour principle, alpha-hedrin, from the seeds of Nigella sativa. *Planta Med* 2001;67(1):29-2.

[15] Ansari AA, Hassan S, Kenne L, Atta-ur-Rehman, Wehler T. Structural studies on a saponin isolated from Nigella sativa. *Phytochemistry* 1988; 27 (12): 3977-9.

[16] Al-Naggar TB, Gomez-Serranillos MP, Carretero ME, Villar AM.Neuropharmacological activity of Nigella sativa L. extracts. *J Ethnopharmacol.* 2003 Sep;88(1):63-8.

[17] Zedlitz S, Kaufmann R, Boehncke WH.Allergic contact dermatitis from black cumin (Nigella sativa) oil-containing ointment. *Contact Dermatitis.* 2002 Mar;46(3):188..

[18] Zaoui A, Cherrah Y, Mahassini N, Alaoui K, Amarouch H, Hassar M.Acute and chronic toxicity of Nigella sativa fixed oil. *Phytomedicine.* 2002 Jan;9(1):69-74.

[19] Al-Jishi SA, Abuo Hozaifa B.Effect of Nigella sativa on blood hemostatic function in rats. *J Ethnopharmacol.* 2003 Mar;85(1):7-1 .

[20] Burits M, Bucar F. Antioxidant activity of Nigella sativa essential oil. Phytother Res. 2000 Aug;14(5):323-8. Institute of Pharmacognosy.

[21] Badary OA, Taha RA, Gamal el-Din AM, Abdel-Wahab MH.Thymoquinone is a potent superoxide anion scavenger. *Drug Chem Toxicol.* 2003 May;26(2):87-98.

[22] Mahmood MS, Gilani AH, Khwaja A, Rashid A, Ashfaq MK.The in vitro effect of aqueous extract of Nigella sativa seeds on nitric oxide production. *Phytother Res.* 2003 Sep;17(8):921-4.

[23] Abdel-Wahhab MA, Aly SE.Antioxidant property of Nigella sativa (black cumin) and Syzygium aromaticum (clove) in rats during aflatoxicosis. *J Appl Toxicol.* 2005 May-Jun;25(3):218-23..

[24] Farah N, Benghuzzi H, Tucci M, Cason Z. The effects of isolated antioxidants from black seed on the cellular metabolism of A549 cells. *Biomed Sci Instrum.* 2005;41:211-6.

[25] Kanter M, Coskun O, Korkmaz A, Oter S. Effects of Nigella sativa on oxidative stress and beta-cell damage in streptozotocin-induced diabetic rats. *Anat Rec A Discov Mol Cell Evol Biol.* 2004 Jul;279(1):685-91.

[26] Kanter M, Meral I, Yener Z, Ozbek H, Demir H. Partial regeneration/proliferation of the beta-cells in the islets of Langerhans by Nigella sativa L. in streptozotocin-induced diabetic rats.*Tohoku J Exp Med.* 2003 Dec;201(4):213-9.

[27] Fararh KM, Atoji Y, Shimizu Y, Shiina T, Nikami H, Takewaki T. Mechanisms of the hypoglycaemic and immunopotentiating effects of Nigella sativa L. oil in streptozotocin-induced diabetic hamsters. *Res Vet Sci.* 2004 Oct;77(2):123-9.

[28] Rchid H, Chevassus H, Nmila R, Guiral C, Petit P, Chokairi M, Sauvaire Y. Nigella sativa seed extracts enhance glucose-induced insulin release from rat-isolated Langerhans islets. *France. Fundam Clin Pharmacol.* 2004 Oct;18(5):525-9.

[29] Fararh KM, Atoji Y, Shimizu Y, Takewaki T.Isulinotropic properties of Nigella sativa oil in Streptozotocin plus Nicotinamide diabetic hamster. *Res Vet Sci.* 2002 Dec;73(3):279-8.

[30] Le PM, Benhaddou-Andaloussi A, Elimadi A, Settaf A, Cherrah Y, Haddad PS. The petroleum ether extract of Nigella sativa exerts lipid-lowering and insulin-sensitizing actions in the rat. *J Ethnopharmacol.* 2004 Oct;94(2-3):251-9.

[31] Meral I, Yener Z, Kahraman T, Mert N. Effect of Nigella sativa on glucose concentration, lipid peroxidation, anti-oxidant defence system and liver damage in experimentally-induced diabetic rabbits. *J Vet Med A Physiol Pathol Clin Med.* 2001 Dec;48(10):593-9.

[32] Ali BH. The effect of Nigella sativa oil on gentamicin nephrotoxicity in rats. *Am J Chin Med.* 2004;32(1):49-55. .

[33] Al-Ghamdi MS. Protective effect of Nigella sativa seeds against carbon tetrachloride-induced liver damage. *Am J Chin Med.* 2003;31(5):721-8.

[34] Turkdogan MK, Ozbek H, Yener Z, Tuncer I, Uygan I, Ceylan E. The role of Urtica dioica and Nigella sativa in the prevention of carbon tetrachloride-induced hepatotoxicity in rats. Turkey. *Phytother Res.* 2003 Sep;17(8):942-6.

[35] el-Dakhakhny M, Mady NI, Halim MA.Nigella sativa L. oil protects against induced hepatotoxicity and improves serum lipid profile in rats. *Arzneimittelforschung.* 2000 Sep;50(9):832-6. Egypt.

[36] Daba MH, Abdel-Rahman MS. Hepatoprotective activity of thymoquinone in isolated rat hepatocytes. *Toxicol Lett.* 1998 Mar 16;95(1):23-9.USA

[37] Thymoquinone protects against carbon tetrachloride hepatotoxicity in mice via an antioxidant mechanism. *Biochem Mol Biol Int.* 1999 Jan;47(1):153-9.

[38] Turkdogan MK, Agaoglu Z, Yener Z, Sekeroglu R, Akkan HA, Avci ME.The role of antioxidant vitamins (C and E), selenium and Nigella sativa in the prevention of liver fibrosis and cirrhosis in rabbits: new hopes. *Dtsch Tierarztl Wochenschr.* 2001 Feb;108(2):71-3. Turkey.

[39] Awad EM. In vitro decreases of the fibrinolytic potential of cultured human fibrosarcoma cell line, HT1080, by Nigella sativa oil. *Phytomedicine.* 2005 Jan;12(1-2):100-7.

[40] Salim EI, Fukushima S. Chemopreventive potential of volatile oil from black cumin (Nigella sativa L.) seeds against rat colon carcinogenesis. *Nutr Cancer.* 2003;45(2):195-202

[41] Gali-Muhtasib H, Diab-Assaf M, Boltze C, Al-Hmaira J, Hartig R, Roessner A, Schneider-Stock R. Thymoquinone extracted from black seed triggers apoptotic cell death in human colorectal cancer cells via a p53-dependent mechanism. *Int J Oncol.* 2004 Oct;25(4):857-66.

[42] El-Mahdy MA, Zhu Q, Wang QE, Wani G, Wani AA. Thymoquinone induces apoptosis through activation of caspase-8 and mitochondrial events in p53-nullmyeloblastic leukemia HL-60 cells. *Int J Cancer.* 2005 May 19; [Epub ahead of print]

[43] Salomi NJ, Nair SC, Jayawardhanan KK, Varghese CD, Panikkar KR. Antitumour principles from Nigella sativa seeds. *Cancer Lett.* 1992 Mar 31;63(1):41-6., India.

[44] Kumara SS, Huat BT.Extraction, isolation and characterisation of antitumor principle, alpha-hederin, from the seeds of Nigella sativa. *Planta Med.* 2001 Feb;67(1):29-32. Singapore.

[45] Worthen DR, Ghosheh OA, Crooks PA.The in vitro anti-tumor activity of some crude and purified components of blackseed, Nigella sativa L. *Anticancer Res.* 1998 May-Jun;18(3A):1527-32. USA.

[46] Islam SN, Begum P, Ahsan T, Huque S, Ahsan M.Immunosuppressive and cytotoxic properties of Nigella sativa. *Phytother Res.* 2004 May;18(5):395-8.

[47] Hosseinzadeh H, Parvardeh S, Nassiri-Asl M, Mansouri MT. Intracerebroventricular administration of thymoquinone, the major constituent of Nigella sativa seeds, suppresses epileptic seizures in rats. *Med Sci Monit.* 2005 Apr;11(4):BR106-10. Epub 2005 Mar 24.

[48] Hosseinzadeh H, Parvardeh S. Anticonvulsant effects of thymoquinone, the major constituent of Nigella sativa seeds, in mice. *Phytomedicine.* 2004 Jan;11(1):56-64.

[49] Harvey RA, Champe PC, Mycek MJ. *Lippncotts illustrated reviews: Pharmacology* ed.2000 Lippincott Williams and Wilkins,pp 450-451.

[50] Mansour M, Tornhamre S. Inhibition of 5-lipoxygenase and leukotriene C4 synthase in human blood cells by thymoquinone. *J Enzyme Inhib Med Chem.* 2004 Oct;19(5):431-6.

[51] El-Dakhakhny M, Madi NJ, Lembert N, Ammon HP.Nigella sativa oil, nigellone and derived thymoquinone inhibit synthesis of 5-lipoxygenase products in polymorphonuclear leukocytes from rats. *J Ethnopharmacol.* 2002 Jul;81(2):161-4.

[52] Al-Majed AA, Daba MH, Asiri YA, Al-Shabanah OA, Mostafa AA, El-Kashef HA.Thymoquinone-induced relaxation of guinea-pig isolated trachea. *Res Commun Mol Pathol Pharmacol.* 2001;110(5-6):333-45.

[53] Kirui PK, Cameron J, Benghuzzi HA, Tucci M, Patel R, Adah F, Russell G. Effects of sustained delivery of thymoqiunone on bone healing of male rats. *Biomed Sci Instrum.* 2004;40:111-6.

[54] Houghton PJ, Zarka R, de las Heras B, Hoult JR. Fixed oil of Nigella sativa and derived thymoquinone inhibit eicosanoid generation in leukocytes and membrane lipid peroxidation. *Planta Med Feb* 1995; 61 (1): 33-6.

[55] Al-Ghamdi MS. Anti-inflammatory, analgesic and anti-pyretic activity of Nigella sativa. *J Ethnopharmacol* 2001; 76: 45-8.

[56] Abdel-Fattah AM, Matsumoto K, Watanabe H. Antinociceptive effects of Nigella sativa oil and its major component, thymoquinone, in mice. *Eur J Pharmacol* 2000; 14 (1): 89-97.

[57] Hanafy MS, Hatem ME.Studies on the antimicrobial activity of Nigella sativa seed (black cumin). *J Ethnopharmacol.* 1991 Sep;34(2-3):275-8.

[58] Morsi NM.Antimicrobial effect of crude extracts of Nigella sativa on multiple antibiotics-resistant bacteria. *Acta Microbiol Pol.* 2000;49(1):63-74.

[59] Salem ML, Hossain MS.Protective effect of black seed oil from Nigella sativa against murine cytomegalovirus infection. *Int J Immunopharmacol.* 2000 Sep;22(9):729-40.

[60] Haq A, Abdullatif M, Lobo PI, Khabar KS, Sheth KV, Al-Sedairy ST. Nigella sativa: Effect on human lympocytes and polymorphonuclear leucocyte phagocytic activity. *Immunopharmacology* 1995; 30 (2): 147-50.

[61] Haq A, Lobo Pl, Al-Tufail M, Rama NR, Al-Sedairy ST. Immunomodulatory effect of *Nigella sativa* proteins fractionated by ion exchange chromatography. *Int J Immunopharmacol* 1999; 21 (4): 283-5.

[62] Swamy SM, Tan BK. Cytotoxic and imunopotentiating effects of ethanolic extract of Nigella sativa L seeds. *J Ethnopharmacol* 2000; 70 (1): 1-7.

SECTION 2: GINSENGS

Overview

There are several varieties of ginseng: Asian ginseng (Panax ginseng), American Ginseng (Panax quinquefolius), and Siberian ginseng (Eleutherococcus Chinensis) are the most common (plant family Araliacae). Commonly, ginseng refers to "true" ginseng, Panax ginseng C.A. Meyer

Technically Siberian ginseng does not belong in the same genus as Asian or American ginseng and does not contain the same ingredients. The roots of Asian and American ginseng contain several triterpene glycosides known as ginsenosides (saponins). that are believed to contribute to its beneficial properties.

The most commonly used and researched of the ginsengs is Panax ginseng, also called Korean ginseng. The main active components of ginseng are ginsenosides, which are triterpene saponins. The majority of published research on the medicinal activity of Panax ginseng has focused on ginsenosides which have been shown to have a variety of beneficial effects, including anti-inflammatory, antioxidant, anti-diabetic and anticancer effects. In experimental animal studies a protective effects on the nervous system have also been shown including protective effect against brain ischemia, neurodegeneration and chemical induced neurotoxicity.

Results of clinical research studies demonstrate that Panax ginseng may improve psychologic function, cognitive performance overall, Panax ginseng appears to be well tolerated, although caution is advised about concomitant use with some pharmaceuticals, such as warfarin, oral hypoglycemic agents, insulin, and phenelzine.

Beneficial Effect of Ginseng in Diabetes

The only example of an approved antidiabetic drug that was developed from a plant source with a long history of use for diabetes is the biguanide Metformin from French lilac (Galega officinalis).Experimental and clinical data are beginning to emerge supporting a beneficial antidiabetic effect for ginseng (Panax spp.).

1-Anti-Diabetic Activity in ob/ob Mice

In experimental studies, both panax ginseng root and ginseng berry showed anti-diabetic activity in ob/ob mice, which exhibit profound obesity and hyperglycemia that phenotypically resemble human type-2 diabetes.

Ginseng root extract (150 mg/kg body weight) and ginseng berry extract (150 mg/kg body wt.) significantly decreased fasting blood glucose from 195 mg/dl to 143 +/- 9.3 mg/dl and 150 +/- 9.5 mg/dl on day 5, respectively (both $P < 0.01$ compared with the vehicle). On day 12, although fasting blood glucose level did not continue to decrease in the root group (155 +/- 12.7 mg/dl), the berry group became normoglycemic (129 +/- 7.3 mg/dl; $P < 0.01$). Using the intraperitoneal glucose tolerance test. On day 0, basal hyperglycemia was exacerbated by intraperitoneal glucose load, and failed to return to baseline after 120 min.

After 12 days of treatment with ginseng root extract (150 mg/kg body wt.), the area under the curve (AUC) showed some decrease (9.6%). However, after 12 days of treatment with ginseng berry extract (150 mg/kg body wt.), overall glucose exposure improved significantly, and the AUC decreased 31.0% (P < 0.01). In addition, we observed that body weight did not change significantly after ginseng root extract (150 mg/kg body wt.) treatment, but the same concentration of ginseng berry extract significantly decreased body weight (P < 0.01). Compared to ginseng root, ginseng berry exhibits more potent anti-hyperglycemic activity, and only ginseng berry shows marked anti-obesity effects in ob/ob mice [1].

2-Antioxidant Activities of wild Panax Ginseng Leaf Extract Intake in Streptozotocin (STZ)-Induced Diabetic Rats (WGLE)

In STZ induced hyperglycemia, 4 weeks of WGLE supplementation was associated with lower blood glucose levels: in animals fed 40 mg/kg (266 mg/dL) and 200 mg/kg (239 mg/dL) than those in no-WGLE fed diabetic rats (464 mg/dL). The concentration of blood TBARS, which are considered the main products of glucose oxidation in blood, was also lowered by WGLE supplementation indicating that WGLE supplementation is involved in suppressing a sudden increase in blood glucose levels and a consequent decrease in TBARS levels in diabetic rats. TBARS levels in the liver, kidney and spleen of WGLE-fed diabetic groups were also significantly lower than in the control diabetic group indicating that oral administration of WGLE effectively suppresses lipid peroxidation that occurs in the organs of diabetic rats. Antioxidant activities of WGLE supplementation further extend in suppressing activities of antioxidant related enzymes, such as glutathione peroxidase, catalase and superoxide dismutase, in organs of diabetic rats. WGLE supplementation is detoxifying free radicals that are produced excessively in diabetic-induced complications [2].

3- Ginseng Therapy in Non-Insulin-Dependent Diabetic Patients

In a double-blind placebo-controlled study, 36 newly diagnosed NIDDM patients were treated for 8 weeks with ginseng (100 or 200 mg) or placebo. Ginseng therapy elevated mood, improved psychophysical performance, and reduced fasting blood glucose (FBG) and body weight. The 200-mg dose of ginseng improved glycated hemoglobin, serum PIIINP, and physical activity. Placebo reduced body weight and altered the serum lipid profile but did not alter FBG [3].

4-Effects of Dietary and Natural Plant Constituent Supplementation on Glucose Homeostasis

Effects of dietary and natural plant constituent supplementation on glucose homeostasis and the progress of diabetes were studied in db/db mice, a typical non-insulin-dependent model. In five different experimental diets were as follows: control diet, 0.5% mulberry leaf water extract diet, 0.5% Korean red ginseng diet, 0.5% banana leaf water extract diet, and 0.5% combination diet (mulberry leaf water extract/Korean red ginseng/banana leaf water extract, 1:1:1).

Mulberry leaf water extract, Korean red ginseng, banana leaf water extract, and the combination of above herbs effectively reduced blood glucose, insulin, TG, and percent HbA1c in study animals (p<0.05).in association with increased expressions of liver PPAR-alpha mRNA and adipose tissue PPAR-gamma mRNA in animals fed diets supplemented with dietary mulberry, Korean red ginseng, and banana

The expression of liver LPL mRNA was also increased with experimental diets containing herbs. The efficacy was highest in animals fed the combination diet for all of the markers used. These results suggest that mulberry leaf water extract, Korean red ginseng, banaba leaf water extract, and the combination of these fed at the level of 0.5% of the diet significantly increase insulin sensitivity, and improve hyperglycemia possibly through regulating PPAR-mediated lipid metabolism [4].

Protective Effect on the Nervous System

1- Memory Enhancing and Neuroprotective Effects of Selected Ginsenosides in Amnesia Models

The effects of ginsenosides Rg3(R), Rg3(S) and Rg5/Rk1 (a mixture of Rg5 and Rk1, 1:1, w/w), which are components isolated from processed P, when orally administered for 4 days, significantly ameliorated the memory impairment (assessed using a passive avoidance test) in mice induced by the single oral administration of ethanol. The memory impairment induced by the intraperitoneal injection of scopolamine was also significantly recovered by ginsenosides Rg3(S) and Rg5/Rk1. Among the three ginsenosides, Rg5/Rk1 enhanced the memory function of mice most effectively in both the ethanol and scopolamine-induced amnesia models. Moreover, the latency period of the Rg5/Rk1-treated mice was 1.2 times longer than that of the control (no amnesia) group in both models, implying that Rg5/Rk1 may also exert beneficial effects in the normal brain. The effects of these ginsenosides on the excitotoxic and oxidative stress-induced neuronal cell damage in primary cultured rat cortical cells. The excitotoxicity induced by glutamate or N-methyl-D-aspartate (NMDA) was dramatically inhibited by the three ginsenosides. Rg3(S) and Rg5/Rk1 exhibited a more potent inhibition of excitotoxicity than did Rg3(R). In contrast, these ginsenosides were all ineffective against the H_2O_2- or xanthine/xanthine oxidase-induced oxidative neuronal damage. Ginsenosides Rg3(S) and Rg5/Rk1 significantly reversed the memory dysfunction induced by ethanol or scopolamine, and their neuroprotective actions against excitotoxicity may be attributed to their memory enhancing effects [5].

2- Protective Effect Against Brain Ischemia

A possible protective action of Korean ginseng tea (KGT) prepared from the roots of Panax ginseng, against hypoperfusion/reperfusion induced brain injury(stroke) has been demonstrated, using rat global and focal models of ischemia. Varied biochemical/enzymatic alterations, produced subsequent to the application of middle cerebral artery and bilateral carotid artery occlusion followed by reperfusion viz. increase in lipid peroxidation and decrease in glutathione, glutathione reductase, catalase, glutathione-S-transferase, glutathione peroxidase and superoxide dismutase, were markedly reversed and restored to near normal levels in the groups pre-treated with KGT 350mg/kg given orally for 10 days.

A possible therapeutic potential in cerebrovascular diseases (CVD) including stroke has been suggested remembering that the present treatment strategies for CVD are far from adequate [6].

A neuroprotective activity of ginseng roots has been shown in 5-min ischemic gerbils using a step-down passive avoidance task and subsequent neuron and synapse counts in the hippocampal CA1 region.

Oral administration of red ginseng powder for 7 days before the induced ischemia significantly prevented the ischemia-induced decrease in response latency, as determined by the passive avoidance test, and rescued a significant number of ischemic hippocampal CA1 pyramidal neurons in a dose-dependent manner. Intraperitoneal injections of crude ginseng saponin for 7 days before the induced ischemia exhibited a similar neuroprotective effect.

Crude ginseng non-saponin had a significant but less potent protective effect against impaired passive avoidance task and degeneration of hippocampal CA1 neurons. Pure ginsenosides Rb1, Rg1 and Ro: Ginsenoside Rb1 significantly prolonged the response latency of ischemic gerbils and rescued a significant number of ischemic CA1 pyramidal neurons, whereas ginsenosides Rg1 and Ro were ineffective. Post- ischemic treatment with red ginseng powder crude ginseng saponin or ginsenoside Rb1 was ineffective. The neuroprotective activities of red ginseng powder, crude ginseng saponin and ginsenoside Rb1 were confirmed by electron microscopy counts of synapses in individual strata of the CA1 field of ischemic gerbils pretreated with the drugs. Red ginseng powder and crude ginseng saponin are effective in preventing delayed neuronal death, and that ginsenoside Rb1 is one of the neuroprotective molecules within ginseng root [7].

3- Protective Effects of Ginseng Components in on 3-Nitropropionic Acid- Induced Degeneration

*In 3-nitropropionic acid (3-NP) induced neurodegeneration which is an inhibitor of succinate dehydrogenase which is produced by treatment with 3-nitropropionic acid (90 mg/kg) over a 5-day period resulting in severe impairment of movement and loss of neurons in the striatum Pre-treatment with a preparation of ground leaves and stems, which contains greater levels of ginsenosides than ground root, improved the behavioral score and reduced the volume of the striatal lesion in contrast to pretreatment with whole ginseng which has no protective effect.

A partial purification of American ginseng was performed to concentrate the putative protective components: Rb1, Rb3, and Rd (termed Rb extract). Pre-treatment with the Rb extract significantly reduced the 3-nitropropionic acid-induced motor impairment and cell loss in the striatum, and it completely prevented any mortality. Significant effects on motor function, mortality, and the striatal lesion volume also were measured in animals pretreated with the individual ginsenosides, Rb1, Rb3, or Rd. Partial purification of whole ginseng to concentrate the neuroprotective components was necessary to demonstrate that some of the ginsenosides components have neuroprotective activity [8].

*The precise cause of neuronal cell death in Huntington's disease (HD) is not known. Systemic administration of 3-nitropropionic acid (3-NP), an irreversible succinate dehydrogenase inhibitor, not only induces a cellular ATP depletions but also causes a selective striatal degeneration similar to that seen in HD. Recent accumulating reports have shown that ginseng saponins (GTS), the major active ingredients of Panax ginseng, have protective effects against neurotoxin insults. In the present study, we examined in vitro and in vivo effects of ginseng saponins on striatal neurotoxicity induced by repeated treatment of 3-NP in rats. Here, we report that systemic administration of ginseng saponins produced significant protections against systemic 3-NP- and intrastriatal malonate-induced lesions in rat striatum with dose-dependent manner. GTS also improved significantly 3-NP-caused behavioral impairment and extended survival. However, GTS itself had no effect on 3-NP-induced inhibition of succinate dehydrogenase activity. To explain the mechanisms underlying in vivo protective effects of GTS against 3-NP-induced striatal degeneration, we examined in vitro effect of GTS against 3-NP-caused cytotoxicity using cultured rat striatal neurons. We found that GTS inhibited 3-NP-induced intracellular Ca(2+) elevations. GTS restored 3-NP-caused mitochondrial transmembrane potential reduction in cultured rat striatal neurons. GTS also prevented 3-NP-induced striatal neuronal cell deaths with dose-dependent manner. The EC(50) was 12.6 +/- 0. 7microg/ml. These results suggest that in vivo protective effects of GTS against 3-NP-induced rat striatal degeneration might be achieved via in vitro inhibition of 3-NP-induced intracellular Ca(2+) elevations and cytotoxicity of striatal neurons [9].

4- In Vivo Protective Effect of Ginsenosides

In vivo protective effect of ginsenosides has been shown on kainic acid (KA)-induced neurotoxicity in rat hippocampus using the methods of acid fuchsin (AF) staining and heat-shock protein-70 (HSP-70) immunoreactivity to detect neuronal death and stress, respectively. Pretreatment of ginsenosides (50 or 100 mg/kg for 7 days) via intraperitoneal administration significantly attenuated KA (10 mg/kg intra-peritoneally)-induced cell death by decreasing AF-positive neurons in both CA1 and CA3 regions of rat hippocampus compared with KA treatment alone. Pretreatment of ginsenosides (50 or 100 mg/kg for 7 days) via intra-peritoneal administration also significantly suppressed KA-induced induction of HSP-70 in both regions of rat hippocampus. Ginsenosides are effective in protecting hippocampal CA1 and CA3 cells against kainic acid induced neurotoxicity [10].

5- Ginsenoside Rg1 Protective Effect in 1-Methyl-4-Phenyl-1,2,3,6-Tetrahydropyridine (MPTP)-Induced Substantia Nigra Neuron Lesion

In Parkinson disease mice model induced in C57-BL mice by giving 1-methyl-4-phenyl-1,2,3,6-tetrahydropyridine (MPTP) . Pre-treatments of C57-BL mice with different doses of Rg1 or N-acetylcystein C (NAC) were found to protect against MPTP-induced substantia nigra neurons loss. Rg1 or NAC prevented Glutathione (GSH) reduction and T-SOD activation in substantia nigra, and attenuated the phosphorylations of JNK and c-Jun following MPTP treatment. The antioxidant property of Rg1 along with the blocking of JNK signaling cascade might contribute to the neuroprotective effect of ginsenoside Rg1 against MPTP [11].

6- Partially Purified Extract that Concentrates the Rb Ginsenosides (Rb extract) has been shown to have a Dose-Dependent Anticonvulsant Effect in all three Models of Chemically Induced Seizures

One hour after treatment with normal saline, or one of the three ginseng preparations, seizures were induced in adult, male, Sprague-Dawley rats with kainic acid (KA; 10 mg/kg), pilocarpine (300 mg/kg, preceded by methylscopolamine, 1 mg/kg, s.c.), or pentylenetetrazole (PTZ, 50 mg/kg). Time to onset of seizure activity, duration of seizure activity for PTZ, seizure severity, and weight change for KA and pilocarpine were determined for each animal. The brains from animals who had received KA or pilocarpine were examined for severe neuronal stress, by using immunoreactivity for heat-shock protein (HSP)72. The Rb extract had a dose-dependent anticonvulsant effect in all three models of chemically induced seizures: increasing the latency to the seizures; decreasing the seizure score, weight loss, and subsequent neuronal damage after pilocarpine; and shortening the seizure duration and reducing mortality after PTZ. The Rb extract also significantly reduced the effects of KA, including completely blocking behavioral seizures. The root preparation increased the mortality rate after administration of pilocarpine, but had no other significant effects. The leaves/stems preparation, at 120 mg/kg, reduced the weight loss after pilocarpine, but had no other significant effects. Ginseng extract made from either the root or leaves/stems is ineffective against chemically induced seizures. A partial purification of the whole extract that concentrates the Rb1 and Rb3 ginsenosides has significant anticonvulsant properties [12].

Improvement of Cognitive Performance During Sustained Mental Activity

Panax ginseng improves performance and subjective feelings of mental fatigue during sustained mental activity in healthy adult volunteers. This effect could possibly be attributed to the acute gluco-regulatory properties of the extract [13].

Using a double-blind, placebo-controlled, balanced crossover design, 30 healthy young adults completed a 10 min test battery at baseline, and then six times in immediate succession commencing 60min after the day's treatment (placebo, 200mg G115 or 400mg G115). The 10 min battery comprised a Serial Threes subtraction task (2min); a Serial Sevens task (2min); a Rapid Visual Information Processing task (5min); then a 'mental fatigue' visual analogue scale. Blood glucose was measured prior to each day's treatment, and before, during and after the post-dose completions of the battery. Both the 200mg and 400mg treatments led to significant reductions in blood glucose levels at all three post-treatment measurements (p 0.005 in all cases). The most notable behavioral effects were associated with 200mg of ginseng and included significantly improved Serial Sevens subtraction task performance and significantly reduced subjective mental fatigue throughout all (with the exception of one time point in each case) of the post-dose completions of the 10min battery (p 0.05).

Effects on Psychologic Function and Physical Performance in Man

Clinical trials investigating the effects of Panax ginseng on various psychologic parameters were contradictory For every study showing a positive benefit in terms of energy levels and/or physical or mental performance, there is at least one other study showing no benefits. Part of the discrepancy in results from well-controlled studies may have to do with differences between the ginseng extracts used in various studies (non-standardized extracts with unknown quantities of active components).

However, in one study [14] of 112 healthy volunteers older than 40 years, the administration of 400 mg per day of the standardized ginseng product Gerimax for eight weeks resulted in better and faster simple reactions and abstract thinking, but no change in concentration, memory, or subjective experience.

The results of two small studies [15,16] each including about 30 young, healthy volunteers who received 200 mg of G115 daily for eight weeks, showed improvement in certain psychomotor functions (i.e., better attention, processing, and auditory reaction time), social functioning, and mental health. However, some of the effects present at the fourth week disappeared by the eighth week [16].

A study of 384 postmenopausal women who were randomized to receive placebo or ginseng for 16 weeks showed improvements in three subsets of a Psychological General Well-Being index [18]. [Evidence level A, randomized controlled trial (RCT)] In addition, a small study [19] of 20 healthy young volunteers who received a single 400-mg dose of ginseng found improvement in cognitive performance, secondary memory performance, speed of performing memory tasks, and accuracy of attentional tasks. However, another study [18] showed no effect on positive affect, negative affect, or total mood disturbance in 83 young healthy volunteers who took 200 to 400 mg per day of G115 for eight weeks.

Most of the clinical studies investigating the value of Panax ginseng in enhancing physical performance have shown no clinical effect [20] One study [21] on the use of 200 mg per day of G115 in 19 healthy adult women showed no change in physical work performance, energy metabolic responses, or oxygen uptake.

Similarly, a study of 31 healthy men who took 200 or 400 mg of G115 daily for eight weeks found no change in physiologic or psychologic responses to submaximal or maximal exercise [22]. Evidence level B, lower quality RCT] In another study [23], a different product standardized to 7 percent ginsenosides and administered at 200 mg per day was given to 28 healthy young adults for 21 days. No ergogenic effects were demonstrated, including no change in maximal oxygen consumption, exercise time, workload, plasma lactate level, hematocrit, or heart rate.

Anti Cancer Effect of Ginseng Component

In experimental studies ginseng and various ginseng components (ginsenoside-Rb1, ginsenoside Rg3, Ginsenoside-Rb2, Ginsenoid Rh2 saponins) and some metabolites demonstrated an inhibitory effects on various experimentally induced tumors in animals including colon, liver, brain, lung and skin cancers and also in experimental human cancer models including breast, prostate, and renal cancers. Preliminary clinical studies has shown that Panax ginseng inhibits the recurrence of AJCC stage III gastric cancer and shows immunomodulatory activities during postoperative chemotherapy, after a curative resection with D2 lymph node dissection. A significant reduction in the risk of cancer development among those who regularly consumed ginseng has been reported in a case-control studies. In face of this accumulating evidence largely obtained from experimental studies and early clinical reports, ginseng extracts and its synthetic derivatives should be examined for their preventive effect on various types of human cancers.

1- Inhibitory Effect on Adenocarcinoma of the Small Intestine

Inhibitory effects of white a ginseng has been shown on tumor development using medium-term liver and multi-organ carcinogenicity bioassay systems. No modifying potential of the ginseng preparations were evident in terms of the numbers or areas of glutathione S-transferase placental form (GST-P)-positive foci in rat livers. White ginseng, although not its red counterpart, was found to decrease the incidences of adenocarcinoma of the small intestine and colon in the medium-term multi-organ carcinogenesis model, without any affect on the numbers of aberrant crypt foci (ACF). Ginseng may have inhibitory effects on the progression stage of rat intestinal carcinogenesis, but the influence is not strong. Ginseng did not appear to have promoting or inhibitory effects in other organs under the present experimental conditions. Possible application on ginseng for chemoprevention of colon cancer in humans, can be concluded given the lack of obvious adverse effects [24].

2- Inhibitory Effect on Colon Carcinogenesis in Rats

Colorectal cancer remains the second leading cause of cancer deaths in the United States. Efforts to prevent colon cancer have targeted early detection through screening and chemoprevention. The inhibitory effects of ginseng on the development of 1,2 dimethylhydrazine (DMH)-induced aberrant crypt foci (ACF) in the colon has been studied in rats. Male, 6-week-old rats were injected with DMH once a week for 4 weeks. Rats in Groups 1 and 2 were fed diets containing red and white ginseng, respectively, at a dose of 1% for 5 weeks, starting one week before the first treatment of DMH. Animals in Groups 3 and 4 received red or white ginseng for 8 weeks starting after DMH treatment. Group 5 served as a carcinogen control group. Numbers of ACF with at least four crypts were significantly reduced in the colon of Group 2 treated with red ginseng combined with DMH. Moreover, rats were injected with DMH 4 times at one-week intervals. They were also fed diets containing 1% red or white ginseng or the control diet throughout 30 days of the experiment. Treatment with red ginseng resulted in a significant decrease of 5- bromo-2'-deoxyuridine labeling indices in colonic crypts comprising ACF. These findings suggest that dietary administration of red ginseng in combination with DMH suppresses colon carcinogenesis in rats, and the inhibition may be associated, in part, with inhibition of cell proliferation, acting on ACF in the colonic mucosa [25].

In an other experiment groups of 10 F344 rats were fed ginseng powder at a dose of 0.5 g/kg or 2 mg/kg for 5 weeks. During weeks 2 and 3 rats were injected with 10 mg/kg azoxymethane to induce aberrant crypt foci (ACF). Controls (n=10) did not receive azoxymethane (AOM). Rats were killed by CO_2 overdose and ACF counted in the rat colon.

In 8 week post-initiation experiments ginseng powder inhibited the progression of established ACF, indicating a cytostatic effect. This may be due to an anti-inflammatory effect [26].

3- Anti brain Tumors in Rat

The potential role of ginsenoside Rh2 (G-Rh2) in brain tumor has been shown in rat C6 gliomal cell line G-Rh2 induced many apoptotic manifestations in C6 gliomal cells as evidenced by changes in cell morphology, generation of DNA fragmentation, activation of caspase and production of reactive oxygen species (ROS). As a result, co treatment with antioxidants or a broad-spectrum caspase inhibitor, N-benzyloxycarbonyl-Val-Ala-Asp-fluoromethylketone effectively attenuated G-Rh2-induced cell death. However, specific cleavage of poly(ADP-ribose)polymerase into 85 kDa protein was not detected as demonstrated in many other apoptotic paradigms. Expression levels of Bcl-2 and Bax remained unchanged following G-Rh2 treatment. Furthermore, G-Rh2-induced cell death in C6 gliomal cells over expressing antiapoptotic protein, Bcl-X(L), was comparable to that in parental cells. G-Rh2-induced cell death is mediated by the generated ROS and the activation of caspase pathway in a Bcl-X(L)-independent manner [27].

4- Anticarcinogenic Effect on the Development of Liver Cancer

Anticarcinogenic effect of red ginseng (Panax ginseng C.A. Meyer) on the development of liver cancer induced by diethyl nitrosamine (DEN) in rats was studied, in preventive and curative groups. In the preventive group, the rats were given with DEN concomitantly with red ginseng fluid, and in the curative group, the rats were administered with red ginseng fluid after they developed liver cancer nodules induced by DEN. The result of the preventive group revealed that the developmental rate of liver cancer in the experimental group was 14.3%, while 100% in the control group, with the difference being statistically significant. DNA, RNA, glycogen, gamma-GT, SDH, and 5'-NT were maintained at relatively normal level in experimental group, and decreased or increased in the control group. The result of curative group showed that hepatoma nodules of the DEN-red ginseng group I were smaller than those of control group I, the structure of hepatic tissue was well preserved, the area with gamma-GT positive was smaller, and the ultrastructure of hepatocytes was normal [28]. Oral administration of red ginseng extracts (1% in diet for 40 weeks) resulted in the significant suppression of spontaneous liver tumor formation in C3H/He male mice. Average number of tumors per mouse in control group was 1.06, while that in red ginseng extracts-treated group was 0.33 (p<0.05). Incidence of liver tumor development was also lower in red ginseng extracts-treated group, although the difference from control group was not statistically significant. The administration of white ginseng extracts was proven to suppress tumor promoter-induced phenomena in vitro and in vivo [29].

5- Phytoestrogen and Inhibitory Effects in Breast Cancer

A component of Panax ginseng, ginsenoside-Rb1, acts by binding to estrogen receptor The estrogenic activity of ginsenoside-Rb1 in a transient transfection system using estrogen-responsive luciferase plasmids in MCF-7 cells. Ginsenoside-Rb1 activated the transcription of the estrogen-responsive luciferase reporter gene in MCF-7 breast cancer cells at a concentration of 50 microM. Activation was inhibited by the specific estrogen receptor antagonist ICI 182,780, indicating that the estrogenic effect of ginsenoside-Rb1 is estrogen receptor dependent. Ginsenoside-Rb1 induced estrogen-responsive gene c-fos by semi-quantitative RT-PCR assays and Western analyses. Ginsenoside-Rb1 increased c-fos both at mRNA and protein levels. However, ginsenoside-Rb1 failed to activate the glucocorticoid receptor, the retinoic acid receptor, or the androgen receptor in CV-1 cells transiently transfected with the corresponding steroid hormone receptors and hormone responsive reporter plasmids. Ginsenoside-Rb1 acts a weak phytoestrogen, presumably by binding and activating the estrogen receptor [30].

American ginseng (Panax quinquefolius L.) purportedly alleviates menopause symptoms because of putative estrogenicity American ginseng (AG) extract in MCF-7 breast cancer cells, induced the estrogen- regulated gene pS2 by Northern AG and estradiol equivalently induced RNA expression of pS2. AG, in contrast to estradiol, caused a dose-dependent decrease in cell proliferation ($P < 0.005$). AG had no adverse effect on the cell cycle while estradiol significantly increased the proliferative phase (percent S-phase) and decreased the resting phase (G(0)-G(1) phase) ($P < 0.005$). Concurrent use of AG and breast cancer therapeutic agents resulted in a significant ($P < 0.005$) suppression of cell growth for most drugs evaluated. In vitro use of AG and breast cancer therapeutics synergistically inhibited cancer cell growth [31].

6- Anti-Proliferative Activity on Human Prostate Carcinoma LNCaP Cell Line

In a study of the anti-proliferative activity of ginsenosides using human prostate carcinoma LNCaP cell line, ginsenoside Rg3 displayed growth inhibitory activity. The cells lost its adherent property after incubation in the presence of 250 microM of ginsenoside for 48h. The expression of biomarker genes, including prostate specific antigen (PSA), androgen receptor (AR) and 5alpha-reductase (5alphaR), and that of the proliferating cell nuclear antigen (PCNA), were suppressed. Ginsenoside Rg3 induced classic apoptotic morphology and interfered with the expression of apoptosis-related genes, bcl-2 and caspase-3, in LNCaP cells, as demonstrated by fluorescence microscopy, flow cytometry and reverse transcriptase-polymerase chain reaction. Ginsenoside Rg3 activated the expression of cyclin-kinase inhibitors, p21 and p27, arrested LNCaP cells at G1 phase, and subsequently inhibited cell growth through a caspase3-mediated apoptosis mechanism [32].

7- Invasiveness Inhibition on Endometrial Cancer Cell Lines Ishikawa

Ginsenoside-Rb2 derived from ginseng inhibited invasiveness to the basement membrane of endometrial cancer cell lines Ishikawa. HHUA and HEC-1-A cells. These cells dominantly expressed matrix metalloproteinase (MMP)-2 (gelatinase A) among MMPs by zymography. Ginsenoside-Rb2 suppressed the expression and activity of MMP-2, but did not alter the expression of tissue inhibitors of metalloproteinase (TIMP)-1 and TIMP-2 in the cells. Therefore, ginsenoside-Rb2 might inhibit invasiveness to the basement membrane via MMP-2 suppression in some endometrial cancers, and can be used as a medicine for inhibition of secondary spreading of uterine endometrial cancers.The average life span the DEN-red ginseng group II and the DEN control group II were 72.8 and 42.3 days, respectively [33].

8- Anticarcinogenic Effects on Lung Adenoma in Newborn N: GP (S) Mice

Anticarcinogenic effects of fresh, white, and red ginseng (Panax ginseng C A Meyer) roots and their saponins have been shown in lung adenoma in newborn N:GP(S) mice induced by a subcutaneous injection of benzo(a)pyrene 0.5 mg. After weaning, ginseng powders or extracts were given in the drinking water for 6 wk. In the 9th wk the incidence and multiplicity of lung adenoma were counted. Anticarcinogenic effects were found in 6-year-dried fresh ginseng, 5- and 6-year white ginseng, and 4-, 5-, and 6-year-red ginseng powders. Anticarcinogenic effects were also found in 6-year-dried fresh ginseng, 5- and 6-year-white ginseng, and 4-, 5-, and 6-year-red ginseng extracts. The content of major ginsenosides Rb1, Rb2, Rc, Rd, Re, Rf, Rg1 showed a little higher tendency in fresh or white ginsengs than red ginseng. This tendency was increased as the cultivation ages were increased. But there was no relationship was found between ginsenoside contents and preparation types or cultivation ages. Long-cultivated ginseng and red ginseng contain a higher amount of Anticarcinogenic components [34].

9- Antitumor Activity of Ginseng Metabolite Against Human Myeloid Leukemia (HL-60), Pulmonary Adenocarcinoma (PC-14), Gastric Adenocarcinoma (MKN-45) and Hepatoma (HepG2) Cell Lines

The in vitro antitumor activity of a novel ginseng saponin metabolite, 20-O-beta-D-glucopyranosyl-20(S)-protopanaxadiol (IH-901), has been demonstrated against four human cancer cell lines and one subline resistant to cisplatin (CDDP). The growth inhibitory activity of the compound was estimated by MTT tetrazolium assay. The mean concentrations of IH-901 needed to inhibit the proliferation of the cells by 50% (IC50) were 24.3, 25.9, 56.6 and 24.9 microM against human myeloid leukemia (HL-60), pulmonary adenocarcinoma (PC-14), gastric adenocarcinoma (MKN-45) and hepatoma (HepG2) cell lines, respectively. These values are higher than that of CDDP. In the CDDP-resistant PC/DDP cell line, the IC50 values of IH-901 and CDDP were 20.3 and 60.8 microM, respectively. IH-901 is not cross-resistant to CDDP in this cell line and could be a candidate for the treatment of CDDP resistant pulmonary cancer [35].

10- Anti-Tumor-Promoting Activity on two-stage Carcinogenesis of Mouse Skin Tumors

The extract of the roots of Panax notoginseng (Araliaceae) exhibited a significant anti-tumor-promoting activity on two-stage carcinogenesis of mouse skin tumors induced by 7,12-dimethylbenz[a]anthracene (DMBA) as an initiator and a mycotoxin, fumonisin B1, as a non-12-O-tetradecanoylphorbol-13-acetate (non-TPA) type promoter. Further, the extract exhibited the anti-tumor-initiating activity on two-stage carcinogenesis of mouse skin tumors induced by a nitric oxide donor, (+/-)-(E)-methyl-2-[(E)-hydroxyimino]-5-nitro-6-methoxy-3-hexen amide (NOR-1) as an initiator and TPA as a promoter [36].

11- Hypersensitization of Multidrug-Resistant Breast Cancer Cells to Paclitaxel

Rh2 is a ginsenoside extracted from ginseng inhibited cell growth by G1 arrest at low concentrations and induced apoptosis at high concentrations in a variety of tumor-cell lines, possibly through activation of caspases. The growth arrest and apoptosis may be mediated by 2 separate mechanisms. Apoptosis is not dependent on expression of the wild-type p53 nor the caspase 3. In addition, the apoptosis induced by Rh2 was mediated through glucocorticoid receptors. Most interestingly, Rh2 can act either additively or synergistically with chemotherapy drugs on cancer cells. Hypersensitized multidrug-resistant breast cancer cells to paclitaxel. Rh2 possesses strong tumor-inhibiting properties, and potentially can be used in treatments for multidrug-resistant cancers, especially when it is used in combination with conventional chemotherapy agents [37].

12- Anti-Proliferative Effects on Human Renal Cancer Cell Lines

Anti-proliferative effects of lipid soluble Panax ginseng components has been demonstrated on human renal cancer cell lines. Petroleum ether extract of Panax ginseng roots (GX-PE) or its partially purified preparation (7:3 GX) was added to cultures of three human renal cell carcinoma (RCC) cell lines, A498, Caki-1, and CURC II. Proliferation of RCC cells was estimated by a [3H]thymidine incorporation assay and cell cycle distribution was analyzed by flow cytometry. GX-PE, 7:3 GX, panaxydol and panaxynol inhibited proliferation of all three RCC cell lines in a dose dependent manner in vitro with an order of potency, 7:3 GX > panaxydol > panaxynol = GX-PE. Additive effect of interleukin 4 was also demonstrated, most prominently in Caki-1 which responded poorly to GX-PE alone. Analysis of cell cycle in CURC II and Caki-1 treated with GX-PE demonstrated increase in G1 phase population and corresponding decrease in S phase population. The present study demonstrated that proliferation of human RCC cell lines were inhibited by lipid soluble components of Panax ginseng roots by blocking cell cycle progression at G1 to S phase transition [38].

13- Inhibitory Effect on AJCC Stage III Gastric Cancer

Red ginseng powder from Panax ginseng C.A. Meyer inhibits the recurrence of AJCC stage III gastric cancer and shows immunomodulatory activities during postoperative chemotherapy, after a curative resection with D2 lymph node dissection. Flow cytometric analyses for peripheral T-lymphocyte subsets showed that the red ginseng powder restored CD4 levels to the initial preoperative values during postoperative chemotherapy. Depression of CD3 during postoperative chemotherapy was also inhibited by the red ginseng powder ingestion. This study demonstrated a five-year disease free survival and overall survival rate that was significantly higher in patients taking the red ginseng powder during postoperative chemotherapy versus control (68.2% versus 33.3%, 76.4% versus 38.5%, respectively, $p <$ 0.05). In spite of the limitation of a small number of patients (n = 42), these findings suggest that red ginseng powder may help to improve postoperative survival in these patients. Additionally, red ginseng powder may have some immunomodulatory properties associated with CD3 and CD4 activity in patients with advanced gastric cancer during postoperative chemotherapy [39].

14- Inhibition growth of Human Ovarian Cancer Cells (HRA) in Vitro and in nude Mouse

Ginsenoside Rh2 (Rh2), isolated from an ethanol extract of the processed root of Panax ginseng CA Meyer, inhibits growth of human ovarian cancer cells (HRA) in vitro and in nude mouse. Rh2 inhibited proliferations of various established human ovarian cancer cell lines in a dose-dependent manner between 10 and 60 microM in vitro and induced apoptosis at around the IC50 dose. When HRA cells were inoculated s.c. into the right flank of nude mice, all mice formed a palpable tumor within 14 days. Although i.p. administration of Rh2 alone hardly inhibited the tumor growth, when Rh2 was combined with cis-diamminedichloroplatinum(II) (CDDP) the tumor growth was significantly inhibited, compared to treatment with CDDP alone. When mice were treated p.o. with Rh2 daily (but not weekly), the tumor growth was significantly ($P<0.01$) inhibited, compared to CDDP treatment alone. When Rh2 was combined with CDDP, the degree of tumor growth retardation was not potentiated. The survival time was significantly ($P<0.05$) longer than that of medium alone-treated controls or the group treated with CDDP alone. p.o. administration of Rh2 has a dose-dependent inhibitory effect on the tumor growth. I.p. and weekly administration of CDDP had more potent antitumor activity in the order of 1 mg/kg, 2 mg/kg and 4 mg/kg, whereas p.o. and daily administration of Rh, (0.4 to 1.6 mg/kg) not only had antitumor activity comparable to that of 4 mg/kg CDDP, but also resulted in a significant increase of the survival. Doses of Rh2 used in this study did not result in any adverse side-effects as confirmed by monitoring hematocrit values and body weight, unlike 4 mg/kg CDDP, which had severe side-effects. It is noteworthy that p.o. but not i.p. treatment with Rh2 resulted in induction of apoptotic cells in the tumor in addition to augmentation of the natural killer activity in spleen cells from tumor-hearing nude mice. In view of the toxicity of CDDP, Rh2 alone would seem to warrant further evaluation for treatment of recurrent or refractory ovarian tumor [40].

15- A Significant Reduction in the Risk of Cancer Development among those who Regularly Consumed Ginseng in a Case-Control Studies

A case-control studies have shown a significant reduction in the risk of cancer development among those who regularly consumed ginseng. A prospective cohort study evaluated the preventive effect of ginseng against cancer on a population residing in a ginseng cultivation area on the basis of the result of case-control studies. This study was conducted in Kangwha-eup from August 1987 to December 1992. 4634 people over 40 years old who completed a questionnaire on ginseng intake were studied. In an attempt to obtain detailed information about ginseng intake, we asked them to specify their age at initial intake, their frequency and duration of ginseng intake, the kind of ginseng, etc. Multiple logistic regression was used to estimate relative risks (RR) when controlling simultaneously for covariates. Ginseng consumers had a decreased risk (RR = 0.40, 95% confidence interval [CI]: 0.28-0.56) compared with non-consumers. On the type of ginseng, the RR was 0.31 (95% CI: 0.13-0.74) for fresh ginseng extract consumers and 0.34 (95% CI: 0.20-0.53) for consumers of multiple combinations. There was no cancer death among 24 red ginseng consumers. There was a decreased risk with a rise in the frequency of ginseng intake, showing a dose-response relationship. The RR of ginseng consumers were 0.33 (95% CI:

0.18-0.57) in gastric cancer and 0.30 (95% CI: 0.14-0.65) in lung cancer. Among ginseng preparations, fresh ginseng extract consumers were significantly associated with a decreased risk of gastric cancer (RR = 0.33, 95% CI: 0.12-0.88). Panax ginseng C.A. Meyer has non-organ specific preventive effect against cancer, providing support for the previous case-control studies [41].

In 905 pairs case-control study, 62% had a history of ginseng intake compared to 75% of the controls, a statistically significant difference (p<0.01). The odds ratio (OR) for cancer in relation to ginseng intake was 0.56. In extended case-control study with 1987 pairs, the ORs for cancer were 0.37 in fresh ginseng extract users, 0.57 in white ginseng extract users, 0.30 in white ginseng extract users, 0.30 in white ginseng powder users, and 0.20 in red ginseng users. Those who took fresh ginseng slices, fresh ginseng juice, and white ginseng tea, however, did not show decrease in the risk. Overall, the risk decreased as the frequency and duration of ginseng intake increased. With respect to the site of cancer, the ORs for cancers of the lip, oral cavity, pharynx, esophagus, stomach, colorectal, liver, pancreas, larynx, lung and ovary were significantly reduced by ginseng intake. Smokers with ginseng intake showed lower ORs for cancers of lung, lip, oral cavity and pharynx and liver than those without ginseng intake. In 5 yr follow- up cohort study conducted in the ginseng cultivation area, Kangwha-eup, ginseng intakers had significantly lower risk than non-intakers. As for the type of ginseng, cancer risk significantly decreased among intakers of fresh ginseng extract, alone or together with other ginseng preparations. Among 24 red ginseng intakers, no cancer death occurred during the follow-up period. The risk for stomach and lung cancers was significantly reduced by ginseng intake, showing a statistically significant dose-response relationship in each follow-up year. Panax ginseng C.A. Meyer has been established as non-organ specific cancer preventive, having dose response relationship [42].

16- Chemopreventive, Antimutagenic, and Radioprotective Effects

Chemopreventive action and antimutagenic effects of a standardized Panax Ginseng extract (EFLA400, processed Panax ginseng extract containing a high titer of ginsenoside Rg3 (>3.0% w/w) known as Phoenix ginseng) have been demonstrated in Swiss albino mice. The oral administration of EFLA400 at 1, 3 and 10 mg/kg body weight at pre, peri and post-initiational phases, showed significant reductions in the number, size and weight of the papillomas. A significant reduction in tumor incidence (71.41 +/- 6.73%, 72.19 +/- 4.54% and 70.46 +/- 0.38% at 1, 3 and 10 mg/kg body weight, respectively) was observed in animals in the EFLA400 treated group compared with 100% tumor incidence in the control group. The cumulative number of papillomas during an observation period of 16 weeks was significantly reduced in the EFLA400 treated group (24 +/- 0.94, 16 +/- 1.41 and 11 +/- 1.41 at 1, 3 and 10 mg/kg body weight, respectively). However, the average latent period was significantly increased from 10.81 +/- 0.1 weeks in the control group to 12.39 +/- 0.28 weeks in the treated group (10 mg/kg body weight). The average tumor weight was recorded as 128.55 +/- 8.48, 116.00 +/- 8.48 and 57.5 +/- 3.29 mg in 1, 3 and 10 mg/kg body weight EFLA400 treated groups respectively. Chromosomal aberrations and micronuclei induction was also evaluated in bone marrow cells. These genotoxicity end-points were compared with papilloma occurrence at the same dose levels of carcinogen and ginseng. In the EFLA400 treated groups significantly reduced frequencies of chromosomal aberrations and micronuclei induced by DMBA and croton oil were observed. However, the maximum decrease in the frequencies of chromosomal aberrations and micronuclei were recorded in the 10 mg/kg body weight EFLA400 treated group than that of the 1 and 3 mg/kg body weight EFLA400 treated animals [43].

RADIOPROTECTIVE POTENTIAL OF GINSENG

A majority of potential Radioprotective synthetic compounds have demonstrated limited clinical application owing to their inherent toxicity. The radioprotective effects of ginseng on mammalian cells have been reported both in vitro and in vivo.The water-soluble extract of whole ginseng appears to give a better protection against radiation-induced DNA damage than does the isolated ginsenoside fractions. Since free radicals play an important role in radiation-induced damage, the underlying radioprotective mechanism of ginseng could be linked, either directly or indirectly, to its antioxidative capability by the scavenging free radicals responsible for DNA damage. In addition, ginseng's radioprotective potential may also be related to its immunomodulating capabilities. Ginseng appears to be a promising radioprotector for therapeutic or preventive protocols capable of attenuating the deleterious effects of radiation on human normal tissue, especially for cancer patients undergoing radiotherapy [44].

Effect on the Immune System

A study [45] of 227 healthy volunteers demonstrated that daily administration of 100 mg of G115 for 12 weeks enhanced the efficacy of polyvalent influenza vaccine. The patients who received ginseng had a lower incidence of influenza and colds, higher antibody titers, and higher natural killer cell activity levels. Another study [46] in 60 healthy volunteers showed enhanced chemotaxis, phagocytosis, increased total lymphocyte count, and increased numbers of T helper cells in those who received G115 in a dosage of 100 mg twice daily for eight weeks. In a study of 75 patients with acute exacerbation of chronic bronchitis who were treated with antibiotics or antibiotics plus ginseng, those in the ginseng group showed faster bacterial clearance [47].

In 45 patients with erectile dysfunction, use of ginseng improved erectile function, sexual desire, and intercourse satisfaction [48].

The antioxidant activity of Korean red ginseng (KRG) and its effect on erectile function have been studied in non-insulin-dependent diabetes mellitus (NIDDM) rats. Oxidative stress is an important factor in vascular complications of diabetes. In a total of 84 male Sprague-Dawley rats, NIDDM was induced by an intraperitoneal injection of 90 mg/kg of Streptozotocin on day 2 after birth. According to the diabetic period, they were classified as either short-term (22 weeks, n = 32) or long-term (38 weeks, n = 32) diabetics. Of those, 20 (10 short-term and 10 long-term) were fed 30 mg/kg of KRG three times weekly for 1 month. The remaining diabetic rats (22 short-term and 22 long-term) and their age-matched controls (n = 10 each for each group) were fed a normal diet. Erectile function was measured after electrostimulation of the cavernous nerve. The intracavernous pressure after nerve stimulation and cavernous glutathione level were significantly lower in the long-term than the short-term diabetics with a normal diet and were markedly decreased compared with their age-matched controls (P <0.01 and P <0.05, respectively). The malondialdehyde content was markedly increased in the short-term diabetics compared with the controls (P <0.05). In contrast, erectile function was not impaired in the diabetic group treated with KRG. Furthermore, both glutathione and malondialdehyde levels in those treated with KRG were comparable to their age-matched controls. Oxidative stress to cavernous tissue may be a contributory factor in erectile dysfunction in diabetics. KRG may preserve potency in the NIDDM rats through its antioxidant activity [49].

Adverse Effects, Drug Interactions, and Contraindications

Interpretation of documented adverse effects and drug interactions can be difficult because of the variety of available ginseng formulations, and because the exact amount of ginseng in these products may not be identified. Possible drug interactions have been reported between P. ginseng and warfarin, phenelzine and alcohol. P. ginseng monopreparations are rarely associated with adverse events or drug interactions.

Advances in the development of standardized extracts for both Panax ginseng (G-115) and Panax quinquefolius (CNT-2000) have and will continue to assist in the assessment of efficacy and safety standards for ginseng products.

Panax ginseng generally is well tolerated, and its adverse effects are mild and reversible. reported side effects include nausea, diarrhea, euphoria, insomnia, headaches, hypertension, hypotension, mastalgia, and vaginal bleeding. Panax ginseng may interact with caffeine to cause hypertension, and it may lower blood alcohol concentrations. It also may decrease the effectiveness of warfarin. Concomitant use of Panax ginseng and the monoamine oxidase inhibitor phenelzine may result in manic-like symptoms. Contraindications to the use of Panax ginseng include high blood pressure, acute asthma, acute infections, and nose bleeds or excessive menstruation. These effects appear to occur primarily with high dosages or prolonged use [50,51,52,53].

One female patient experienced menometrorrhagia (abnormal uterine bleeding) and sinus tachycardia with occasional atrial premature beats.in association with use of both oral and topical ginseng for cosmetic reasons. Arrhythmia stopped 10 days after stoping taking ginseng, smoking, and drinking coffee [54].

REFERENCES

[1]   Dey L, Xie JT, Wang A, Wu J, Maleckar SA, Yuan CS.Anti-hyperglycemic effects of ginseng: comparison between root and berry. *Phytomedicine*. 2003;10(6-7):600-5. USA.

[2]   Jung CH, Seog HM, Choi IW, Choi HD, Cho HY. Effects of wild ginseng (Panax ginseng C.A. Meyer) leaves on lipid peroxidation levels and antioxidant enzyme activities in streptozotocin diabetic rats. *J Ethnopharmacol*. 2005 Apr 26;98(3):245- South Korea.

[3]   Sotaniemi EA, Haapakoski E, Rautio A.Ginseng therapy in non-insulin-dependent diabetic patients. *Diabetes Care*. 1995 Oct;18(10):1373-5   Finland.

[4]   Park MY, Lee KS, Sung MK.Effects of dietary mulberry, Korean red ginseng, and banana on glucose homeostasis in relation to PPAR-alpha, PPAR-gamma, and LPL mRNA expressions. *Life Sci*. 2005 Jun 22; [Epub ahead of print]

[5]   Bao HY, Zhang J, Yeo SJ, Myung CS, Kim HM, Kim JM, Park JH, Cho J, Kang JS.Memory enhancing and neuroprotective effects of selected ginsenosides. *Arch Pharm Res*. 2005 Mar;28(3):335-42. Korea.

[6]   Shah ZA, Gilani RA, Sharma P, Vohora SB.Cerebroprotective effect of Korean ginseng tea against global and focal models of ischemia in rats. *J Ethnopharmacol*. 2005 Jun 18; [Epub ahead of print India].

[7]   Wen TC, Yoshimura H, Matsuda S, Lim JH, Sakanaka M.Ginseng root prevents learning disability and neuronal loss in gerbils with 5-minute forebrain ischemia. *Acta Neuropathol (Berl)*. 1996;91(1):15-22.Japan

[8]   Lian XY, Zhang Z, Stringer JL.Protective effects of ginseng components in a rodent model of neurodegeneration. *Ann Neurol*. 2005 May;57(5):642-8.USA.

[9]   Kim JH, Kim S, Yoon IS, Lee JH, Jang BJ, Jeong SM, Lee JH, Lee BH, Han JS, Oh S, Kim HC, Park TK, Rhim H, Nah SY.Protective effects of ginseng saponins on 3-nitropropionic acid-induced striatal degeneration in rats. *Neuropharmacology*. 2005 Apr;48(5):743-56.Seoul, Republic of Korea.

[10]   Lee JH, Kim SR, Bae CS, Kim D, Hong H, Nah S. Protective effect of ginsenosides, active ingredients of Panax ginseng, on kainic acid-induced neurotoxicity in rat hippocampus. *Neurosci Lett*. 2002 Jun 7;325(2):129-33. South Korea.

[11]   Chen XC, Zhou YC, Chen Y, Zhu YG, Fang F, Chen LM.Ginsenoside Rg1 reduces MPTP-induced substantia nigra neuron loss by suppressing oxidative stress. *Acta Pharmacol Sin*. 2005 Jan;26(1):56-62. China.

[12]   Lian XY, Zhang ZZ, Stringer JL.Anticonvulsant activity of ginseng on seizures induced by chemical convulsants. *Epilepsia*. 2005 Jan;46(1):15-22. USA.

[13]   Reay JL, Kennedy DO, Scholey AB.Single doses of Panax ginseng (G115) reduce blood glucose levels and improve cognitive performance during sustained mental activity. *J Psychopharmacol*. 2005 Dec;19(4):357-65. UK.

[14]   Wesnes KA, Ward T, McGinty A, Petrini O. The memory enhancing effects of a Ginkgo biloba/ Panax ginseng combination in healthy middle-aged volunteers. *Psychopharmacology* 2000;152:353-61.

[15]   Sorensen H, Sonne J. A double-masked study of the effects of ginseng on cognitive functions. *Curr Ther Res Clin Exp* 1996;57:959-68.

[16]   D'Angelo L, Grimaldi R, Caravaggi M, Marcoli M, Perucca E, Lecchini S, et al. A double-blind, placebo-controlled clinical study on the effect of a standardized ginseng extract on psychomotor performance in healthy volunteers. *J Ethnopharmacol* 1986;16:15-22.

[17]   Ellis JM, Reddy P. Effects of Panax ginseng on quality of life. *Ann Pharmacother* 2002;36:375-9.

[18]   Wiklund IK, Mattsson LA, Lindgren R, Limoni C. Effects of a standardized ginseng extract on quality of life and physiological parameters in symptomatic postmenopausal

women: a double-blind, placebo-controlled trial. Swedish Alternative Medicine Group. *Int J Clin Pharmacol Res* 1999;19:89-99.

[19] Pieralisi G, Ripari P, Vecchiet L. Effects of a standardized ginseng extract combined with dimethylaminoethanol bitartrate, vitamins, minerals, and trace elements on physical performance during exercise. *Clin Ther* 1991;13:373-82.

[20] Cardinal BJ, Engels HJ. Ginseng does not enhance psychological well-being in healthy, young adults: results of a double-blind, placebo-controlled, randomized clinical trial. *J Am Diet Assoc* 2001; 101:655-60.

[21] Bahrke MS, Morgan WR. Evaluation of the ergogenic properties of ginseng: an update. *Sports Med* 2000;29:113-33.

[22] Engels HJ, Said JM, Wirth JC. Failure of chronic ginseng supplementation to affect work performance and energy metabolism in healthy adult females. *Nutr Res [United States]* 1996;16:1295-1305.

[23] Engels HJ, Wirth JC. No ergogenic effects of ginseng (Panax ginseng C.A. Meyer) during graded maximal aerobic exercise. *J Am Diet Assoc* 1997; 97:1110-5.

[24] Ichihara T, Wanibuchi H, Iwai S, Kaneko M, Tamano S, Nishino H, Fukushima S. White, but not Red, Ginseng Inhibits Progression of Intestinal Carcinogenesis in Rats. *Asian Pac J Cancer Prev.* 2002;3(3):243-250. Japan.

[25] Fukushima S, Wanibuchi H, Li W.Inhibition by ginseng of colon carcinogenesis in rats. *J Korean Med Sci.* 2001 Dec;16 Suppl:S75-80.Japan

[26] Wargovich MJ.Colon cancer chemoprevention with ginseng and other botanicals. *J Korean Med Sci.* 2001 Dec;16 Suppl:S81-6. USA.

[27] Kim HE, Oh JH, Lee SK, Oh YJ.Ginsenoside RH-2 induces apoptotic cell death in rat C6 glioma via a reactive oxygen- and caspase-dependent but Bcl-X(L)-independent pathway. *Life Sci.* 1999;65(3):PL33-40 Korea.

[28] Wu XG, Zhu DH, Li X. Anticarcinogenic effect of red ginseng on the development of liver cancer induced by diethylnitrosamine in rats. *J Korean Med Sci.* 2001 Dec;16 Suppl:S61-5. China.

[29] Nishino H, Tokuda H, Ii T, Takemura M, Kuchide M, Kanazawa M, Mou XY_et al Cancer chemoprevention by ginseng in mouse liver and other organs. *J Korean Med Sci.* 2001 Dec;16 Suppl:S66-9. Japan.

[30] Lee YJ, Jin YR, Lim WC, Park WK, Cho JY, Jang S, Lee SK.Ginsenoside-Rb1 acts as a weak phytoestrogen in MCF-7 human breast cancer cells. *Arch Pharm Res.* 2003 Jan;26(1):58-63. Korea.

[31] Duda RB, Zhong Y, Navas V, Li MZ, Toy BR, Alavarez JG.American ginseng and breast cancer therapeutic agents synergistically inhibit MCF-7 breast cancer cellgrowth. *J Surg Oncol.* 1999 Dec;72(4):230-9. USA.

[32] Liu WK, Xu SX, Che CT.Anti-proliferative effect of ginseng saponins on human prostate cancer cell line. *Life Sci.* 2000 Aug 4;67(11):1297-306. Hong Kong,

[33] Fujimoto J, Sakaguchi H, Aoki I, Toyoki H, Khatun S, Tamaya T.Inhibitory effect of ginsenoside-Rb2 on invasiveness of uterine endometrial cancer cells to the basement membrane. *Eur J Gynaecol Oncol.* 2001;22(5):339-41 Japan.

[34] Yun TK, Lee YS, Kwon HY, Choi KJ.Saponin contents and anticarcinogenic effects of ginseng depending on types and ages in mice. *Zhongguo Yao Li Xue Bao.* 1996 Jul;17(4):293-8. Korea.

[35] Lee SJ, Sung JH, Lee SJ, Moon CK, Lee BH.Antitumor activity of a novel ginseng saponin metabolite in human pulmonary adenocarcinoma cells resistant to cisplatin. *Cancer Lett.* 1999 Sep 20;144(1):39-43. South Korea.

[36] Konoshima T, Takasaki M, Tokuda H.Anti-carcinogenic activity of the roots of Panax notoginseng. II. *Biol Pharm Bull.* 1999 Oct;22(10):1150-2. Japan

[37] Jia WW, Bu X, Philips D, Yan H, Liu G, Chen X, Bush JA, Li G. Rh2, a compound extracted from ginseng, hypersensitizes multidrug-resistant tumor cells to chemotherapy. *Can J Physiol Pharmacol.* 2004 Jul;82(7):431-7. Canada.

[38] Sohn J, Lee CH, Chung DJ, Park SH, Kim I, Hwang WI. Effect of petroleum ether extract of Panax ginseng roots on proliferation and cell cycle progression of human renal cell carcinoma cells. *Exp Mol Med.* 1998 Mar 31;30(1):47-51. Korea.

[39] Suh SO, Kroh M, Kim NR, Joh YG, Cho MY. Effects of red ginseng upon postoperative immunity and survival in patients with stage III gastric cancer. *Am J Chin Med.* 2002;30(4):483-94. Korea.

[40] Nakata H, Kikuchi Y, Tode T, Hirata J, Kita T, Ishii K, Kudoh K, Nagata I, Shinomiya N.Inhibitory effects of ginsenoside Rh2 on tumor growth in nude mice bearing human ovarian cancer cells. *Jpn J Cancer Res.* 1998 Jul;89(7):733-40.

[41] Yun TK, Choi SY. Non-organ specific cancer prevention of ginseng: a prospective study in Korea. *Int J Epidemiol.* 1998 Jun;27(3):359-64.

[42] Yun TK, Choi SY, Yun HY. Epidemiological study on cancer prevention by ginseng: are all kinds of cancers preventable by ginseng? *J Korean Med Sci.* 2001 Dec;16 Suppl:S19-27.

[43] Panwar M, Kumar M, Samarth R, Kumar A.Evaluation of chemopreventive action and antimutagenic effect of the standardized Panax ginseng extract, EFLA400, in Swiss albino mice. *Phytother Res.* 2005 Jan;19(1):65-71. India.

[44] Lee TK, Johnke RM, Allison RR, O'brien KF, Dobbs LJ Jr. Radioprotective potential of ginseng. *Mutagenesis.* 2005 Jun 14; [Epub ahead of print] USA.

[45] Allen JD, McLung J, Nelson AG, Welsch M. Ginseng supplementation does not enhance healthy young adults' peak aerobic exercise performance. *J Am Coll Nutr* 1998;17:462-6.

[46] Scaglione F, Cattaneo G, Alessandria M, Cogo R. Efficacy and safety of the standardized Ginseng extract G115 for potentiating vaccination against the influenza syndrome and protection against the common cold [corrected]. *Drugs Exp Clin Res* 1996;22:65-72.

[47] Scaglione F, Ferrara F, Dugnani S, Falchi M, Santoro G, Fraschini F. Immunomodulatory effects of two extracts of Panax ginseng C.A. Meyer. *Drugs Exp Clin Res* 1990;16:537-42.

[48] Hong B, Ji YH, Hong JH, Nam KY, Ahn TY. A double-blind crossover study evaluating the efficacy of korean red ginseng in patients with erectile dysfunction: a preliminary report. *J Urol* 2002;168: 2070-3.

[49] Ryu JK, Lee T, Kim DJ, Park IS, Yoon SM, Lee HS, Song SU, Suh JK. Free radical-scavenging activity of Korean red ginseng for erectile dysfunction in non-insulin-dependent diabetes mellitus rats. *Urology*. 2005 Mar;65(3):611

[50] World Health Organization. WHO monographs on selected medicinal plants. Geneva: World Health Organization, 1999.

[51] Yun TK, Choi SY. Non-organ specific cancer prevention of ginseng: a prospective study in Korea. *Int J Epidemiol* 1998;27:359-64.

[52] Coon JT, Ernst E. Panax ginseng: a systematic review of adverse effects and drug interactions. *Drug Saf* 2002;25:323-44.

[53] Kitts D, Hu C.Efficacy and safety of ginseng. *Public Health Nutr.* 2000 Dec;3(4A):473-85.

[54] Kabalak AA, Soyal OB, Urfalioglu A, Saracoglu F, Gogus N. Menometrorrhagia and tachyarrhythmia after using oral and topical ginseng. *J Womens Health (Larchmt).* 2004 Sep;13(7):830-3.Turkey.

SECTION 3: CAFFEINE

Overview

Caffeine (1,3,7-trimethylxanthine) is one of 3 xanthines (theophylline and theobromine) that occur in plants. Caffeine is the most widely consumed central nervous system (CNS) stimulant throughout the world. Its found in highest concentrations in coffee, but also present in tea, cola drinks, choclate candy and cocoa. Coffee contains approximately 1.3% caffeine and a cup of coffee contains 100-150 mg.Caffeine is has a stimulant effect on the cerebral cortex and medullary centers and also on the myocardium. The stimulant effect on the myocardium has been attributed to phosodiaestrase inhibition and blockade of the adenosine receptors. Caffeine has also a weak diuretic effect mainly due to reduced tubular reabsorption of sodium. Caffeine is known to improve physical performance, however it has been suggested that the improvement consists of restoration of the impaired performance by fatigue rather than improving the normal maximum performance. This effect on physical performance is considered to be due to a delay in the onset of fatigue, inattentiveness and sleepiness The administration of caffeine is not without risks. A large dose of caffeine has a positive intropic and chronotropic on the heart, increasing contractility and heart rate. This effect may trigger premature ventricular contraction and may be harmful in patients with angina.

The Antioxidant Activity of Roasted Coffee Residues

The antioxidant activity of roasted coffee residues has been demonstrated experimentally. Extraction with four solvents (water, methanol, ethanol, and n-hexane) showed that water extracts of roasted coffee residues (WERCR) produced higher yields and gave better protection for lipid peroxidation. WERCR showed a remarkable protective effect on oxidative damage of protein.

In addition, WERCR showed scavenging of free radicals as well as the reducing ability and to bind ferrous ions, indicating that WERCR acts as both primary and secondary antioxidants. The HPLC analyses showed that phenolic acids (chlorogenic acid and caffeic acid) and nonphenolic compounds [caffeine, trigonelline, nicotinic acid, and 5-(hydroxymethyl) furfuraldehyde] remained in roasted coffee residues. These compounds showed a protective effect on a liposome model system. The concentrations of flavonoids and polyphenolic compounds in roasted coffee residues were 8,400 and 20,400 ppm, respectively. In addition, the Maillard reaction products (MRPs) remaining in roasted coffee residues were believed to show antioxidant activity. Roasted coffee residues have excellent potential for use as a natural antioxidant source because the antioxidant compounds remained in roasted coffee residues [3].

Caffeine Inhibit HIV-1 Replication

Human immunodeficiency virus type I (HIV-1) DNA integration is an essential step of viral replication. It has been suggested recently that this stage of HIV-1 life-cycle triggers a cellular DNA damage response and requires cellular DNA repair proteins for its completion. These include DNA-PK (DNA-dependent protein kinase), ATR (ataxia telangiectasia and Rad3-related), and, at least in some circumstances, ATM (ataxia telangiectasia mutated). Host cell proteins may constitute an attractive target for anti-HIV-1 therapeutics, since development of drug resistance against compounds targeting these cellular cofactor proteins is unlikely. It has been show that an inhibitor of ATR and ATM kinases, caffeine, can suppress replication of infectious HIV-1 strains, and provide evidence that caffeine exerts its inhibitory effect at the integration step of the HIV-1 life-cycle. Caffeine-related methylxanthines including the clinically used compound, theophylline, act at the same step of the HIV-1 life-cycle as caffeine and efficiently inhibit HIV-1 replication in primary human cells. The possibility of therapeutic approaches targeting host cell proteins [4].

Beneficial Effect of Caffeine on Brain Function

L-Arginine metabolism in the brain is very important for normal brain function. In addition to brain protein synthesis, arginine is a substrate for the production of urea, creatine, nitric oxide, agmatine, glutamic acid, ornithine, proline and polyamines, many of these compounds are very important in brain function. In experiment protocol on male Wistar rats weighing about 200 g. Caffeine was added to the drinking water in gradually increasing amounts, from 2 g/l over the first 3 days, to 4 g/l over the last 7 days. A control group was given drinking water without caffeine. The level of lipid peroxidation, arginase and diamine oxidase (DAO) activity in the brain was measured. Arginase and diamine oxidase were decreased in animals treated with caffeine. The level of lipid peroxidation (MDA) was decreased also. The inhibitory effect of caffeine on arginase activity indicates that caffeine provides more arginine for consumption in other metabolic pathways and the moderate short-term consumption of caffeine may be beneficial for brain function [5].

Protective Effect in Brain Trauma

It has been demonstrated that ethanol exerts dose-dependent effects, both beneficial and detrimental, on the outcome of traumatic brain injury (TBI). Recently, it has been reported that co-administration of caffeine (10 mg/kg) and a low amount of alcohol (0.65 g/kg; caffeinol) reduces cortical infarct volume up to 80%, and improves motor coordination, following a rodent model of reversible common carotid/middle cerebral artery occlusion. However, the protective effects of caffeinol following other CNS insults, nor its influence on cognitive function, have been examined. Using a controlled cortical impact model of brain injury, the effect of caffeinol administration on TBI-associated motor and cognitive deficits was assessed. When given 15 min following injury, caffeinol reduced cortical tissue loss and improved working memory. However, no influence on motor skills, Morris water maze performance or associative learning and memory was observed. Delayed administration (6 h post-injury) of caffeinol containing a dose of ethanol (1 g/kg) previously demonstrated to improve motor performance eliminated the working memory benefit and cortical protection. The early administration of caffeine may be beneficial in lessening some of the deficits and cortical tissue loss associated with brain trauma [6].

Protective Effect Against Parkinson Disease

Epidemiological studies have consistently demonstrated an inverse association between coffee consumption and Parkinson's disease (PD). Caffeine consumption is associated with a reduced risk of Parkinson's disease in men but not in women. This gender difference may be due to an interaction between caffeine and use of postmenopausal estrogens. The relation between coffee consumption and Parkinson's disease mortality was studied among participants in the Cancer Prevention Study II, a cohort of over 1 million people enrolled in 1982. Causes of deaths were ascertained through death certificates from January 1, 1989, through 1998. Parkinson's disease was listed as a cause of death in 909 men and 340 women. After adjustment for age, smoking, and alcohol intake, coffee consumption was inversely associated with Parkinson's disease mortality in men (p(trend) = 0.01) but not in women (p = 0.6). In women, this association was dependent on postmenopausal estrogen use; the relative risk for women drinking 4 or more cups (600 ml) of coffee per day compared with nondrinkers was 0.47 (95% confidence interval: 0.27, 0.80; p = 0.006) among never users and 1.31 (95% confidence interval: 0.75, 2.30; p = 0.34) among users. Caffeine reduces the risk of Parkinson's disease but this hypothetical beneficial effect may be prevented by use of estrogen replacement therapy [7].

A beneficial effect of caffeine at a dose comparable to that of human exposure has been shown in a model of PD. Unilateral intrastriatal 6-hydroxydopamine (6-OHDA)-lesioned rats were pretreated with caffeine (20 mg/kg; i.p.) 1 h before surgery and treated twice a day (10 mg/kg) for 1 month. Apomorphine-induced rotations and number of Nissl-stained neurons of substantia nigra pars compacta (SNC) were counted. Caffeine administration for 1 month could attenuate the rotational behavior in lesioned rats and protect the neurons of SNC against 6-OHDA toxicity [8].

Neuroprotective Effects of Caffeine Against Neurodegeneration in (AD)

In a case-control study 54 patients with probable Alzheimer's disease AD fulfilling the National Institute of Neurologic and Communicative Disorders and Stroke and the AD and Related Disorders Association criteria, in a Dementia Clinics setting. Controls were 54 accompanying persons, cognitively normal, matched for age (+/-3 years) and sex. Patients with AD had an average daily caffeine intake of 73.9 +/- 97.9 mg during the 20 years that preceded diagnosis of AD, whereas the controls had an average daily caffeine intake of 198.7 +/- 135.7 mg during the corresponding 20 years of their lifetimes ($P < 0.001$, Wilcoxon signed ranks test). Using a logistic regression model, caffeine exposure during this period was found to be significantly inversely associated with AD (odds ratio=0.40, 95% confidence interval=0.25-0.67), whereas hypertension, diabetes, stroke, head trauma, smoking habits, alcohol consumption, non-steroid anti-inflammatory drugs, vitamin E, gastric disorders, heart disease, education and family history of dementia were not statistically significantly associated with AD. Caffeine intake was associated with a significantly lower risk for AD, independently of other possible confounding variables. These results, if confirmed with future prospective studies, may have a major impact on the prevention of AD [9].

Adenosine is a neuromodulator in the nervous system and it has recently been observed that pharmacological blockade or gene disruption of adenosine A(2A) receptors confers neuroprotection under different neurotoxic situations in the brain. The coapplication of either caffeine (1-25 micro M) or the selective A(2A) receptor antagonist, 4-(2-[7-amino-2(2-furyl)(1,2,4)triazolo (2,3-a)(1,3,5)triazin-5-ylamino]ethyl)phenol (ZM 241385, 50 nM), but not the A receptor antagonist, 8-cyclopentyltheophylline (200 nM), prevented the neuronal cell death caused by exposure of rat cultured cerebellar granule neurons to fragment 25-35 of beta-amyloid protein (25 micro M for 48 h), that by itself caused a near three-fold increase of propidium iodide-labeled cells. In vitro evidence suggested that adenosine A(2A) receptors may be the molecular target responsible for the observed beneficial effects of caffeine consumption in the development of Alzheimer's disease [10].

Cognitive and Mood Improvements of Caffeine

In placebo-controlled, double-blind, balanced crossover the acute cognitive and mood effects of caffeine in habitual users and habitual non-users of caffeine have been studied Following overnight caffeine withdrawal, 24 habitual caffeine consumers (mean=217 mg/day) and 24 habitual non-consumers (20 mg/day) received a 150 ml drink containing either 75 or 150 mg of caffeine or a matching placebo, at intervals of > or =48 h. Cognitive and mood assessments were undertaken at baseline and 30 min post-drink. There were no baseline differences between the groups' mood or performance. Following caffeine, there were significant improvements in simple reaction time, digit vigilance reaction time, numeric working memory reaction time and sentence verification accuracy, irrespective of group. Self-rated mental fatigue was reduced and ratings of alertness were significantly improved by caffeine independent of group. There were also group effects for rapid visual information processing false alarms and spatial memory accuracy with habitual consumers outperforming non-consumers. There was a single significant interaction of group and treatment effects on jittery ratings. Separate analyses of each groups' responses to caffeine revealed overlapping but differential responses to caffeine. Caffeine tended to benefit consumers' mood more while improving performance more in the non-consumers [11].

The beneficial effect of caffeine on mood and cognitive function was attributed to counteracting reductions in the turnover of central noradrenaline [12]. Twenty-four healthy volunteers were given either clonidine (200 microg) or placebo and consumed coffee containing caffeine (1.5 mg/kg) or placebo. The test battery was then repeated 30 min, 150 min and 270 min later. A second cup of coffee (with the same amount of caffeine as the first) was consumed 120 min after the first cup. The results showed that clonidine reduced alertness, impaired many aspects of performance and slowed saccadic eye movements; caffeine removed many of these impairments. Both clonidine and caffeine influenced blood pressure (clonidine reduced it, caffeine raised it) but the effects appeared to be independent, suggesting that separate mechanisms were involved. In addition, there were some behavioural effects of caffeine that were independent of the clonidine effect (e.g. effects on speed of encoding of new information) and these may reflect other neurotransmitter systems (e.g cholinergic effects). Caffeine counteracts reductions in the turnover of central noradrenaline.

Coffee Consumption Associated with a Lower Risk of Clinical Type 2 Diabetes

Coffee is a major source of caffeine, which has been shown to acutely reduce sensitivity to insulin, but also has potentially beneficial effects.The association between coffee consumption and risk of clinical type 2 diabetes in a population-based cohort of 17111 has been studied. Dutch men and women aged 30-60 years. During 125774 person years of follow-up, 306 new cases of type 2 diabetes were reported. After adjustment for potential confounders, individuals who drank at least seven cups of coffee a day were 0.50 (95% CI 0.35-0.72, p=0.0002) times as likely as those who drank two cups or fewer a day to develop type 2 diabetes. Coffee consumption was associated with a substantially lower risk of clinical type 2 diabetes [13].

A Beneficial Effect of Coffee in Xerostomia

A positive effect of coffee in xerostomia has been reported.10 patients underwent a trial treatment with Cappuccino coffee. All of them (8 university lecturers and 2 clerks) aged from 60 to 69 (average 63) years old, used a tricyclic antidepressant because of insomnia as a monosymptomatic type of depression or insomnia as a dominant symptom in the course of depression. One, evening dose of doxepine was from 150 to 250 (average 225) mg, causing xerostomia next day usually between 9-15 o'clock. The five-minute--chewing of 15.0 g of Cappuccino coffee increased the amount of saliva, decreased xerostomia and improved the ability of speech. The beneficial effect of coffee lasted from 0.5 to 4 (average about 2) hours [14].

Risks Associated with Caffeine

Caffeine Intake has been Associated with Risk of Osteoporosis, Breast Cancer, Endometriosis, and Fibrocystic Breast Disease

At high doses (equivalent to more than 2 cups of coffee or four cans of caffeinated soda daily), caffeine intake was positively associated with plasma estrone before and after adjustment for confounders ($r = 0.26$, $p = 0.05$). Sex hormone-binding globulin levels were positively associated with increasing caffeine intake (adjusted $r = 0.09$, $p = 0.03$). The positive association of caffeine with estrone and its inverse association with bioavailable testosterone suggest that caffeine's reported association with several chronic conditions may be mediated by an effect on endogenous sex steroids [15].

Women from an established epidemiologic cohort had measures of BMD and gave a medical and behavioral history that included caffeinated coffee and daily milk intake between the ages of 12 and 18 years, 20 and 50 years, and 50 years of age and older. In a community-based population of older women, in Rancho Bernardo, Calif.ornia, 980 postmenopausal women aged 50 to 98 years (mean age, 72.7 years) participated between 1988 and 1991. Bone density at the hip and lumbar spine was measured by dual energy x-ray absorptiometry. There was a statistically significant graded association between increasing lifetime intake of caffeinated coffee and decreasing BMD at both the hip and spine, independent of age, obesity, parity, years since menopause, and the use of tobacco, alcohol, estrogen, thiazides, and calcium supplements. Bone density did not vary by lifetime coffee intake in women who reported drinking at least one glass of milk per day during most of their adult lives. Lifetime caffeinated coffee intake equivalent to two cups per day is associated with decreased bone density in older women who do not drink milk on a daily basis [16].

Cardiovascular Risk

Intake of coffee has been suggested as a cardiovascular risk factor; however, definitive data are lacking. Acute intake of coffee or beverages containing caffeine can increase blood pressure, heart minute volumes, and cardiac index, as well as activate the sympathetic nervous system in nonhabitual coffee drinkers. Interestingly, this is not observed in habitual coffee drinkers. Restriction of coffee or caffeinated beverages is no longer indicated in the seventh report of the Joint National Committee on Prevention, Detection, Evaluation, and Treatment of High Blood Pressure (JNC 7) guidelines for the treatment of hypertension. In fact, no clear association between coffee and the risk of hypertension, myocardial infarction, or other cardiovascular diseases has been demonstrated. In contrast to early studies, recent research indicates that habitual moderate coffee intake does not represent a health hazard and may even be associated with beneficial effects on cardiovascular health [17].

A study investigated the relation between coffee drinking and the hypertensive status in twenty-two normotensive and 26 hypertensive, nonsmoking men and women, with a mean age of 72.1 years (range, 54 to 89 years). After 2 weeks of a caffeine-free diet, subjects were randomized to continue with the caffeine-free diet and abstain from caffeine-containing drinks or drink instant coffee (5 cups per day, equivalent to 300 mg caffeine per day) in addition to the caffeine-free diet for an additional 2 weeks. Change in systolic and diastolic blood pressures (SBP, DBP) determined by 24-hour ambulatory BP monitoring showed significant interactions between coffee drinking and hypertension status. In the hypertensive group, rise in mean 24-hour SBP was greater by 4.8 (SEM, 1.3) mm Hg (P=0.031) and increase in mean 24-hour DBP was higher by 3.0 (1.0) mm Hg (P=0.010) in coffee drinkers than in abstainers. No significant differences were observed between abstainers and coffee drinkers in the normotensive group for 24-hour, daytime, or nighttime SBP or DBP. In older men and women with treated or untreated hypertension, ABP increased in coffee drinkers and decreased in abstainers. Therefore restriction of coffee intake may be beneficial in older hypertensive individuals [18].

On the other hand, a randomized controlled intervention in 171 healthy non-smokers over the age of 50 years, compared the effects of coffee-drinking with abstaining from caffeine in normotensives , untreated hypertensives and subjects on drug treatment for hypertension . In normotensive coffee drinkers there was a significant reduction in the postprandial fall in supine systolic BP of 4.1 mmHg (+/- s.e.m. 1.1) and in standing systolic BP of 5.2 +/- 1.6 mmHg. Among untreated hypertensived. abstainers showed a significant attenuation of the postprandial fall in supine, but not standing, systolic BP. Among treated hypertensives who were tea drinkers the postprandial fall decreased for supine systolic BP by 3.8 +/- 1.2 mmHg (P = 0.029) and for standing systolic BP by 5.2 +/- 2.1 mmHg. 7. Both tea and coffee were potentially beneficial in decreasing postprandial falls in systolic BP, but coffee drinking may increase fasting diastolic pressures in untreated hypertensives [19].

REFERENCES

[1]   Ashton CH.Caffeine and health. *BMJ* 1987;295:1293.
[2]   Sutherland EW, Rall TW.The relation of adenosine-3,5 phosphate to the action of catecholamines.In: *Adrenergic mechanisms.Ciba foundation and committee for symposium on drug action.*1960 Little brown &Co.
[3]   Yen WJ, Wang BS, Chang LW, Duh PD.Antioxidant properties of roasted coffee residues *Agric Food Chem.* 2005 Apr 6;53(7):2658-63. Taiwan, China.
[4]   Nunnari G, Argyris E, Fang J, Mehlman KE, Pomerantz RJ, Daniel R. Inhibition of HIV-1 replication by caffeine and caffeine-related methylxanthines. *Virology.* 2005 May 10;335(2):177-84. USA.
[5]   Dash PK, Moore AN, Moody MR, Treadwell R, Felix JL, Clifton GL. Post-trauma administration of caffeine plus ethanol reduces contusion volume and improves working memory in rats. USA

[6]   Nikolic J, Bjelakovic G, Stojanovic I.Effect of caffeine on metabolism of L-arginine in the brain. *Mol Cell Biochem.* 2003 Feb;244(1-2):125-8. Yugoslavia.

[7]   Ascherio A, Weisskopf MG, O'Reilly EJ, McCullough ML, Calle EE, Rodriguez C, Thun MJ.Coffee consumption, gender, and Parkinson's disease mortality in the cancer prevention study II cohort: the modifying effects of estrogen. *Am J Epidemiol.* 2004 Nov 15;160(10):977-84. USA.

[8]   Joghataie MT, Roghani M, Negahdar F, Hashemi L. Protective effect of caffeine against neurodegeneration in a model of Parkinson's disease in rat: behavioral and histochemical evidence. *Parkinsonism Relat Disord.* 2004 Dec;10(8):465-8. Iran.

[9]   Maia L, de Mendonca A.Does caffeine intake protect from Alzheimer's disease? *Eur J Neurol.* 2002 Jul;9(4):377-82.Portugal.

[10]   Dall'Igna OP, Porciuncula LO, Souza DO, Cunha RA, Lara DR. Neuroprotection by caffeine and adenosine A2A receptor blockade of beta-amyloid neurotoxicity. *Br J Pharmacol.* 2003 Apr;138(7):1207-9.

[11]   Haskell CF, Kennedy DO, Wesnes KA, Scholey AB.Cognitive and mood improvements of caffeine in habitual consumers and habitual non-consumers of caffeine. *Psychopharmacology (Berl).* 2005 Jun;179(4):813-25. Epub 2005 Jan UK.

[12]   Smith A, Brice C, Nash J, Rich N, Nutt DJ. Caffeine and central noradrenaline: effects on mood, cognitive performance, eye movements and cardiovascular function. *J Psychopharmacol.* 2003 Sep;17(3):283-92 UK

[13]   van Dam RM, Feskens EJ.Coffee consumption and risk of type 2 diabetes mellitus. *Lancet.* 2002 Nov 9;360(9344):1477-8. Netherlands.

[14]   Chodorowski Z. Cappuccino. Coffee treatment of xerostomia in patients taking tricyclic antidepressants: preliminary report. *Przegl Lek.* 2002;59(4-5):392-3.

[15]   Ferrini RL, Barrett-Connor E.Caffeine intake and endogenous sex steroid levels in postmenopausal women. The Rancho Bernardo Study. *Am J Epidemiol.* 1996 Oct 1;144(7):642-4. USA.

[16]   Barrett-Connor E, Chang JC, Edelstein SL.Coffee-associated osteoporosis offset by daily milk consumption. The Rancho Bernardo Study. *JAMA.* 1994 Jan 26;271(4):280-3.

[17]   Sudano I, Binggeli C, Spieker L, Luscher TF, Ruschitzka F, Noll G, Corti R. Cardiovascular effects of coffee: is it a risk factor? *Prog Cardiovasc Nurs.* 2005 Spring;20(2):65-9. Switzerland.

[18]   Rakic V, Burke V, Beilin LJ..Effects of coffee on ambulatory blood pressure in older men and women: A randomized controlled trial. *Hypertension.* 1999 Mar;33(3):869-73.

[19]   Rakic V, Beilin LJ, Burke V.Effect of coffee and tea drinking on postprandial hypotension in older men and women. *Clin Exp Pharmacol Physiol.* 1996 Jun-Jul;23(6-7):559-63.

In: Nutrition Research Advances

Editor: Sarah V. Watkins, pp. 207-222

ISBN 1-60021-516-5

© 2007 Nova Science Publishers, Inc.

Chapter VII

COFFEE LIPID CLASS
VARIATION DURING STORAGE

Gulab N. Jham[1], Vidigal Muller[1] and Paulo Cecon[2]

Universidade Federal de Viçosa, [1]Labarótorio de Pesquisas de Produtos Naturais (LPPN),
[2]Departamentos de Química and Informática, Viçosa, MG 36.570-000, Brazil.

ABSTRACT

Despite little literature on coffee lipids, it has been hypothesized that they lower coffee quality through hydrolysis of the triacylglycerols during storage releasing free fatty acids, which are in turn oxidized to produce compounds producing off-flavour. Coffee is stored for extended periods by small producers in Brazil to fetch better market prices. As a part of our coffee-breeding program aiming to improve the quality of Brazilian coffee, we plan to evaluate the role of lipids during storage, developing initially methods (TLC-thin layer chromatography, HLPC-LSD-high performance liquid chromatography with light sensitive detection and HPLC with refractive index detection) for their determination. In this study experiments were carried out to evaluate the variation of lipid classes (free fatty acids, fatty acids after oil hydrolysis, triacylglycerols-TAG and terpene esters-TE) during coffee storage. Three types of coffee beans (immature, random mixture and cherry) picked in Viçosa, MG, Brazil (a region traditionally considered to be a producer of low quality coffee), were dried by two widely used procedures (dryer and open air cement patio) and stored on wood shelves in a house without neither temperature nor humidity control for 19 months. We tried to reproduce storage conditions used by small farmers in Brazil. At 4, 7, 10, 13, 16 and 19 months of storage, a part of samples was withdrawn and lipid classes were analyzed using the methods developed in our laboratory. The experiment consisted of thirty-six treatments in a randomised block design with three repetitions. The following treatments (T) were used: immature coffee beans dried in a dryer (T_1) and on a patio (T_2); a random mixture of coffee beans dried in a dryer (T_3) and on a patio (T_4) and cherry coffee beans dried in a dryer (T_5) and on a patio (T_6). In these treatments, samples were stored for four months followed by analysis of lipid classes. The procedure was repeated for immature, random and cherry coffee beans after 7, 10, 13, 16 and 19 months of storage corresponding to treatments T_7-T_{12}, T_{13}-T_{18}, T_{19}-T_{24}, T_{25}-T_{30} and T_{31}-T_{36}, respectively. Lipid class data were statistically analyzed through variance and regression. The qualitative factors (type of coffee and type of drying) and the averages were compared by the Tukey test at 5% probability. The quantitative factor (months of storage) and the averages were chosen based on the significance of regression coefficients using the t test at 5% probability and determination coefficients (r^2). While apparently random variation was observed in a few cases, no effects of storage time, storage type and coffee type were found on the lipid classes. These results contradict literature studies where a small number of samples were studied utilizing short storage times.

1. INTRODUCTION

Most Brazilian coffee produced for internal consumption is considered to be of low quality. A number of factors such as poor post-harvesting practices (Informe Agropecuário, 1997), fungal contamination (Zambolin et al., 1996) and the presence of undesired compounds (Spadone et al., 1990) have been reported as possible causes. Despite little literature on coffee lipids, it has been hypothesized that they lower coffee quality through hydrolysis of the triacylglycerols during storage releasing free fatty acids, which are in turn oxidized to produce compounds producing off-flavour. Degradation of free amino acids, sugars and oxidation of lipids in coffee stored for one year has been reported with coffee quality loss (Multon et al., 1973). Increased free fatty acids content has been associated to long storage in subtropical conditions and may be due to enzymatic activity. The latter is assumed also to be a cause of flavour deterioration (Wajda & Walczky, 1978). In a simulated study, linoleic acid (L), which is susceptible to oxidation, was reported to be reduced in rancid beans with respect to fresh beans; while palmitic acid (P) remained unaltered (Fourney et al., 1982). Higher concentrations of free fatty acids in *robusta* than in *arabica* coffee beans were linked to rough processing or storage conditions (Speer et al., 1993).

In Brazil, coffee is often stored over extended periods of times by small producers to obtain better prices. However, the long-term storage effects on coffee quality and chemical composition have been little studied (Multon et al., 1973; Wajda & Walczky, 1978; Speer et al., 1993). No such studies have been carried out under Brazilian conditions. Such studies are very important since it is known that small variations in storage temperature and humidity may have profound influence on coffee quality (Illy & Viani, 1995).

Our coffee breeding program aims to study the role of lipids in coffee quality and initially methods were developed for their determination. We reported lipid classes and the TAG molecular species by TLC (thin layer chromatography) (Nikolova-Damyanova et al., 1998). HPLC-LSD (high performance liquid chromatography-light sensitive detector) (Jham et al., 2003) and HPLC-RID (high performance liquid chromatography-refractive index detector) (Jham et al., 2005) methods were reported for the identification and determination of relative % of individual TAG molecular species in eight coffee types. More recently, liquid chromatography-mass spectrometry (LC-MS) (Segall et al., 2005) for determination of coffee TAGs has also been reported. In addition, effects of coffee type and drying procedures on lipid classes and TAG molecular species by TLC were reported on a few coffee samples (Jham et al., 2001). We now report the variation of coffee lipid classes (free fatty acids, fatty acids after oil hydrolysis, triacylglycerols-TAGs and terpene esters-TE) of three type of coffee beans (immature, random mixture and cherry) dried by two widely used procedures (dryer and open air cement patio) stored for nineteen months in Viçosa in the State of Minas Gerais, Brazil.

2. METHODS AND MATERIALS

2.1. Coffee Samples

The details have been described before (Nikanva-Dayanova et al., 1998) and hence will be briefly described. About 10 kg of coffee (Catuaí Vermelho, *Coffea arabica* L) were harvested in Viçosa, MG by the "derriça" method (coffee beans were hand-removed from the tree and allowed to drop on the floor covered with cloth). From this sample, a random mixture was obtained by separating 5 kg and the rest was used to obtain immature and cherry beans by placing the coffee sample in a tank containing 50 L of water. The dry beans floated immediately and were separated while the immature and cherry beans remained at the bottom of the tank. After draining the water tank, the immature and the cherry beans were hand-separated and allowed to air-dry for 20 h. The three types of coffee beans (immature, random mixture and cherry) were divided in roughly six equal parts and dried by two methods (dryer and patio). A dryer prototype developed by the Agricultural Engineering Dept. of Universidade Federal de Viçosa was used for drying with the air temperature at 45°C for several hours until humidity was 11% (Jham et al., 2003, 2005). For patio drying, coffee samples were spread on a cement floor and dried for several days until a humidity of 14% was attained. All samples were stored in jute bags on wooden racks in a house without control of neither temperature nor humidity. After 4, 7, 10, 13 and 19 months of storage, about 1 kg of each of the coffee samples was withdrawn, lipids extracted and analysed (oil, acidity, TAGs and fatty acids after hydrolysis). Treatments used in this study are described in Table 1.

2.2. Chemical Analysis

2.2.1. Oil Extraction

The oil was extracted from the coffee beans in a Soxhlet extractor for 6 h using hexane as the solvent. The solvent was evaporated at 40^{0}C in a rotatory evaporator, dried over anhydrous sodium sulphate, filtered, re-evaporated, weighed, stored at -10°C. The samples were thawed to room temperature for chemical analysis (acidity, free fatty acids and fatty acids after hydrolysis and main lipid classes-TE and triacylglycerols).

Table 1. Description of the treatments (T) used in the study

T	Description
T_1	Immature coffee beans dried in a dryer and analyzed after four months of storage
T_2	Immature coffee beans dried on a patio and analyzed after four months of storage
T_3	Random mixture of coffee beans dried in a dryer and analyzed after four months of storage
T_4	Random mixture of coffee beans dried on a patio and analyzed after four months of storage
T_5	Cherry coffee beans dried in a dryer and analyzed after four months of storage
T_6	Cherry coffee beans dried on a patio and analyzed after four months of storage
T_7	Immature coffee beans dried in a dryer and analyzed after seven months of storage
T_8	Immature coffee beans dried on a patio and analyzed after seven months of storage
T_9	Random mixture of coffee beans dried in a dryer and analyzed after seven months of storage
T_{10}	Random mixture of coffee beans dried on a patio and analyzed after seven months of storage
T_{11}	Cherry coffee beans dried in a dryer and analyzed after seven months of storage
T_{12}	Cherry coffee beans on a patio and analyzed after seven months of storage
T_{13}	Immature coffee beans dried in a dryer and analyzed after ten months of storage
T_{14}	Immature coffee beans obtained dried on a patio and analyzed after ten months of storage
T_{15}	Random mixture of coffee beans dried in a dryer and analyzed after ten months of storage
T_{16}	Random mixture of coffee beans dried on a patio and analyzed after ten months of storage
T_{17}	Cherry coffee beans obtained dried in a dryer and analyzed after ten months of storage
T_{18}	Cherry coffee beans dried on a patio and analyzed after ten months of storage
T_{19}	Immature coffee beans dried in a dryer and analyzed after thirteen months of storage
T_{20}	Immature coffee beans dried on a patio and analyzed after thirteen months of storage
T_{21}	Random mixture of coffee beans dried in a dryer and analyzed after thirteen months of storage
T_{22}	Random mixture of coffee beans dried on a patio and analyzed after thirteen months of storage
T_{23}	Cherry coffee beans dried in a dryer and analyzed after thirteen months of storage
T_{24}	Cherry coffee beans dried on a patio and analyzed after thirteen months of storage
T_{25}	Immature coffee beans obtained dried in a dryer and analyzed after sixteen months of storage
T_{26}	Immature coffee beans on a patio and analyzed after sixteen months of storage
T_{27}	Random mixture of coffee beans dried in a dryer and analyzed after sixteen months of storage
T_{28}	Random mixture of coffee beans dried on a patio and analyzed after 16 months of storage
T_{29}	Cherry coffee beans dried in a dryer and analyzed after sixteen months of storage
T_{30}	Cherry coffee beans obtained dried on a patio and analyzed after sixteen months of storage
T_{31}	Immature coffee beans dried in a dryer and analyzed after nineteen months of storage
T_{32}	Immature coffee beans dried on a patio and analyzed after nineteen months of storage
T_{33}	Random mixture of coffee beans dried in a dryer and analyzed after nineteen months of storage
T_{34}	Random mixture of coffee beans dried on a patio and analyzed after nineteen months of storage
T_{35}	Cherry coffee beans dried in a dryer and analyzed after nineteen months of storage
T_{36}	Cherry coffee beans dried on a patio and analyzed after nineteen months of storage

2.2.2. Coffee Oil Acidity

Titrable acidity was determined by Association of Official Analytical Chemists method (1984) expressing it as oleic acid using 0.5g of sample and using 0.01 mol/L for titration.

2.2.3. Identification of the Main Lipid Classes by Analytical Silica Gel TLC

Reference mixture of lipid classes was prepared by mixing equal aliquots of 10% solutions of docosane, cholesteryl_oleate, methyl oleate, oleyl alcohol, cholesterol, 1,3-diolein, 1-monoolein-rac-glycerol, L-α dioleylphosphatidyl choline (all purchased form Sigma-Aldrich Chemie GmbH, Germany), triacylglycerol fraction from sunflower oil in dichloromethane. A reference TAG mixture was prepared by mixing equal quantities of TAGs from lard and sunflower oils. To this mixture 100 g kg^{-1} of tristearin was added to increase the proportion of the trisaturated TAG (SSS; S, saturated acyl residue). This mixture was used to identify the TAGs from SSS to DDD (D, dienoic acyl residues). Pure TAG fractions with known composition from tangerine and linseed oils (Tarandjiiska et al., 1996) were used to identify the TAGs.

The lipid class composition was determined by analytical silica gel TLC. An aliquot of the 1% lipid solution in dichloromethane was applied on 4 cm x 19 cm glass plates (ca 0.200 mm thick layer). The lipid classes were identified by comparison with a reference lipid mixture (20 µL of 1% solution in dichloromethane), which was applied alongside each plate. The plates were developed with ca. 4 ml petroleum ether-acetone, 100:8 (by volume). The lipid zones were detected by spraying with 50% ethanolic sulphuric acid and heating at 200°C on a metal plate with temperature control.

2.2.4. Isolation, Purification and Quantification of Lipid Classes by Preparative Silica Gel TLC

An aliquot of the 10% stock solution was applied on 20 cm x 20 cm plates (ca. 1 mm thick layer) and developed with petroleum ether-acetone 100:8 (by volume). The separated zones were detected by spraying the edge of each plate with 2,7-dichlorofluorescein. Partial acylglycerols, free fatty acids and polar lipids, which migrated below the sterols in this system, were collected jointly, and the components were isolated on a second preparative silica TLC plate with mobile phase light petroleum-acetone-acetic acid (70:30:1, by volume). All zones form the two plates were scrapped, transferred to small glass columns and eluted with ethyl ether. The solvent was evaporated under stream of nitrogen and the residue was weighed in small glass containers (of known weight) to a constant weight.

2.2.5. Quantitative (%) Fatty Acid Composition of Oil by Gas Chromatography (GC)

Hydrolysis of the oil and methylation were carried out as described (Jham et al., 1982). The fatty acid methyl esters were identified by standards. A Shimadzu gas chromatograph, model 17-A fitted with FID, auto sampler and an integration system was used. Fused silica capillary columns (30 m x 0.25 mm; film thickness of 0.25 µm) coated with the Carbowax stationary phase were purchased from Supelco. The GC oven temperature was increased from 60°C to 240°C at a rate of 6°C/min.

2.3. TAG Determination

The detailed procedures for the identification of individual coffee TAG by HPLC-LSD (Jham et al., 2003) and HPLC-RID were described (Jham et al., 2005). A LC-MS procedure to determine the TAG composition has also been described (Segall et al., 2005). In these procedures, crude oil was injected into the HPLC and the individual TAG identified with standards and literature procedures (Christy, 1987, Nikolova-Damyanova et al., 1990). With the LSD, a linear gradient of acetonitrile (solvent A) and dichloromethane-dichloroethane (8:2, v/v) (solvent B) was generated from 55% A to 65% B over 40 minutes. The flow rate was 0.5 mL/min. The mobile phase with RID was acetonitrile/acetone (1:1, v/v) at a flow rate of 2 mL/min. A Techsphere ODS column (5 μm, 250 x 4.6 mm id, HPLC Technology, Herts, England) equipped with a Techsphere ODS guard-column (5 μm, 10 x 4.6 mm, HPLC Technology, Herts, England) was used in both cases.

2.4. Statistical Analysis

The experiment was arranged in subdivided parcels, with the parcels in a 3x2 factorial scheme [(three types of coffee beans-immature, random mixture and cherry coffee beans) and two types of drying procedures-dryer and patio)] and the sub parcels being storage time (4, 7, 10, 13, 16 and 19 months) in a completely randomised design with 3 repetitions. Data on lipid classes (acidity, fatty acid after hydrolysis, TE and TAG) were statistically analysed through variance and regression. The qualitative factors (type of coffees and types of drying) the averages were compared by the Tukey test at 5% probability. The quantitative factor (months of storage) and the models were chosen based on the significance of regression coefficients using the t test at 5% probability and determination coefficient (r^2) and the biological phenomenon.

3. RESULTS AND DISCUSSION

The storage conditions used in this study attempted to simulate the conditions used by small coffee producers. Hence, a simple house with wooden racks without control of the temperature nor humidity was utilized.

3.1. Coffee Oil Acidity

No effect of storage time on acidity the coffee types or type of drying was noted, i.e., as the storage time increased the coffee acidity did not change (Table 2). However, a significant effect of coffee type was noted on acidity, with higher values being obtained for cherry coffee beans as compared to immature coffee beans (Table 3). A higher coffee acidity was verified for patio drying than for conventional drying (Table 4). Unfortunately, comparisons of our results with the literature values will be difficult since no such studies have been conducted. However, it is generally empirically accepted that cherry coffee beans are considered to have lower acidity than the immature coffee beans.

Table 2. Adjusted regression equations for coffee acidity as a function of storage time for three types of coffee and two types of drying

Type of coffee beans	Adjusted equation
Immature	$\hat{Y} = 3.99$
Random mixture	$\hat{Y} = 4.53$
Cherry beans	$\hat{Y} = 5.22$
Type of drying	
Conventional	$\hat{Y} = 3.65$
Patio	$\hat{Y} = 5.51$

Table 3. Average acidity* for the three types of coffees as a function of storage time

Storage time (months)	Immature coffee beans	Random mixture of coffee beans	Cherry coffee beans
4	3.57 c	4.02 b	4.60 b
7	3.80 b	4.02 b	4.93 a
10	4.41 c	4.97 b	5.52 a
13	4.50 c	510 b	5.78 a
16	3.70 c	4.52 b	5.15 a
19	3.92 c	4.57 b	5.37 a

*Averages followed by same small letter in a column do not differ by the Tukey test at 5% probability.

Table 4. Average acidity* for combinations of storage time and drying

Storage time (months)	Type of drying	
	Dryer	Patio
4	3.17 b	4.98 a
7	3.39 b	5.10 a
10	3.95 b	5.98 a
13	4.24 b	6.05 a
16	3.54 b	5.37 a
19	3.64 b	5.60 a

*Averages followed by same small letter in a column do not differ by the Tukey test at 5% probability.

3.2. Oil

The % oil obtained in this study is in agreement with the literature value (8.7-12.2%) reported for crude coffee beans (Belitz & Grosh, 1988) and our study (Nikalova-Damyanova et al., 1998).

No effect of storage time was noted for any of the coffee types or drying types with the average % oil being $\hat{Y}$ =10.82. However, the quantity of oil behaved differently with respect to coffee type and drying type. For all the coffee types studied, a higher oil value was found for conventional drying as compared to patio drying. In relation to type of drying, a higher % of oil was obtained for immature coffee beans than for cherry beans (Table 5).

Table 5. Average oil* (%) as a function of coffee bean type and storage type

Type of coffee beans	Type of drying	
	Dryer	Patio
Immature	12.02 aA	10.50 bA
Random mixture	11.27 aB	10.46 bA
Cherry	10,70 aC	9.95 bB

*Averages followed by same small letter in a column do not differ by the Tukey test at 5% probability.

Table 6. Adjusted regression equations for the % of palmitic acid (P) and linoleic acid (L) as a function of storage time, coffee type and drying

Type of coffee beans	Type of drying	Variable	Adjusted equations
Immature	Dryer	P	$\hat{Y}$ = 38.23
Immature	Patio	P	$\hat{Y}$ = 40.19
Random mixture	Dryer	P	$\hat{Y}$ = 39.87
Random mixture	Patio	P	$\hat{Y}$ = 37.87
Cherry	Dryer	P	$\hat{Y}$ = 40.86
Cherry	Patio	P	$\hat{Y}$ 41.91
Immature	Dryer	L	$\hat{Y}$ = 40.05
Immature	Patio	L	$\hat{Y}$ = 39.68
Random mixture	Dryer	L	$\hat{Y}$ = 37.77
Random mixture	Patio	L	$\hat{Y}$ = 36.73
Cherry	Dryer	L	$\hat{Y}$ = 37.38
Cherry	Patio	L	$\hat{Y}$ = 39.40

3.3. Fatty Acid (FA) Composition of Coffee Oil after Lipid Hydrolysis

The fatty acids identified in all oils after hydrolysis were miristic (14:0), palmitic (16:0), palmitoleic (16:1), stearic (18:0), oleic (cis 9-18:1), linoleic acid (cis 9,12-18:2), linolenic (cis 9,12, 15-18:32) , arahidic (20:0) and bechenic (22:0) acids The major acids were the P and L acids (~40% each) corresponding to about 80% of the total FA. These results are in agreement with the literature studies (Kaufmann & Hamsagar, 1963; Speer et al., 1993) and with our study (Nikalova-Damyanova et al., 1998).

No effect of storage time in any of the coffee types and storage types was observed on the relative % of both P and L, i.e., as the storage time increased the % of the acids did not change (Table 6). After seven months of storage, for immature coffee beans there was no effect of type of drying for P and L acids (Tables 7 and 8). However, cherry coffee beans presented higher % of P for all storage times and types of drying. In general, immature coffee beans presented the highest % for all storage and drying types. This result was not in agreement with that of Fourney et al., 1982 who reported through simulated experiments that the % of L, susceptible to oxidation was reduced in rancid beans with respect to fresh beans while that of P remained practically unaltered.

Table 7. Average palmitic acid (%)* as a function of storage time, type of coffee and drying

Type of coffee beans	Storage time (months)					
	4		7		10	
	Type of drying					
	Dryer	Patio	Dryer	Patio	Dryer	Patio
Immature	38.43 bB	42.80aA	35.96bB	42.40abA	40.76aA	38.83aA
Random mixture	41.46 aA	35.80bB	43.00aA	39.80bB	39.00aA	36.80aA
Cherry	40.36abB	43.23aA	43.30aA	44.30aA	40.29aA	38.50aA

Type of coffee beans	Storage time (months)					
	13		16		19	
	Type of drying					
	Dryer	Patio	Dryer	Patio	Dryer	Patio
Immature	37.16bA	38.41bA	41.60aA	41.91aA	35.46A	36.80bA
Random mixture	41.16aA	36.60bB	33.70bB	40.66aA	38.10abA	37.57bA
Cherry	40.70aA	41.50aA	39.83aB	42.70aA	40.66aA	41.23

*Averages followed by same small letter in a column do not differ by the Tukey test at 5% probability.

3.4. Triacylglycerols (TAGs) and Terpene Esters (TE)

The methodology used for lipid class analysis is presented is presented in Figure 1 (Jham et al., 2004). The most abundant class was the TAGs (~75%) followed by substantial amounts of terpene esters (~14%) (Table 9). In addition, all samples contained small amounts of sterol esters, partial acylglycerols, polar lipids, free fatty acids and unidentified material. These results were in agreement with our previous studies (Nikalova-Damyanova et al., 1998) and literature study (Kaufmann & Hamsagar, 1962). Small amounts (0.5%-2.5%) of free fatty acids have been reported in coffee (Speer et al., 1993), although their origin was not discussed.

No effects of bean type, drying type nor storage time was noted on the TAGs composition, although some apparently random variation was observed. This result was in agreement with our previous study (Jham et al., 2001) where a small number of samples were evaluated. It has been hypothesized in the literature that the TAGs are degraded during storage releasing free fatty acids, which are in turn oxidized to produce compounds responsible for off-flavour. Degradation of free amino acids, sugars and oxidation of lipids in coffee stored for one year has been reported along with loss of the coffee quality (Multon et al., 1973, Wajda & Walczky, 1978).

No effects of bean type, drying type and storage time were noted on the TE (Table 10) composition. The chemical structure of the TE has not been yet determined.

**Table 8. Average linoleic acid* (%) as a function
of storage time, type of coffee and drying**

Type of coffee	Storage time (months)					
	4		7		10	
	Type of drying					
	Dryer	Patio	Dryer	Patio	Dryer	Patio
Immature	40.83 aA	40.86 aA	43.16 aA	38.80 bB	39.13 aA	40.00 aA
Random mixture	38.00 bA	35.63 bB	37.16 bA	36.36 cA	38.63 aA	38.30 aA
Cherry	37.50 bB	41.50 aA	36. 19 bB	41.74 aA	37.31 aB	39.89 aA

Type of coffee	Storage time (months)					
	13		16		19	
	Type of drying					
	Dryer	Patio	Dryer	Patio	Dryer	Patio
Immature	39.83 aA	40.80 aA	38.5 0abA	37.36 aA	38.83 aA	40.27 aA
Random mixture	36.60 bA	36.78 bA	39.56 aA	35.86 abB	36.70 aA	37.44 bA
Cherry	37.70 abB	41.63 aA	37.00 bA	33.9 4bB	38.60 aA	38.21 abA

*Averages followed by same small letter in a column do not differ by the Tukey test at 5% probability.

Table 9. Average TAG (%) for the three types of coffee

Type of coffee beans	TAG
Immature	73.18 a
Random mixture	72.91 a
Cherry beans	72.95 a

*Averages followed by the same letter in a column indicate no significant difference at 5% probability by the Scot-Knott test.

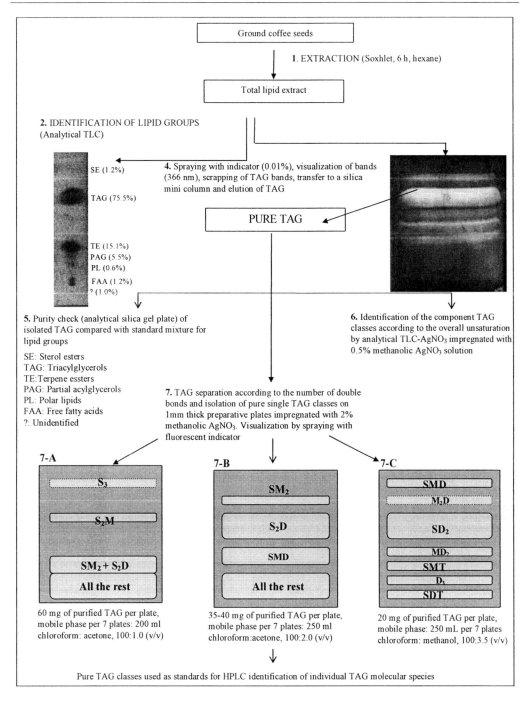

Figure 1. Fluxogram for the separation of coffee triacylglycerols.

3.5. TAG Molecular Species of Crude Coffee Oils

The average TAG composition (%) of six coffee samples obtained with a crude hexane extract using LSD is presented in Table 11. Twelve TAG molecular species were identified in all the samples with a representative % composition being LLL (5.88%), StLLn (1.88%), OLL (4.93%), PLL (26.92%), OOL (1.05%), StLL (5.15%), POL (11.38%), PPL (25.98%), POO+ALL (1.43%), PStL (9.67%), PPO (2.38%) and PStO (3.64%) (in order of elution, Ln-linolenic, L-linoleic, O-oleic, P-palmitic and St-stearic acid residues). A solvent gradient was utilized to separate the TAG molecular species (Figure 2). As reported, the TAG molecular species did not vary with coffee type and drying type (Jham et al., 2003).

Table 10. Average terpene esters *(%) as a function of storage time, type of coffee and drying

Type of coffee beans	Storage time (months)					
	4		7		10	
	Type of drying					
	Dryer	Patio	Dryer	Patio	Dryer	Patio
Immature	14.13 a	15.10 a	13.43aa	14.83 a	14.10 a	14.43 a
Random mixture	15.10 a	15.26 a	14.30 a	14.63 a	14.60 a	14.96 a
Cherry	14.87 a	15.20 a	14.73 a	14.83 a	13.50 a	14.50 a

Type of coffee beans	Storage time (months)					
	13		16		19	
	Type of drying					
	Dryer	Patio	Dryer	Patio	Dryer	Patio
Immature	13.17 a	14.53 a	14.60 a	14.67 a	14.91 a	15.00 a
Random mixture	15.44 a	13.46 a	13.90 a	14.70 a	15.65 a	15.10 a
Cherry	14.34 a	14.60 a	14.67 a	14.86 a	14.71 a	15.00 a

*Averages followed by same small letter in a column do not differ by the Tukey test at 5% probability.

Table 11. Average TAG* composition (%) of six coffee samples obtained with a crude hexane extract using a light sensitive detector LSD**

T	LLL	StLLn	OLL	PLL	OOL	StLL	POL	PPL	POO+ALL	PStL	PPO	PStO
T_1	5.88 a	1.83 a	4.93 a	26.92 a	1.05 a	5.15 a	11.38 a	25.98 a	1.43 a	9.67 a	2.38 a	3.64 a
T_3	5.69 a	1.90 a	5.23 a	26.74 a	1.42 a	5.41 a	11.41 a	25.15 a	1.35 a	9.71 a	2.35 a	3.58 a
T_5	6.41 a	1.71 a	5.30 a	26.89 a	0.98 a	5.28 a	11.16 a	25.18 a	1.63 a	9.58 a	2.05 a	3.64 a
T_2	6.45 a	1.75 a	5.60 a	27.18 a	0.81 a	5.79 a	11.25 a	23.90 a	1.31 a	9.88 a	2.88 a	3.75 a
T_3	5.92 a	1.84 a	5.65 a	27.54 a	1.66 a	5.28 a	11.88 a	24.80 a	1.63 a	9.84 a	2.87 a	3.02 a
T_6	5.68 a	1.92 a	5.52 a	26.88 a	1.53 a	4.94 a	11.91 a	25.33 a	1.56 a	9.71 a	2.33 a	3.62 a

*Averages followed by same small letter in a column do not differ by the Tukey test at 5% probability;
**Jham et al. 2003;
T: See Table 1 for the treatment description;
Ln-linolenic, L-linoleic, O-oleic, P-palmitic and St- stearic acid residues

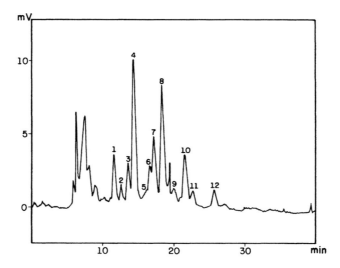

Figure 2. Typical chromatogram obtained on analysis of a crude hexane extract using a light sensitive detector Peaks 1 to 12 are LLL, SLLn, OLL, PLL, OOL, StLL, POL, PPL, POO + ALL, PStL, PPO and PStO (Ln-linolenic, L-linoleic, O-oleic, P-palmitic and St- stearic acid residues). The five peaks eluting before peak 1 corresponded to the more polar compounds (free acids, monacylglycerols and diacylglycerols) found in the crude coffee extract (Nikolova-Damyanova, B., Velikova, & Jham, 1998).

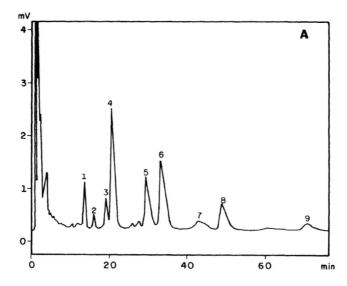

Figure 3. Typical chromatogram obtained on analysis of a crude hexane extract using a refractive index detector. Peaks 1-9 correspond to LLL, StLLn, OLL, PLL, StLL + POL, PPL + OOL, ALL, PStL + POO and PStO (Ln-linolenic, L-linoleic, O-oleic, P-palmitic and St-stearic acid residues).

Preparative silver ion thin-layer chromatography (Ag-TLC) was also utilized for the preparative isolation of TAG classes according to the degree of unsaturation (Jham et al., 2005, Figure 2). These were used as standards to identify TAGs species from eight coffee samples evaluate effects of bean type, drying procedures and geographic origin on the TAG composition by means of RP-HPLC using a refractive index detector (RID).

Table 12. Comparison of average TAG composition* (%) of six coffee samples obtained with a crude hexane extract using a refractive index detector (RID) and a light sensitive detector (LSD)**

T***	% TAG composition in crude hexane										
	LLL		StLLn		OLL		PLL		StLL+POL		
	RID	LSD	RID	LSD	RID	LSD	RID	LSD	RID	LSD****	
										StLL	POL
T₁	5.78 abA	5.85 bA	2.06	1.83	5.15	5.69	29.72	27.89	14.80	5.00	10.93
	(1, 2)	(1, 3)	(2, 2)	(2, 3)	(3, 2)	(3, 3)	(4, 2)	(4, 3)	(5, 2)	(6, 3)	(7, 3)
T₃	6.05 aA	5.69 bB	1.82	1.86	5.05	5.50	29.32	27.92	15.76	5.21	11.01
T₅	5.88 abB	6.41 aA	2.26	1.78	5.00	5.48	29.44	28.16	15.53	5.08	10.76
T₂	5.77 bB	5.65 aA	1.90	1.79	4.92	5.69	30.18	27.06	15.13	5.44	11.00
T₃	5.75 abcB	5.68 bA	1.97	1.87	5.28	5.88	29.14	27.14	15.4.8	4.94	11.61
T₆	5.74 abA	5.92 bA	2.04	1.81	5.21	5.65	29.77	26.93	15.16	5.08	11.48
GA*****	-	-	1.95	1.86	5.19B	5.62A	29.46A	27.45B	15.37B	16.35A	
VC(%)	2.54		10.43		4.83		4.28		5.43		

T***	% TAG composition in crude hexane							
	PPL+OOL			PStL+POO			PStO	
	RID	LSD****		RID	LSD****		RID	LSD
		PPL	OOL		PStL	POO		
T₁	22.94	23.08	0.95	9.65	9.65	1.10	3.78 abA	3.62 abA
	(6, 2)	(8, 3)	(5, 3)	(8, 2)	·(10, 3)	(9, 3)	(9, 2)	(12, 3)
T₃	23.72	25.15	1.32	10.90	9.71	1.35	2.99 aB	3.56 abA
T₅	22.54	22.18	0.98	11.96	9.58	1.63	3.38 abA	3.62 abA
T₂	23.16	20.90	0.81	11.23	9.88	1.31	2.85 abB	3.77 aA
T₃	22.34	22.53	1.33	11.79	9.71	1.56	3.34 abA	3.55 abA
T₆	22.63	21.46	1.00	10.82	9.84	1.63	3.62 abA	3.01 abB
GA*****	22.75B	23.35A		11.21A	11.17A		-	-
VC(%)	4.20			5.32			9.37	

*Averages followed by at least one lower case letter in the column or upper case letter in the row do not differ by the Tukey test (5% probability);

** Jham et al. 2004;

*** See Table 1 for description of treatments;

****For comparison of statistical data, the sum of TAG molecular species obtained with the LSD was compared to the RID results;

*****No interaction between treatments and detector but differences in two detectors were obtained;

T: treatment; GA: general average; VC: variation coefficient;

Ln=linolenic, L=linoleic, O=oleic, P=palmitic and St= stearic acid residues;

% TAG in the first row followed by two numbers in parentheses represents the peak number in Fig. 2;

PPO (~5%) detected by LSD not considered;

ALL (~5%) detected by RID not considered

Acetonitrile/acetone (1:1, v/v) was used as elution solvent. The following nine TAGs species were identified in all the coffee samples: LLL (5.78%), SLLn (2.06%), OLL (5.15%), PLL (29.72%), StLL + POL (14.80%), PPL + OOL (22.94%), ALL, PStL + POO (9.65%) and PStO (3.78%). In agreement with our previous studies, no effects of bean type, drying procedures and geographic origin on the TAG composition were found. It has been demonstrated that although resolution with RP-HPLC/RID was poorer as compared to the previously described RP-HPLC-light scattering detector (RP-HPLC/LSD) approach, in general the results were in good agreement. Thus, despite the limitation of the RP-HPLC/RID, the method is suitable for monitoring the TAG composition of coffee stored over prolonged period of time or to determine relative percentage of the resolved TAGs.

4. CONCLUSION

Although variation in lipid class was noted in some treatments, it appeared to be random. Hence, it appears that the lipid classes do not vary during storage using the methodology in this study. However, a more detailed study, using HPLC should be conducted to determine the variation of individual TAGs during storage. In order to draw definite conclusions, these studies should be conducted simultaneously with cup quality tests. The role of volatile compounds in coffee quality should also be investigated.

REFERENCES

Association of Official Analytical Chemists. *Official Methods of Analysis*. (1984). 4th ed., 1-1141.

Belitz, H. D. & Grosh, W. (1988). *Food Chemistry*. Berlin, Springer Verlag.

Christie, W. W. (1987). *High Performance liquid Chromatography and Lipids*. Oxford, Pergamon.

Fourney, G. E., Cros, E. & Vicent, J. C. (1982). Estudo preliminaire de l'oxydation de l'huile de café. In: *Proc. 10th ASIC Coll.*, 235-246.

Illy, A. & Viani, R. (1995). *Expresso coffee: The Chemistry of Quality*, London, Academic.

González, A. G., Pablos, F., Martín, M. J., León-Camacho, C. & Valdenebro, M. S. (2001). HPLC analysis of tocopherols and triglycerides in coffee and their use as authentication parameters. *Food Chemistry, 73*, 93-101.

Informe Agropecuário (1997). Qualidade do Café. 18, 1-76.

Jham, G. N., Teles, F. F. F. & Campos, L. 1982. Use of aqueous HCl/MeOH as esterification reagent for analysis of fatty acids derived from soybean lipids. *Journal of American Oil Chemists Society, 59*, 132-133.

Jham, G. N., Velikova, R. Muller H., Nikolova-Damyanova, B. & Cecon, P. R. (2001). Lipid classes and triacylglycerols in coffee samples from Brazil: effects of coffee type and drying procedures. *Food Research International, 34*, 111-115.

Jham, G. N., Nikolova-Damyavova, B., Viera, M., Natalino, R. & Rodrigues, A. C. (2003). Determination of triacylglycerol composition of eight coffee samples by RP-HPLC. *Phytochemical Analysis, 13*, 99-104.

Jham, G. N., Velikova, R., Nikolova-Damyavova, B., Rabelo. S. C., Silva, J. C. T., Souza, P. K., Moreira, M.V. & Cecon, P. R. (2005). Preparative silver ion TLC/RP-HPLC determination of coffee triacylglycerol molecular species. *Food Research International, 38*: 121-126.

Kaufmann, H. P. & Hamsagar, R. S. (1962). Zur Kentnis der Lipoide der Kaffeebohne. I: Ueber Fettsaure des Cafestols. *Fette Seifen Anstrichmiffel, 64,* 206-213.

Multon, J. L., Poisson, B. & Cachaginer, M. (1973). Evolution de plusieurs caratéristiquers d'un café Arabica au cours d'un stockage expérimental effectuéà 5 humidités relatives et 4 températures différentes. In: *Proc. 6th ASIC Coll.,* 268-277.

Nikolova-Damyanova, B., Velikova, R. & Jham, G. N. (1998). Lipid classes, fatty acid composition and triacylglycerol molecular species in crude coffee beans harvested in Brazil. *Food Research International, 31,* 479-486.

Nikolova-Damyanova B, Christie W. W, Herslof, B. (1990). The structure of the triglycerides of meadowfoam oil. *Journal of the American Oil Chemists Society, 67,* 503-507.

Segall, S. D., Artz, W. E., Raslan, D. S., Jham, G. N. & Takahashi, J. A. (2005). TAG Composition of Coffee Beans (*Coffea canephora* L.) by Reversed-Phase High Performance Liquid Chromatography and Tandem Mass Spectroscopy. In preparation.

Spadone, J. C., Takeoke, G. & Liardon, R. (1990). Analytical investigation of Rio off-flavor in green coffee. *Journal of Agriciculture and Food Chemistry, 38,* 226-233.

Speer, K., Sehat, N. & Montang A. (1993). Fatty acids in coffee. In: *Proc. 15th ASIC Coll.,* 583-592.

Wajda, P. & Walczyk, D. (1978). Relationship between acid values of extracted fatty matter and age of green coffee bean. *Journal of Science Food Agriculture, 29,* 237-245.

Tarandjiiska, R., Marekov, I., Nikolova-Damyanova, B. & Amidzhin, B. (1996). Determination of molecular species of triacylglycerols classes and molecular species in seed oils with high content of linolenic fatty acids. *Journal of Science and Food Agriculture, 72,* 403-410.

Zambolim, L., Sondahl, M. & Fernandes, N. T. (1996). *Microorganismos associados à qualidade de bebida de café. Relatório Anual sobre a Qualidade da Bebida.* Universidade Federal de Viçosa, Viçosa – MG. 1-55.

In: Nutrition Research Advances
Editor: Sarah V. Watkins, pp. 223-240

ISBN 1-60021-516-5
© 2007 Nova Science Publishers, Inc.

Chapter VIII

MATERNAL DIET THROUGH PREGNANCY –THE KEY TO FUTURE GOOD HEALTH OF THE NEXT GENERATION?

Michael E Symonds, Helen Budge, Alison Mostyn,
Terence Stephenson and David S Gardner

Centre for Reproduction and Early Life, Institute of Clinical Research, University
Hospital, Nottingham, NG7 2UH, United Kingdom.

ABSTRACT

Epidemiological studies on historical and contemporary populations indicate that the intra-uterine environment is a major factor contributing to later health and disease in the resulting offspring. These findings are supported by experimental studies which indicate that both macro and micronutrient deficiencies or excesses can have substantial long-term health implications for the offspring. In this chapter we will consider the extent to which changes in maternal diet, lifestyle and age can interact to substantially impact on the future health of the offspring. The impact of both increasing and decreasing maternal dietary intake, either throughout pregnancy, or at defined stages of development will be covered. Focus will be on the interaction between the maternal diet and her endocrine status with respect to placental development and later function. This will be related to key stages in development from the time of conception through to early adulthood and its impact on cardiovascular control systems, kidney development and metabolic homeostasis. Critically, we will consider the extent to which a mismatch between diet in utero and that available during lactation or early childhood can mean individuals are programmed to later obesity and cardiovascular disease including diabetes.

INTRODUCTION

There are an extensive number of publications based on a range of populations across the world showing that different aspects of maternal size, shape and nutrition in conjunction with weight at birth and subsequent growth trajectory can have a substantial influence on an individual's later health and well being [1-4]. As historical cohort studies introduce many different relationships between their wide range of variables, it is not surprising that an array of animal models have been utilised in order to examine the potential mechanisms behind these findings. Such studies have focused on both the short and longer term consequences of manipulating the maternal diet either throughout pregnancy, or at defined stages, and have enabled substantial advances to be made within the field [5,6]. At the same time, they have resulted in a number of controversies [7-9] which, whilst of academic interest in their own right, have also enabled further breakthroughs to be made. One example is the potential role of the stress hormone cortisol in mediating the effects of an adverse maternal environment on fetal development [5]. In the rodent, in which the offspring are born immature with an undeveloped hypothalamic-pituitary-adrenal axis, changes in maternal or postnatal cortisol concentrations have a pronounced effect on offspring behaviour [10]. Apart from infants that were growth retarded in utero [11], whether the same outcomes are found in humans or large mammals, which are born with a mature hypothalamic-pituitary-adrenal axis at birth, remains debatable.

The aim of this chapter is to attempt to integrate findings from relevant large and small animal studies in order to summarize potential nutritionally mediated mechanisms in key windows of development. These can then be targeted in order to substantially affect the long term health of that individual. We will not cover every nutrient, animal model or organ as these have been well reviewed recently, for example in the extensive review by McMillen & Robinson [12].

The majority of epidemiological studies have used birth weight as a main outcome measure, largely because this data is easily and routinely recorded and, therefore, more readily available. Surprisingly, the continuum of birth weights has not been regarded as a whole but have been arbitrarily divided into sub groups and related to different aspects of adult health [1]. Despite this potential limitation, where additional information on the shape and size of individual babies has been obtainable it has revealed that there are additional contributing factors to later health. Thus, infants who were either long and thin, or short and fat, appear to be at potentially increased risk of different adult diseases [13,14]. In addition, although largely neglected in more recent studies, a mismatch between placental and fetal weights has been shown to be an important marker of later hypertension [15].

MATERNAL NUTRITION AND LONG TERM HEALTH OUTCOMES

It is well established from a substantial number of earlier animal studies that quite severe reductions in maternal dietary intake [16] or placental nutrient supply to the fetus can result in intra-uterine growth retardation [17]. To date, a majority of animal experiments have, therefore, focussed on the impact of maternal nutrient restriction on fetal growth and later outcomes [12]. More recently, however, as an increased number of animal experiments have been conducted, it has become apparent that there is not a simple relationship between maternal food intake and fetal growth or weight at birth [18]. Indeed, in some models the same apparent gross changes in maternal diet can result in both an increase and decrease in birth weight between studies [19].

It is not only the magnitude of any nutritional intervention that determines long term outcomes, but also its timing and duration. This concept is well supported from retrospective studies examining a comparatively small proportion of the Dutch population exposed to a 3-4 month period of famine during World War II – known as the 'Dutch Hunger Winter' or 'Dutch Famine of 1944'. These ongoing epidemiological investigations have illustrated that the very different outcomes in the adult offspring are dependent upon the period during pregnancy when the mother was exposed to the famine, as summarised in Figure 1 [20]. Exposure during only the first trimester of pregnancy gave rise to offspring with increased risk of coronary heart disease [21] whereas being subjected to the famine in the second trimester increased the risk of renal disease [22]. In contrast, famine exposure during late gestation tended to impact upon intermediary metabolism, in particular, glucose-insulin homeostasis [23].

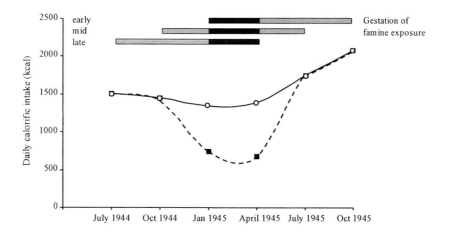

Figure 1. Summary of the relationship between time of exposure to famine during pregnancy and long term adverse outcome. Black bars represent period of famine during gestation (grey bars).

These differential effects can be readily explained when considering the chronological development of system and/or organ growth in the fetus. Cardiovascular growth has a priority early in gestation when there is minimal tissue growth but establishment of the fetal heart and its circulatory system. In contrast, development of nephron number is normally set towards the end of mid gestation [24], whilst adipose and muscle growth, which are both highly insulin sensitive tissues, occur primarily in late gestation [25]. As will now be considered in more detail, findings from the Dutch Famine are supported by cumulative evidence using large animal models in which a comparable 50% reduction in food intake [5] was imposed over the same relative stages of pregnancy. Investigations of this type are also of relevance to contemporary populations in which a 50% variation in maternal food intake between the upper and lower quartiles have been recorded through gestation [26].

MATERNAL NUTRIENT RESTRICTION IN EARLY GESTATION AND PROGRAMMING OF THE CARDIOVASCULAR SYSTEM

The early period of gestation is coincident with conception, embryogenesis and implantation or uterine attachment (Figure 2). The major physiological control system that appears to be reset following a global reduction in maternal food intake over this period of gestation is the central regulation of blood pressure control. In this regard, offspring born to mothers nutrient restricted between 0-30 days gestation have smaller brains [27] and show behavioral differences as young adults [28]. At the same time, although resting and stimulated blood pressure is unaffected, nutrient restricted offspring show a marked leftward shift in their baroreflex function curve [27] which, in humans, is an established precursor of later hypertension [29,30]. In contrast to the renal effects seen with more prolonged nutrient restriction in later gestation [31], there is no effect on nephron number, kidney shape or size, or its endocrine sensitivity to growth factors or cortisol [32]. In contrast, neither placental mass or body composition at either mid [32] or late fetal gestation [33,34], nor in young adulthood, is altered [27]. It is, therefore, not surprising that during adulthood these individuals have normal glucose homeostasis, the same amount of adipose tissue and similar plasma cortisol profiles as controls [35].

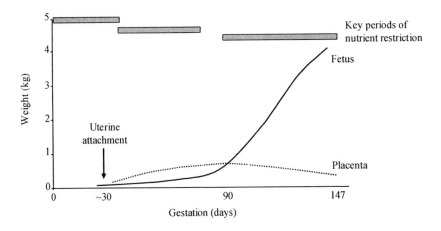

Figure 2. Summary of the main developmental windows during the reproductive period in which manipulation of the maternal diet significantly modulates placental and fetal development. Filled bars represent windows of developmental plasticity corresponding to the key periods of nutritional manipulation identified in the text.

What is also notable about these findings is that any long term outcomes are not gender specific and occur in the absence of any differences in birth weight or later growth [27]. These findings, therefore, are in in contrast to studies in rats in which maternal consumption of a diet in which protein, but not energy content is similarly reduced by 50% resulted in higher blood pressure in males but not females [36]. The magnitude of effect may, however, be related to an increased stress response, as blood pressure was measured under conditions of restraint and heating that have themselves been shown to result in elevated blood pressure [37]. Interestingly, the long term rise in blood pressure in females appeared to be related to a transient rise in maternal plasma glucose together with a slower rate of apoptosis within the embyo's inner cell mass [36]. This adverse effect of exposure to high maternal plasma glucose is of particular interest because excess maternal nutrition at the time of conception, leading to elevated plasma glucose, has also been linked to teratogenesis via enhanced oxidative stress [38]. To this extent, the higher maternal plasma glucose observed in dams fed a low protein diet may well relate to the higher carbohydrate content (necessary to maintain the overall energy content [19]) of these diets.

MATERNAL NUTRIENT RESTRICTION IN EARLY TO MID GESTATION AND PROGRAMMING OF KIDNEY DEVELOPMENT

For sheep, as in humans but unlike rodents, kidney development is completed and the adult nephron complement reached before birth. The pronephros develops and degenerates by day 30 of gestation [39], near to the time of implantation or uterine attachment. Over the same time period, the mesonephros becomes functional at ~ day 17 of gestation and the full complement of nephrons is developed by days 27-30. Organ regression then occurs over the next 30 days gestation [39]. At ~ 30 days gestation the metanephros is made up of a mass of metanephric mesenchyme into which the ureteric bud has grown and branched once. Subsequent branchings of the ureteric duct induce the formation of new nephrons until ~ day 130 when the full nephron complement is largely complete [40]. It is not perhaps surprising that the organ whose growth is most affected by maternal nutrient restriction over the period of 28-80 days gestation followed by a restoration of maternal diet up to term, is the kidney [41].

At term, offspring of mothers nutrient restricted between early to mid gestation have a disproportionately larger placenta in conjunction with heavier kidneys that are of different shape and show a persistent reduction in nephron number [31]. These adaptations are accompanied, at birth, with an increase in renal sensitivity to glucocorticoids as a consequence of a greater mRNA abundance of both the glucocorticoid receptor (type 2) and glucocorticoid responsive genes i.e. angiotensinogen 2 type I-receptor [41]. In addition, although 11β-hydroxysteroid dehydrogenase type 2 enzyme activity is enhanced [41], this adaptation does not persist into later life [31] suggesting renal sensitivity to stress is only increased around the time of birth in conjunction with the fetal surge in cortisol [42].

Interestingly, these adaptations in the fetal sheep occur despite a reduction in maternal plasma cortisol, thyroid hormones, leptin and insulin concentrations over the period of nutrient restriction [43,44] (Figure 3). The primary outcome of these changes could be to reduce maternal energy requirements, thereby maintaining maternal and, thus, fetal plasma glucose [43,45]. It may, therefore, be that the accompanying maternal hyperglycaemia [46], together with an increase in glucose supply and uptake by the conceptus [47], represent an important mechanism by which later kidney function is compromised [48,49] as is the case with maternal dexamethasone or cortisol administration early in gestation [48]. Support for this concept is provided by the finding that even when a low protein/high carbohydrate diet is fed to rats throughout gestation the mothers remain hyperglycaemic up to at least 14 days gestation [50]. These offspring go on to have a persistently lower nephron number in later life [51], although this is not necessarily accompanied by raised blood pressure [52,53].

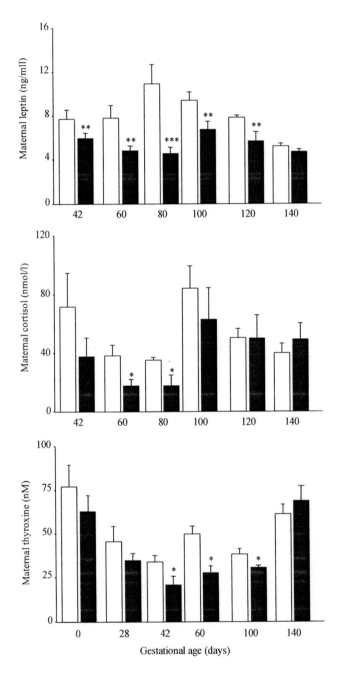

Figure 3. Summary of the primary maternal endocrine adaptations to nutrient restriction between early to mid gestation. Values are means and their standard errors from the same 7 mothers per nutritional group that were sampled hourly by the same individuals at each time point data adapted in part from Bispham et al [43].

Offspring of mothers that were nutrient restricted for part, or all, of early pregnancy do not show an immediate rise in blood pressure [18], indeed this can actually be reduced during juvenile life [31,54]. This contrasts with the long term outcomes of being born to mothers subjected to a large corticosteroid surge early, but not later, in gestation [49] in which blood pressure is persistently raised from as early as 4 months of age [55]. These studies also indicate that males have a higher blood pressure than females irrespective of the prenatal environment although it should be noted that males were castrated at two months of age, whilst females were oophorectomized at one year [48]. This difference is important as blood pressure is not different between intact males and females at six months or one year of age [27,31] (Figure 4).

It should be further noted that pregnant rats administered maternal dexamethasone administration in both early and late gestation exhibit a reduction in food intake [56,57], a similar long term hypertensive outcome in the offspring is seen with maternal food restriction alone [57]. It is, therefore, possible that some of the effects seen in sheep born to mothers given dexamethasone early in gestation [49] may similarly be mediated by a reduction in food intake [5]. Short term administration of dexamethasone also appears to have a very different effect on maternal feeding behaviour compared with long term exposure in which food intake is unaffected [58].

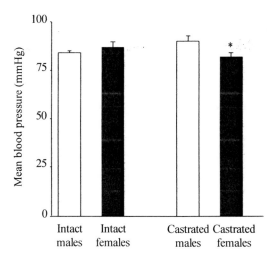

Figure 4. Comparison of blood pressure between young adult males and females that are either intact or following removal of their gonads in early life. Open bars - males; filled bars – females. Adapted from Gardner et al. (27) and Dodic et al. (46). Significant differences between gender in the same study indicated by * P <0.05.

Maternal Nutrient Restriction in Late Gestation and Programming of Adipose Tissue Development and Glucose Homeostasis

A global 50% reduction in maternal food intake in late gestation coincident with the period of maximal fetal growth results in a reduction in fetal but not maternal plasma glucose [59]. This adaptation occurs in conjunction with a transient increase in maternal but not fetal plasma cortisol [59] although the prevailing fetal plasma glucose determines, in part, an individual fetus' cortisol concentration [45]. At the same time, there is a stimulatory plasma glucose threshold below which fetal plasma ACTH is elevated [45]. Despite this apparently heightened responsiveness of the fetal hypothalamic-pituitary axis to glucose and fetuses of nutrient restricted mothers having elevated blood pressure, there is a negative relationship between blood pressure and plasma ACTH [59]. This does, however, indicate a pronounced change in fetal blood pressure regulation that is very different to that seen in late gestation fetuses exposed to maternal nutrient restriction in earlier gestation [60]. Indeed, there is no relationship between fetal plasma ACTH and blood pressure in control fed fetuses and the blood pressure response to both angiotensin II and captopril is unaltered between nutritional groups [59]. Taken together, these findings indicate that maternal nutrient restriction in late gestation only results in a transient change in fetal cardiovascular control as it appears to have no long term outcomes [61], which may explain the lack of any involvement of the renin-angiotensinogen system [59]. The pronounced sensitivity of the fetal brain and cardiovascular control to the prevailing glucose environment at a time of maximal fetal growth perhaps explains the high mortality rate in fetuses of nutrient restricted mothers despite no apparent difference in the oxygen or placental environment [59,62].

The primary organs whose mass is reduced after birth in offspring born to mothers nutrient restricted in late gestation are the liver and adipose tissue [63,64]. Despite this marked reduction in energy reserves at birth, these offspring are able to effectively adapt to the substantial thermal demands following exposure to the extra-uterine environment [65]. In the late gestation fetus, adipose tissue has both brown and white characteristics as the brown adipose tissue specific uncoupling protein (UCP) 1 is highly abundant, as is leptin, a marker of white adipocytes [66]. The major factor determining fetal adipose tissue deposition is fetal glucose supply [67], although surprisingly this does not appear to have a stimulatory effect on mRNA abundance for either UCP1 or leptin [68].

Increasing maternal food intake which elevates maternal plasma glucose [69] and would, therefore, be expected to similarly raise fetal glucose [70] does increase UCP1 content in fetal adipose tissue but does not result in greater adiposity [69]. Reduced maternal food intake during late gestation also reduces the sensitivity of fetal adipose tissue to glucorticoids in conjunction with a reduction in mRNA for both UCP1 and 2 [33,71]. It is therefore perhaps surprising given the close association between adipocyte sensitivity to glucorticoids and later obesity [72] that as young adults these offspring have enhanced fat mass [35]. Other changes within the adipocyte which may be responsible for this adverse adaptation are likely to include an increase in the abundance of the insulin receptor but a reduction in that of glucose transporter 4 [35]. Indeed, as in human diabetes, the molecular basis of insulin resistance appears to lie downstream of the insulin receptor [73]. The finding that glucose transporter 4, the major insulin responsive glucose transporter, was specifically reduced in adipose but not muscle tissue strongly suggests that impaired glucose tolerance in offspring born to late gestationaly nutrient restricted mothers was related to the ability of adipose tissue to take up glucose in an insulin responsive manner [35].

The reduced amount of adipose tissue of neonates born to nutrient restricted mothers is characterised as having a greatly reduced mRNA abundance for leptin (Figure 5) and the long form of the prolactin receptor [65]. Prolactin, acting through its receptor, is one of a number of endocrine stimulatory hormones that acts to ensure UCP1 abundance is maximal at birth [66]. Subsequently, as brown adipose tissue is replaced or becomes white adipose tissue during postnatal development [74], there is a parallel loss of both forms of the prolactin receptor [75]. It is plausible that a combination of reduced leptin secretory capacity, that would be expected to result in lower plasma leptin, and prolactin sensitivity [75] after birth may subsequently delay the rate of loss of UCP1 in these offspring [76]. This may explain why, although UCP1 abundance is reduced at birth in offspring of mothers nutrient restricted in late gestation, there is a marked retention of UCP1 by one month of age [65]. Interestingly, these adaptations have no immediate effect on total fat mass in the growing individual and therefore may be indicative of the very similar nutrient intakes through lactation irrespective of the maternal diet through late pregnancy.

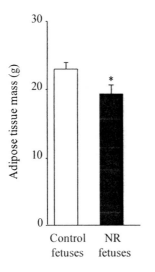 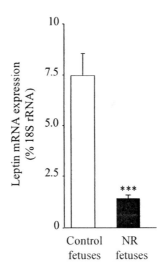

Figure 5. Effect of maternal nutrient restriction (NR) on perirenal adipose tissue mass and leptin mRNA abundance in near term sheep fetuses for which this fat depot constitutes 80% of total fat at term. Values are means with their standard errors and n = 6-8 per nutritional group. Significant differences between nutritional groups at the same age indicated by * P < 0.05; *** P < 0.001.

THE POSTNATAL ENVIRONMENT AND THE POTENTIAL AMPLIFICATION OF THE ADVERSE CARDIOVASCULAR OUTCOMES OF MATERNAL NUTRIENT RESTRICTION THROUGH PREGNANCY

To date, all animal studies investigating the effect of maternal nutritional manipulation through gestation have been conducted on offspring that have been exposed to the same environmental conditions as the mother was exposed to through pregnancy. It is becoming apparent that changes in the diet through lactation both in terms of milk composition and availability can act to amplify the adverse outcomes [77]. This may impact on longevity [78] and fat mass and glucocorticoid sensitivity [79]. It is, therefore, highly likely that a combination of exposure to an adverse in utero environment, in conjunction with conditions of nutritional excess after birth, will result in rapid obesity onset. Such a proposal is supported from epidemiological studies that have focussed attention on contemporary lifestyles with a much greater availability of excess, palatable, energy rich foods [80] and increased prevalence of sedentary behaviour [81].

Although it is generally accepted that the rise in obesity stems from an increase in energy intake, evidence from human longitudinal studies is sparse. Some studies have even suggested that energy intakes have fallen [82], whilst others have shown the expected increase. This may reflect inherent difficulties with self-reported dietary data [83]. Furthermore, whilst the increase in portion sizes in Western Societies [84] has been held responsible, there is little information on the overall effect of this trend on daily energy intake. Nevertheless, excess intake of energy rich foods does appear to be one factor in obesity. This is important because disinhibition of the control of food intake is associated with the presence of obesity in humans [85] and rats fed "cafeteria" [86] or high-fat [87] diets become obese.

We have now gone on to look at the effect of the lactational diet by comparing formula fed offspring with a contemporaneous group reared by their mother. This has been combined with manipulating the post-weaning environment by either maintaining the offspring within a housed enclosure or allowing them to range freely within an adjacent pasture so as to ensure the same climatic conditions. Maintenance within a restricted space resulted in a four fold reduction in 24 hour activity profiles as illustrated in Figure 6. When these activity levels are maintained from the time of weaning up to one year of age, offspring show a substantial increase in fat mass, with the relative fat distribution around the kidneys being promoted by previous nutrient restriction and formula feeding [88]. Furthermore, in previously nutrient restricted individuals, this adaptation was preceded by an elevated plasma cortisol and heart rate but no difference in systolic or diastolic blood pressure (Table 1). Given that when these nutrient restricted offspring are raised under field conditions they actually show a lower blood pressure [31], it appears that the adverse cardiovascular adaptations have been accelerated with a resetting of the hypothalamic-pituitary-adrenal axis. Of particular interest is that the change in the relationship between blood pressure and heart rate has been amplified. This, in conjunction with our previous work [27], would suggest an early onset of hypertension in these offspring.

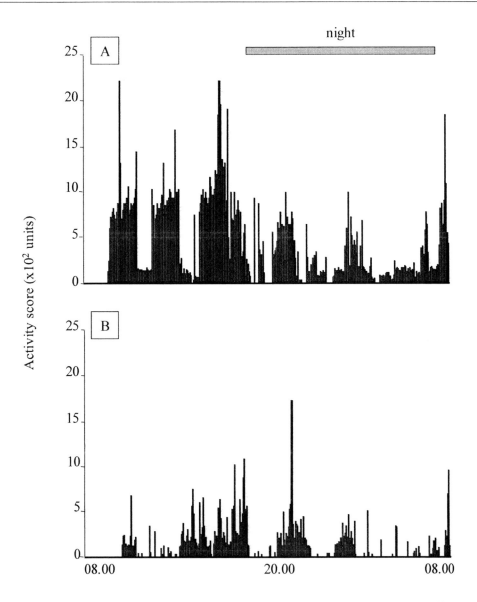

Figure 6. Example of the difference in 24 h activity profiles between young sheep either A) allowed freely to range within a standard pasture or B) maintained within an adjacent housed enclosure so as to ensure the same climatic conditions.

Our current findings complement very recent epidemiological studies indicating that, irrespective of gender, infants who were small at birth and maintained a low body mass index (BMI) up to two years of age, but who subsequently show a pronounced increase in BMI between 2-11 years, have raised fasting insulin concentrations as adults [4]. Critically a significant factor associated with later coronary disease in this group was BMI at both 2 and 11 years of age. It has, therefore, been suggested that those individuals showing more rapid weight gain after 2 years (i.e. after weaning) deposited more fat than muscle, thereby causing insulin resistance.

Table 1. Effect of maternal nutrient restriction between early to mid gestation followed by maintenance of all offspring within a housed enclosure between three to six months of age on basal plasma cortisol concentration plus resting heart rate and blood pressure at six months of age

	Control	Nutrient restricted
Plasma cortisol (nmol/L)	50 ± 13	93 ± 7*
Heart rate (beats/min)	109 ± 4	123 ± 4*
Systolic blood pressure (mmHg)	119 ± 7	124 ± 7

Values are means and their standard errors and n = 8-12 per group and significantly differences from controls indicated by * $P < 0.05$.

CONCLUSION

An increasing amount of epidemiological and experimental research is emphasising the importance of an optimum nutritional environment both during pregnancy and lactation in promoting both maternal and infant health [89,90]. There is now the clear potential to improve long term health and prevent the apparent inevitable rise in childhood and adult obesity by optimising maternal diet and lifestyle. Given the benefits of reducing saturated fat on adult cardiovascular health [91] it is apparent that these types of studies should be extended into improving maternal health particularly before conception.

ACKNOWLEDGEMENTS

The authors acknowledge the support of the British Heart Foundation, the Biotechnology and Biological Sciences Research Council and the European Union Sixth Framework Programme for Research and Technical Development of the European Community – The Early Nutrition Programming Project (FOOD-CT-2005-007036).

REFERENCES

[1]　Barker DJP. *Mothers, Babies and Disease in Later Life*. 2nd Edition. Edinburgh: Churchill Livingstone.; 1998.

[2]　Singhal A. Endothelial dysfunction: role in obesity-related disorders and the early origins of CVD. *Proceedings of the Nutrition Society* 2005;64:15-22.

[3]　Eriksson J, Forsen T, Tuomilehto J, Osmond C, Barker D. Fetal and childhood growth and hypertension in adult life. *Hypertension* 2000;36:790-794.

[4]   Barker D, Osmond C, Forsén T, Kajantie E, Eriksson J. Trajectories of growth among children who have coronary events as adults. *New England Journal of Medicine* 2005;353:1802-1809.

[5]   Symonds ME, Gardner DS, Pearce S, Stephenson T. Endocrine responses to fetal undernutrition: the growth hormone (GH): insulin-like growth factor (IGF) axis. In: Langley-Evans SC, editor. *Fetal Nutrition and Adult Disease - Programming of chronic disease through fetal exposure to undernutrition.* Oxford: CAB International; 2004. p. 353-380.

[6]   Armitage JA, Taylor PD, Poston L. Experimental models of developmental programming: consequences of exposure to an energy rich diet during development. *Journal of Physiology*, London 2005;565:3-8.

[7]   Huxley RH, Sheill AW, Law CM. The role of size at birth and postnatal catch-up growth in determining systolic blood pressure: a systematic review of the literature. *Journal of Hypertension* 2000;18:815-831.

[8]   Singhal A, Lucas A. Early origins of cardiovascular disease: is there a unifying hypothesis? *Lancet* 2004;363:1642-5.

[9]   Susser M, Levin B. Ordeals for the fetal programming hypothesis. *British Medical Journal* 1999;318:885-886.

[10]   Weaver IC, Champagne FA, Brown SE, Dymov S, Sharma S, Meaney MJ, et al. Reversal of maternal programming of stress responses in adult offspring through methyl supplementation: altering epigenetic marking later in life. *Journal of Neuroscience* 2005;25:11045-11054.

[11]   Seckl JR, Meaney MJ. Glucocorticoid programming. *Annals of The New York Academy of Science* 2004;1032:63-84.

[12]   McMillen IC, Robinson JS. Developmental origins of the metabolic syndrome: Prediction, plasticity, and programming. *Physiological Reviews* 2005;85:571-633.

[13]   Barker DJP, Godfrey KM, Osmond C, Bull A. The relation of fetal length, ponderal index and head circumferences to blood pressure and the risk of hypertension in adult life. *Paediatric and Perinatol Epidemiology* 1992;6:35-44.

[14]   Barker DJP, Osmond C, Simmonds SJ, Wield GA. The relation of head size and thinness at birth to death from cardiovascular disease in later life. *British Medical Journal* 1993;306:422-426.

[15]   Barker DJP, Bull AR, Osmond C, Simmonds SJ. Fetal and placental size and risk of hypertension in adult life. *British Medical Journal* 1990;301:259-262.

[16]   Bauer MK, Breier BH, Harding J, Veldhuis JD, Gluckman PD. The fetal somatotrophic axis during long term maternal undernutrition in sheep; evidence of nutritional regulation in utero. *Endocrinology* 1995;136:1250-1257.

[17]   Harding JE, Jones CT, Robinson JS. Studies on experimental growth retardation in sheep. The effects of a small placenta in restricting transport to and growth of the fetus. *Journal of Developmental Physiology* 1985;7:427-442.

[18]   Symonds ME, Budge H, Stephenson T, Gardner DS. Leptin, fetal nutrition and long term outcomes for adult hypertension. *Endothelium* 2005;12:73-79.

[19]   Armitage JA, Khan IY, Taylor PD, Nathanielsz PW, Poston L. Developmental programming of the metabolic syndrome by maternal nutritional imbalance: how strong

is the evidence from experimental models in mammals? *Journal of Physiology*, London 2004;561:355-377.

[20] Ravelli ACJ, Stein ZA, Susser MW. Obesity in young men after famine exposure in utero and early infancy. *New England Journal of Medicine* 1976;295:349-353.

[21] Roseboom TJ, van der Meulen JHP, Osmond C, Barker DJP, Ravelli ACJ, von Montfrans S-T, G.A., et al. Coronary heart disease in adults after perinatal exposure to famine. *Heart* 2000;84:595-598.

[22] Painter RC, Roseboom TJ, van Montfrans GA, Bossuyt PM, Krediet RT, Osmond C, et al. Microalbuminuria in adults after prenatal exposure to the Dutch famine. *Journal of the American Society of Nephrology* 2005;16:189-194.

[23] Ravelli ACJ, van der Meulin JHP, Michels RPJ, Osmond C, Barker DJP, Hales CN, et al. Glucose tolerance in adults after in utero exposure to the Dutch famine. *Lancet* 1998;351:173-177.

[24] Moritz KM, Dodic M, Wintour EM. Kidney development and the fetal programming of adult disease. *Bioassays* 2003:212-220.

[25] Symonds ME, Mostyn A, Stephenson T. Cytokines and cytokine-receptors in fetal growth and development. *Biochemical Society Transactions* 2001;29:33-37.

[26] Godfrey K, Robinson S, Barker DJP, Osmond C, Cox V. Maternal nutrition in early and late pregnancy in relation to placental and fetal growth. *British Medical Journal* 1996;312:410-414.

[27] Gardner DS, Pearce S, Dandrea J, Walker RM, Ramsey MM, Stephenson T, et al. Peri-implantation undernutrition programs blunted angiotensin II evoked baroreflex responses in young adult sheep. *Hypertension* 2004;43:1-7.

[28] Erhard HW, Boissy A, Rae MT, Rhind SM. Effects of prenatal undernutrition on emotional reactivity and cognitive flexibility in adult sheep. *Behavioural Brain Research* 2004;151:25-35.

[29] Ookuwa H, Takata S, Ogawa J, Iwase N, Ikeda T, Hattori N. Abnormal cardiopulmonary baroreflexes in normotensive young subjects with a family history of essential hypertension. *Journal of Clinical Hypertension* 1987;3:596-604.

[30] Eckberg DL. Carotid baroreflex function in young men with borderline blood pressure elevation. *Circulation* 1979;59:632-636.

[31] Gopalakrishnan G, Gardner DS, Dandrea J, Langley-Evans SC, Pearce S, Kurlak LO, et al. Influence of maternal pre-pregnancy body composition and diet during early-mid pregnancy on cardiovascular function and nephron number in juvenile sheep. British *Journal of Nutrition* 2005;94:938-947.

[32] Brennan KA, Gopalakrishnan GS, Kurlak L, Rhind SM, Brooks AN, Rae MT, et al. Impact of maternal undernutrition and fetal number on glucocorticoid, growth hormone and insulin-like growth factor receptor mRNA abundance in the ovine fetal kidney. *Reproduction* 2005;129:151-159.

[33] Budge H, Edwards LJ, McMillen IC, Bryce A, Warnes K, Pearce S, et al. Nutritional manipulation of fetal adipose tissue deposition and uncoupling protein 1 abundance in the fetal sheep; differential effects of timing and duration. *Biology of Reproduction* 2004;71:359-365.

[34] Edwards LJ, McFarlane JR, Kauter KG, McMillen IC. Impact of periconceptional nutrition on maternal and fetal leptin and fetal adiposity in singleton and twin pregnancies. *American Journal of Physiology* 2005;288:R39-R45.

[35] Gardner DS, Tingey K, van Bon BWM, Ozanne SE, Wilson V, Dandrea J, et al. Programming of glucose-insulin metabolism in adult sheep after maternal undernutrition. *American Journal of Physiology* 2005;289:R1407-R1415.

[36] Kwong WY, Wild AE, Roberts P, Willis AC, Fleming TP. Maternal undernutrition during the preimplantation period of rat development causes blastocyst abnormalities and programming of postnatal hypertension. *Development* 2000;127:4195-4202.

[37] Tonkiss J, Trzcinska M, Galler JR, Ruiz-Opazo N, Herrera VL. Prenatal malnutrition-induced changes in blood pressure: dissociation of stress and nonstress responses using radiotelemetry. *Hypertension* 1998;32:108-114.

[38] Wentzel P, Jansson L, Eriksson UJ. Diabetes in pregnancy: uterine blood flow and embryonic development in the rat. *Pediatric Research* 1995;38:598-606.

[39] Wintour EM, Alcorn D, Butkus A, Congiu M, Earnest L, Pompolo S, et al. Ontogeny of hormonal and excretory function of the meso- and metanephros in the ovine fetus. *Kidney International* 1996;50:1624-1633.

[40] Moritz KM, Dodic M, Wintour EM. Kidney development and the fetal programming of adult disease. *Bioessays* 2003;25(3):212-220.

[41] Whorwood CB, Firth KM, Budge H, Symonds ME. Maternal undernutrition during early- to mid-gestation programmes tissue-specific alterations in the expression of the glucocorticoid receptor, 11b-hydroxysteroid dehydrogenase isoforms and type 1 angiotensin II receptor in neonatal sheep. *Endocrinology* 2001;142:2854-2864.

[42] Fowden AL, Li J, Forhead AJ. Glucocorticoids and the preparation for life after birth: are there long-term consequences of the life insurance? *Proceedings of the Nutrition Society* 1998;57:113-122.

[43] Bispham J, Gopalakrishnan GS, Dandrea J, Wilson V, Budge H, Keisler DH, et al. Maternal endocrine adaptation throughout pregnancy to nutritional manipulation: consequences for maternal plasma leptin and cortisol and the programming of fetal adipose tissue development. *Endocrinology* 2003;144:3575-3585.

[44] Clarke L, Heasman L, Juniper DT, Symonds ME. Maternal nutrition in early-mid gestation and placental size in sheep. *British Journal of Nutrition* 1998;79:359-364.

[45] Edwards LJ, Symonds ME, Warnes K, Owens JA, Butler TG, Jurisevic A, et al. Responses of the fetal pituitary-adrenal axis to acute and chronic hypoglycaemia during late gestation in the sheep. *Endocrinology* 2001;142:1778-1785.

[46] Jellyman JK, Gardner DS, Edwards CM, Fowden AL, Giussani DA. Fetal cardiovascular, metabolic and endocrine responses to acute hypoxaemia during and following maternal treatment with dexamethasone in sheep. *Journal of Physiology* 2005;567:673-688.

[47] Wintour EM, Alcorn D, McFarlane A, Moritz K, Potocnik SJ, Tangalakis K. Effect of maternal glucocorticoid treatment on fetal fluids in sheep at 0.4 gestation. *American Journal of Physiology* 1994;266:R1174-R1181.

[48] Dodic M, Hantzis V, Duncan J, Rees S, Koukoulas I, Johnson K, et al. Programming effects of short prenatal exposure to cortisol. *FASEB Journal* 2002;16:1017-1026.

[49] Dodic M, May CN, Wintour EM, Coghlan JP. An early prenatal exposure to excess glucocorticoid leads to hypertensive offspring in sheep. *Clinical Science* 1998;94:149-155.

[50] Fernandez-Twinn DS, Ozanne SE, Ekizoglou S, Doherty C, James L, Gusterson B, et al. The maternal endocrine environment in the low-protein model of intra-uterine growth restriction. *British Journal of Nutrition* 2003;90:815-822.

[51] Welham SJ, Wade A, Woolf AS. Protein restriction in pregnancy is associated with increased apoptosis of mesenchymal cells at the start of rat metanephrogenesis. *Kidney International* 2002;61:1231-1242.

[52] Woods LL, Ingelfinger JR, Rasch R. Modest maternal protein restriction fails to program adult hypertension in female rats. *American Journal of Physiology* 2005;289:R1131-R1136.

[53] Zimanyi MA, Bertram JF, Black MJ. Nephron number and blood pressure in rat offspring with maternal high-protein diet. *Pediatric Nephrology* 2002;17:1000-1004.

[54] Brennan KA, Olson D, Symonds ME. Maternal nutrient restriction alters renal development and blood pressure regulation of the offspring. *Proceeding of The Nutrition Society* 2006:(In press).

[55] Dodic M, Baird R, Hantzis V, Koukoulas I, Moritz K, Peers A, et al. Organs/systems potentially involved in one model of programmed hypertension in sheep. *Clinical and Experimental Pharmacology and Physiology* 2001;28:952-956.

[56] Holness MJ, Sugden MC. Dexamethasone during late gestation exacerbates peripheral insulin resistance and selectively targets glucose-sensitive functions in beta cell and liver. *Endocrinology* 2001;142:3742-3748.

[57] Woods LL, Weeks DA. Prenatal programming of adult blood pressure: role of maternal corticosteroids. *American Journal of Physiology* 2005;289:R955-R962.

[58] Wyrwoll CS, Mark PJ, Mori TA, Puddey IB, Waddell BJ. Prevention of programmed hyperleptinemia and hypertension by postnatal dietary omega-3 fatty acids. *Endocrinology* 2006;147:599-606.

[59] Edwards LJ, McMillen IC. Maternal undernutrition increases arterial blood pressure in the sheep fetus during late gestation. *Journal of Physiology* 2001;533:561-570.

[60] Hawkins P, Steyn C, Ozaki T, Saito T, Noakes DE, Hanson MA. Effect of maternal undernutrition in early gestation on ovine fetal blood pressure and cardiovascular reflexes. *American Journal of Physiology* 2000;279:R340-R348.

[61] Symonds ME, Budge H, Mostyn A, Stephenson T, Gardner DS. Nutritional programming of fetal development: endocrine mediators and long-term outcomes for cardiovascular health. *Current Nutrition and Food Science* 2006;(Submitted).

[62] Symonds ME, Heasman L, Clarke L, Firth K, Owens JA, McMillen IC. Maternal nutrition during late gestation and placental growth. *Contemporary Reviews in Obstetrics and Gynaecology* 1997;9:165-172.

[63] Budge H, Dandrea J, Mostyn A, Evens Y, Watkins R, Sullivan C, et al. Differential effects of fetal number and maternal nutrition in late gestation on prolactin receptor abundance and adipose tissue development in the neonatal lamb. *Pediatric Research* 2003;53:302-308.

[64] Symonds ME, Phillips ID, Anthony RV, Owens JA, McMillen IC. Prolactin receptor gene expression and foetal adipose tissue. *Journal of Neuroendocrinology* 1998;10:885-890.

[65] Pearce S, Budge H, Mostyn A, Korur N, Wang J, Ingleton PM, et al. Differential effects of maternal cold exposure and nutrient restriction on prolactin receptor and uncoupling protein 1 abundance in adipose tissue during development in young sheep. *Adipocytes* 2005;1:57-64.

[66] Symonds ME, Mostyn A, Pearce S, Budge H, Stephenson T. Endocrine and nutritional regulation of fetal adipose tissue development. *Journal of Endocrinology* 2003;179:293-299.

[67] Stevens D, Alexander G, Bell AW. Effects of prolonged glucose infusion into fetal sheep on body growth, fat deposition and gestation length. *Journal of Developmental Physiology* 1990;13:277-281.

[68] Muhlhausler BS, Adam CL, Marrocco EM, Findlay PA, Roberts CT, McFarlane JR, et al. Impact of glucose infusion on the structural and functional characteristics of adipose tissue and on hypothalamic gene expression for appetite regulatory neuropeptides in the sheep fetus during late gestation. *Journal of Physiology* 2005;565:185-195.

[69] Budge H, Bispham J, Dandrea J, Evans L, Heasman L, Ingleton P, et al. Effect of maternal nutrition on brown adipose tissue and prolactin receptor status in the fetal lamb. *Pediatric Research* 2000;47:781-786.

[70] Mühlhäusler BS, Roberts CT, Yuen BSJ, Marrocco E, Budge H, Symonds ME, et al. Determinants of fetal leptin synthesis, fat mass and circulating leptin concentrations in well nourished ewes in late pregnancy. *Endocrinology* 2003;144:4947-4954.

[71] Gnanalingham MG, Mostyn A, Symonds ME, Stephenson T. Ontogeny and nutritional programming of fat mass: potential role of glucocorticoid sensitivity and uncoupling protein-2. *American Journal of Physiology* 2005;289:R1407 - R1415.

[72] Gnanalingham MG, Mostyn A, Gardner DS, Stephenson T, Symonds ME. Developmental regulation of adipose tissue: Nutritional manipulation of local glucocorticoid action and uncoupling protein 2. *Adipocytes* 2005;1:(In press).

[73] Krook A, Bjornholm M, Galuska D, Jiang XJ, Fahlman R, Myers MG, Jr., et al. Characterization of signal transduction and glucose transport in skeletal muscle from type 2 diabetic patients. *Diabetes* 2000;49:284-292.

[74] Clarke L, Buss DS, Juniper DS, Lomax MA, Symonds ME. Adipose tissue development during early postnatal life in ewe-reared lambs. *Experimental Physiology* 1997;82:1015-1017.

[75] Pearce S, Budge H, Mostyn A, Genever E, Webb R, Ingleton P, et al. Prolactin, the prolactin receptor and uncoupling protein abundance and function in adipose tissue during development in young sheep. *Journal of Endocrinology* 2005;184:351-359.

[76] Mostyn A, Bispham J, Pearce S, Evens Y, Raver N, Keisler DH, et al. Differential effects of leptin on thermoregulation and uncoupling protein abundance in the neonatal lamb. *FASEB Journal* 2002;16:1438-1440.

[77] Symonds ME, Gardner DS. Experimental evidence for early nutritional programming of adult health in animals. *Current Opinion in Clinical Nutrition and Metabolic Care* 2006:(In press).

[78] Ozanne SE, Hales CN. Lifespan: Catch-up growth and obesity in male mice. *Nature* 2004;427:411-412.

[79] Boullu-Ciocca S, Dutour A, Guillaume V, Achard V, Oliver C, Grino M. Postnatal diet-induced obesity in rats upregulates systemic and adipose tissue glucocorticoid metabolism during development and in adulthood. *Diabetologia* 2005;54:197-203.

[80] Putman J, Allhouse J, Kantor LS. US per capita food supply trends: more calories, refined carbohydrates and fats. *Food Reviews* 2002;25:2-15.

[81] Sturm R. The economics of physical activity: societal trends and rationales for interventions. *American Journal of Preventative Medicine* 2004;27(Suppl):126-135.

[82] Cavadini C, Siega-Riz AM, Popkin BM. US adolescent food intake trends from 1965 to 1996. *Archives of Disease in Childhood* 2000;83:18-24.

[83] Harnack LJ, Jeffery RW, Boutelle KN. Temporal trends in energy intake in the United States: an ecologic perspective. *American Journal of Clinical Nutrition* 2000;71:1478-1484.

[84] Young LR, Nestle M. The contribution of expanding portion sizes to the US obesity epidemic. *American Journal of Public Health* 2002;92:246-249.

[85] Bellisle F, Clement K, Le Barzic M, Le Gall A, Guy-Grand B, Basdevant A. The eating inventory and body adiposity from leanness to massive obesity: a study of 2509 adults. *Obesity Research* 2004;12:2023-2030.

[86] Petry CJ, Ozanne SE, Wang CL, Hales CN. Early protein restriction and obesity independently induce hypertension in 1-year-old rats. *Clinical Science* 1997;93:147-152.

[87] Khan I, Dekou V, Hanson M, Poston L, Taylor P. Predictive adaptive responses to maternal high-fat diet prevent endothelial dysfunction but not hypertension in adult rat offspring. *Circulation* 2004;110:1097-1102.

[88] Gardner DS, Budge H, Symonds ME. Bottle feeding of sheep alters regional adipose deposition and increases adult fat mass. *Pediatric Research* 2005;58:1028.

[89] Stuebe AM, Rich-Edwards JW, Willett WC, Manson JE, Michels KB. Duration of lactation and incidence of type 2 diabetes. *Journal of the American Medical Association* 2005;294:2601-2610.

[90] Budge H, Symonds ME. Fetal and neonatal nutrition - Lipid and carbohydrate requirements and adaptations to altered supply at birth. In: Winn HN, Gluckman PD, editors. *The Textbook of Perinatal Medicine 2ed.* Great Yarmouth: Taylor & Francis; 2006. p. 1007-1016.

[91] Appel LJ, Sacks FM, Carey VJ, Obarzanek E, Swain JF, Miller ER, 3rd, et al. Effects of protein, monounsaturated fat, and carbohydrate intake on blood pressure and serum lipids: results of the OmniHeart randomized trial. *Journal of the American Medical Association* 2005;294:2455-2464.

INDEX

D

E

F

I

J

N

O

P

Q

T

U

V

W

X

Y

Z